The South African Response to COVID-19

This book analyses the first two years of South Africa's response to the COVID-19 epidemic, from its emergence in early 2020.

Drawing on the perspectives of a range of public health experts, economists and other social scientists, and development practitioners, this book argues that understanding this early response will be essential to moderate and improve future policy thinking around health governance and epidemic readiness. This book provides a systemic analysis of not only the epidemiological progression of COVID-19 in South Africa, but also the socio-political factors that will be key in determining the future of the country as a whole, including health system challenges, socio-economic disparities and inequalities, and variable (often contradictory and tardy) policy responses. Overall, this book exposes Manichean thinking and the spurious policy dichotomies that pitch public health against human rights, economic recovery against viral vector control, and science against ideology, with lessons not just for South Africa, but also for elsewhere on the African continent, and beyond.

This book will be perfect for researchers and practitioners across Public Health, Health Policy, and Global Health, as well as those with an interest in South African politics and development more generally.

Pieter Fourie teaches Political Science at Stellenbosch University, South Africa. He has worked in the field of Global Health since the late 1990s, including at UNAIDS and the AIDS Foundation of South Africa, and he has taught at universities in South Africa and Australia.

Guy Lamb teaches Political Science at Stellenbosch University, South Africa. He serves as a commissioner with the South African National Planning Commission. Between 2012 and 2020, he was the Director of the Safety and Violence Initiative at the University of Cape Town.

Routledge Studies in Health in Africa

Series Editor: Pieter Fourie

The South African Response to COVID-19

The Early Years

Edited by
Pieter Fourie and Guy Lamb

Routledge
Taylor & Francis Group
LONDON AND NEW YORK

First published 2023
by Routledge
4 Park Square, Milton Park, Abingdon, Oxon OX14 4RN

and by Routledge
605 Third Avenue, New York, NY 10158

Routledge is an imprint of the Taylor & Francis Group, an informa business

British Library Cataloguing-in-Publication Data
A catalogue record for this book is available from the British Library

Library of Congress Cataloging-in-Publication Data
Names: Fourie, Pieter, 1972– editor, author. | Lamb, Guy, editor, author.
Title: The South African response to COVID-19 : the early years / edited by Pieter Fourie and Guy Lamb.
Description: New York : Routledge, 2023. | Includes bibliographical references and index.
Identifiers: LCCN 2022056183 (print) | LCCN 2022056184 (ebook) | ISBN 9781032280073 (hardback) | ISBN 9781032280097 (paperback) | ISBN 9781003294931 (ebook)
Subjects: LCSH: COVID-19 Pandemic, 2020—Government policy—South Africa. | COVID-19 Pandemic, 2020—Economic aspects—South Africa. | Emergency management—South Africa.
Classification: LCC RA644.C67 S655 2023 (print) | LCC RA644.C67 (ebook) | DDC 362.1962414400968—dc23/eng/20221121
LC record available at https://lccn.loc.gov/2022056183
LC ebook record available at https://lccn.loc.gov/2022056184

ISBN: 978-1-032-28007-3 (hbk)
ISBN: 978-1-032-28009-7 (pbk)
ISBN: 978-1-003-29493-1 (ebk)

DOI: 10.4324/9781003294931

Typeset in Bembo
by codeMantra

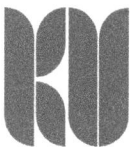

An electronic version of this book is freely available, thanks to the support of libraries working with Knowledge Unlatched (KU). KU is a collaborative initiative designed to make high quality books Open Access for the public good. The Open Access ISBN for this book is 9781003294931. More information about the initiative and links to the Open Access version can be found at www.knowledgeunlatched.org.

Contents

Figures

Tables

Contributors

Laurin Baumgardt is a Doctoral Candidate in the Department of Anthropology at Rice University, United States of America.

Arvin Bhana is a Chief Specialist Scientist in the Health Systems Research Unit at the South African Medical Research Council. He also holds an Honorary Associate Professorship in the School of Nursing and Public Health at the University of KwaZulu-Natal, South Africa.

Pieter Fourie is a Professor in the Department of Political Science at Stellenbosch University, South Africa.

André Janse van Rensburg is a Senior Researcher with the Centre for Rural Health, University of KwaZulu-Natal, South Africa.

Jesal Kika-Mistry is a Doctoral Candidate in the Department of Economics at Stellenbosch University, South Africa. She is a consultant for the Southern Africa Education portfolio at the World Bank.

Guy Lamb is a Senior Lecturer in the Department of Political Science at Stellenbosch University, South Africa.

Keymanthri Moodley is a Distinguished Professor in the Department of Medicine and Director of the Centre for Medical Ethics and Law, Faculty of Health Sciences, Stellenbosch University, South Africa.

Eldridge Moses is a Lecturer in the Department of Economics at Stellenbosch University, South Africa.

Vinothan Naidoo is an Associate Professor in the Department of Political Studies at the University of Cape Town, South Africa.

Warren Parker is a Fellow of the Balsillie School of International Affairs, Waterloo, Canada, and a Senior Research Fellow at the Centre for Communication, Media and Society in the School of Applied Human Sciences, University of KwaZulu-Natal in Durban, South Africa.

Inge Petersen is a Research Professor and Director of the Centre for Rural Health at the University of KwaZulu-Natal, South Africa, as well as a Visiting Professor at the Global Health Institute, University College London.

Steven Robins is a Professor in the Department of Sociology and Social Anthropology at Stellenbosch University, South Africa.

Cindy Steenekamp is a Senior Lecturer in the Department of Political Science at Stellenbosch University, South Africa.

Christiane Struckmann wrote her chapter during her time as a Junior Lecturer in the Department of Political Science at Stellenbosch University, South Africa.

Alan Whiteside is a Fellow of the Balsillie School of International Affairs, Waterloo, Canada, and Professor Emeritus at the University of KwaZulu-Natal, Durban.

Gabrielle Wills is an Education Economist and Researcher with the Research on Socioeconomic Policy group in the Department of Economics at Stellenbosch University, South Africa.

Ingrid Woolard is Dean of the Faculty of Economic and Management Sciences and Professor of Economics at Stellenbosch University, South Africa.

1 The emancipatory catastrophe we need?

Pieter Fourie

Introduction

This book identifies, describes, and tries to make sense of the early South African response to the COVID-19 epidemic. By 'early response', we refer specifically to the first 18 months to two years after the virus first emerged in the country in early 2020. South Africa's early response has had and will continue to have a significant impact on the way the health and public policy response(s) to the epidemic will develop in years to come. We need to understand this early response to moderate and improve policy thinking, specifically regarding 'good' health governance, epidemic readiness, and a responsive health system. This book provides valuable insights and lessons not only in South Africa, but also for the rest of Southern Africa and elsewhere on the African continent.

This book provides the perspectives of a range of public health experts, economists, and other social scientists and development practitioners. Our various chapters provide systemic accounts of not only the epidemiological progression of COVID-19 in South Africa, but specifically of those socio-political sectors that will be key in determining the future of South African society as a whole. As Louis Pasteur famously remarked, 'the pathogen is nothing, the terrain is everything'; this terrain includes health system challenges, massive socio-economic disparities and inequalities, and variable (often contradictory and tardy) policy responses.

This book exposes Manichean thinking and spurious policy dichotomies: public health *versus* human rights; economic recovery *versus* viral vector control; science *versus* ideology and beliefs; and received interventions *versus* home-grown solutions. COVID-19 has exposed weaknesses in pandemic readiness across the world, multilaterally, as well as health system deficits in domestic contexts. As Alex de Waal (2021: 14) states in his recent book *New Pandemics, Old Politics*, 'Covid-19 was the least unexpected pandemic in history'. It is our hope that this book, and its lessons, will contribute to turning COVID-19 into what De Waal (2021: 230) calls 'the emancipatory catastrophe we need'.

Pandemic-driven change – sometimes emancipatory, sometimes catastrophic, often both – has been a feature of human history.

DOI: 10.4324/9781003294931-1

Epidemics and political change in history[1]

From a health perspective, if you live in the developed world and have a regular income, then this is probably the best time in human history to be alive. People in the rich world can now look forward to such long lives that their very longevity has become a key concern – but this is a very recent development. Until Germ Theory became well established in the late 1800s, and until the take-off in medical science after World War II, life for most people was 'nasty, brutish and short'.[2] In fact, in the decade or so after 1945, there was such a strong faith in the ability of medical technology in general, and in antibiotics and vaccines in particular, that the medical community started to speak of a world without any burden of infectious disease. Since the 1970s, a number of old diseases have re-emerged and terrifying epidemics of brand-new pathogens have come to mock any utopian notion of life beyond illness.

History provides good examples and opportunities for natural and social scientists to learn about the diseases and epidemics that made us, that created the world in which we live. Epidemics and other significant systemic shocks to past regimes have been powerful determinants of our civilisation today. Then, as now, some societies have faded away, whilst others flourished, managing to maintain and build their resilience. Robert Baker (2007) considers the scale and impact of a number of diseases and epidemics in history:

- The great influenza (Spanish flu) epidemic of 1918–1920 killed between 50 and 100 million people – most of them young. This makes the Spanish flu the most lethal single-event pandemic in known history. Should its mortality be repeated with the contemporary global population, it would kill in excess of 300 million people.
- AIDS has already killed more than 40 million people, and nearly as many people live with the virus today (UNAIDS, 2022).
- Malaria has been a companion to humans for millennia. In the 20th century alone, malaria claimed between 150 million and 300 million lives, accounting for two to five percent of all deaths (Carter and Mendis, 2002). According to the most recent World Health Organization fact sheet, the estimated number of annual malaria deaths stood at 627,000 in 2020. In the same year, there were an estimated 241 million cases of malaria worldwide – the vast majority of which are in Africa (WHO, 2022a). One consequence of climate change will be a surge in malarial infections globally.
- Cholera killed millions in India immediately after it first appeared in Calcutta in 1817, and humans have been unable to stop its spread. Researchers have estimated that each year there are 1.3–4 million cases and 21,000–143,000 deaths worldwide due to cholera (WHO, 2022b).
- Smallpox killed as many as five million people during the Antonine plague of 165–180 AD and was instrumental in the death of tens of millions of people living in the Americas in the wake of the arrival of Europeans.

- Typhus may have caused the fall of the Athenians in the war against the Peloponnesian League, led by Sparta. Colossal mortality from typhus also occurred during Napoleon's 1815 retreat from Moscow.

Diseases and epidemics are not simply and exclusively biological phenomena that one can approach by biomedicine and public health interventions alone. As Michel Foucault and others[3] remind us, epidemics are political, social, and cultural constructs as much as they are natural entities. Robert Hudson (quoted in Hays, 2009: 3) captures this well, saying that '[d]iseases are not immutable entities but dynamic social constructions that have biographies of their own'. As such, epidemics have the capacity to change the ways in which humans perceive their world, power relations within societies, and the nature of reality itself. For instance, Germ Theory challenged the very idea that disease is some kind of divine retribution or punishment for collective or individual human vice; tuberculosis continues to challenge notions that the poor and their suffering matter less than the rich and their maladies; cholera revolutionised sanitation and the management of waste and water across multiple societies (Evans, 1988).

The Black Death is a particularly good example of a pandemic that had an impact over time, remaking entire societies. It arose in the 14th century, with serial peaks of epidemics up until the 18th century, and even sporadic outbreaks into the modern era. It is said to have killed 34 million people in Europe alone, with similar numbers in Asia. In terms of impact, change, adaptability and, ultimately, resilience in the context of the Black Death, much has been written about the deep, systemic changes to Western European society that came in the wake of the pandemic.

At the most basic level, there was a fundamental and dramatic change in the demography of European society; the Black Death killed between 30 and 60 per cent of everyone in many affected communities. This led to changed conceptions about who was important, how the state could tax the people in its jurisdiction (Cohn, 2007), how divisions of labour had to be adapted in order to maintain the production of food and its commerce, and this ultimately challenged and changed the entire European political economy, contributing to the end of feudalism (Cartwright and Biddiss, 2006). It also led to the challenging of the authority of the Roman Catholic Church, and a questioning of the power of the priests to banish disease. Such a metaphysical shift in conceptions of the cosmos and causal links between the physical and the metaphysical/supernatural worlds eroded the power of religious workers and may have led to secularisation across Europe, sparking the spirit of Enlightenment.

Epidemics continue to act as agents of change in contemporary society, in determining how the world works. Infectious disease continues to kill more people than military or civil strife, but it affects the present in other, profound ways also. When humanity is lucky it even holds the promise of constructive introspection, changing the world for the better and increasing societies' moral fortitude and physical resilience. For instance, improved instruments and global institutions have been put in place to ensure a timely response to epidemics. The World Health Organization was established after World War II and co-ordinates early epidemic detection mechanisms across the world; its International Health Regulations provide important criteria for the management of and general responsiveness to the outbreak of biological threats. Cooper and Kirton (2008) hail these innovations as progress in the human management and political governance of disease globally.

Less directly, but maybe even more importantly, there have been some dramatic cultural advances in human conceptions of disease and epidemics. Contemporary pathogens challenge societies to reflect on what it means to be a good and caring global community, who should care for those who are unable to afford life-saving medical technologies, how one should think about the political control of biotechnologies, and how they are regulated (Fukuyama, 2003). According to McMichael (2004: 1052):

> ... we are living through [... a] great historical transition. This time scale is global and changes are occurring on many fronts. The spread and increased lability of various infectious diseases, new and old, reflect the impacts of demographic, environmental, social, technological and other rapid changes in human ecology. [.... I]t underscores how configurations of social and environmental influences change.

Applying a human ecological approach to contemporary epidemics, Mary Wilson (1995) emphasises that it is critical for societies to remain responsive and adaptable to the emergence and impact of pandemics. In order to do so, she argues that Western societies and states need to move beyond too strict and exclusive a focus on surveillance. This is a timely warning, as surveillance has tended to become the be-all and end-all of a securitised response to epidemics, especially after 9/11.

Her point is not that surveillance in itself is a bad thing – it is critically important and integrated with the International Health Regulations, for instance, which aim to help the international community prevent and respond to acute public health risks that have the potential to cross borders and threaten people worldwide (WHO, 2022c). But surveillance should not become a goal in itself; it should be part of a larger process in which the overall aim is to improve the human condition and to remain responsive to the challenges posed by pathogens and other systemic shocks.

Wilson (1995) suggests that societies should apprehend infectious diseases in their evolutionary and ecological context, and *respond to that context* rather than only formulating short-term responses to recently surveyed outbreaks. Such a response is political, as it will only be possible if we recognise the links between population growth, climatic and environmental change, global migration, and human health and security; develop databases that combine information about climate, demography, population movements, and diseases in humans, animals, and plants; identify markers for regions or populations at high risk of epidemic disease so that we can intervene to reduce the impact of disease; continue efforts to slow population growth; take steps to reduce mass migration and displacement of populations; reduce consumption and pay more attention to land use and production and disposal of toxins and chemicals; take a broader view and longer time frame when analysing the potential impact of interventions; and view human life as part of a constantly evolving biosphere. Each of these activities implies political interpretations and political decisions taken by individuals and political bodies who have the power to act; as Michel Foucault and Susan Sontag (2003) remind us, the very act of observing/surveillance and interpretation is political.

The lessons or 'gifts' of disasters and pandemics in particular seem clear enough when one looks closely, and most particularly when one applies resilience thinking, with a different time frame in mind. As Alex de Waal says above, we should not waste this catastrophe; COVID-19 may be just the inflection point that we need to change the world for the better.

Who will find this book useful?

This book's intended readership includes those working in Public Health, Health Policy-Making, and Global Health – either as academics, as researchers, or as practitioners This includes epistemic communities and communities of practice inside and outside South Africa. Academics will be able to use this for undergraduate and postgraduate teaching, and researchers and policy workers in the field of Public Health and Development may find this a useful text, particularly for its description and explanation of how and why policy responses generally (and the governance response to COVID-19 in South Africa specifically) can influence epidemic morbidity and the mortality. This will be instructive in policy-making and epidemic responses not only in the South African context, but also for understanding linkages in other African contexts. This may serve to improve policy-making in-country, but also policy thinking about disease resilience and the 'good' governance of epidemics elsewhere, including at the global and multilateral levels.

The readership will be mostly based at universities, governments, non-government organisations, development agencies, and multilateral institutions in South Africa, Africa more broadly, in North America, continental Europe, and the United Kingdom. This book is aimed at fairly specialist communities, but the language is made accessible to anyone with an undergraduate background or a good sectoral or popular grasp of the subject matter.

Any course on Public Policy-Making, Global/Public Health, Global Health Governance, or the History of Health would be able to include this book into their syllabus. In terms of academic subject categories, teachers and students of African Studies, Politics, International Relations, Development Studies, Sociology, Social Anthropology, History, and Health Studies may find it particularly useful. Researchers who work in these fields, in national and multilateral government, or policy workers in non-government entities and members of multilateral/health agencies will also be able to use it.

Given the ongoing effects of COVID-19 and the recent and ongoing impacts of Ebola and HIV/AIDS, in the public psyche, as well as in policy communities, the topic of this book should find significant traction in teaching, research, and professional communities. Global Health and Public Health with a focus on 'good health governance' have grown impressively, as fields of study, and as they feed government, non-government, as well as multilateral agency employment – in particular since the explosion in funding for global health since the turn of the millennium – the topic of this book is bound to be taught in cognate courses in many Departments of Politics, International Relations, Development Studies, African Studies, Sociology, Social Anthropology, History, and Health Studies.

This book is useful to policy workers in government, in the overseas development agency environment, or in health-related specialist agencies, in particular as the COVID-19 pandemic has now entered its most divisive political stage: the equitable distribution of vaccines, the reality of under-resourced health systems, and in the face of significant vaccine hesitancy.

What is in the chapters?

In the following 11 chapters, we move from a broad perspective or level of analysis to more focused or sectoral areas of interest.

In Chapter 2, Christiane Struckmann provides a bird's eye view of the progress of the pandemic in South Africa. The chapter notes that the COVID-19 pandemic has disrupted the world in ways few of us have witnessed in our lifetime. In two and half years, 558 million deaths have been recorded worldwide. The economic cost of the pandemic is, however, incalculable. *The Economist* suggests that $10 trillion in GDP was forgone globally in 2020 and 2021. In South Africa, a country with a relatively young population, the COVID-19 case-fatality rate stood at approximately 2.5 per cent, a small number considering the pandemic's socio-economic impact. As of August 2021, South Africa's unemployment rate is the highest in the world; more than half of the country's population lives below the national poverty line. While these numbers are partly a result of the imposition of a very strict lockdown (which, no doubt, saved thousands of lives), they were severely worsened by ineffective leadership, abuse of power, and widespread corruption. Chapter 2 provides a broad overview of the South African government's response to COVID-19 by focussing on a few selected themes: the economic and gendered impact of the pandemic, corruption, and law enforcement. The chapter also maps out how the pandemic unfolded in South Africa.

In Chapter 3, Warren Parker unpacks the uneven South African response to the pandemic. Early on in the pandemic, the World Health Organisation (WHO) and the Chinese government delayed confirmation of human-to-human transmission. A number of countries and territories in East

Asia took action, implementing measures that worked effectively to suppress their initial epidemics. Elsewhere, the pace of response was impeded by the WHO's lack of urgency in declaring a pandemic and stark omissions in prevention guidance that set countries up for failure. South Africa's response to COVID-19 in March 2020 included the declaration of a national state of disaster and the imposition of lockdown measures. But unlike other African countries, various novel approaches were introduced. Nuanced approaches rapidly went awry. The Ministerial Advisory Committee lacked transparency and was overly biomedically focused. The chapter describes the successes and failures during the early phases of South Africa's epidemic response and explores lessons for the future.

In Chapter 4, Alan Whiteside situates the South African epidemic in the global context. A key question is why the disease, and its consequences, vary so greatly from country to country. Up to the end of 2021, most Asian countries and Australia and New Zealand contained the virus. The consequences in Europe and North America were almost uniformly catastrophic. Much of Latin America is believed to be facing a severe, but an under-reported epidemic. Reliable data are hard to come by in most of Africa, but it seemed both caseloads and case-fatality rates are lower. The exception was South Africa where COVID-19 was significantly worse than in the rest of Africa. The pandemic came in waves and the case-fatality rates and apparent seriousness of the disease appear to have diminished. The first part of 2022 saw a different pattern of transmission and the virus and pandemic is in flux. The comparison between COVID-19 and HIV/AIDS has been and will continue to be made. COVID-19 is infinitely more serious than HIV, not in terms of deaths or the case-fatality rate, but in numbers of infections and the disruption it has caused. The chapter traces the evolution of the global epidemics and looks specifically at how the spread in South Africa compares with other parts of the world. It also looks at what was considered 'international best practice' and compares South Africa to this.

Laurin Baumgardt and Steven Robins then, in Chapter 5, zoom in on the South African government's response to COVID as a 'crisis within a crisis'. The response to COVID-19 by means of hard lockdowns and other public health interventions occurred in a time and climate of political instability, uncertainty, and multiple other crises such as police brutality, forced displacements, gender-based violence, chronic inequality, and massive unemployment. By exploring the drastic and urgent government responses to COVID-19, and their embeddedness within these other crises, the authors seek to highlight the contingent and conjunctural relationship between slow, structural, and endemic crises – as well as the spectacular, episodic, and seemingly singular, eruptions of 'crisis', along with their 'blind spots' and tendencies towards restoring social and political stasis. The chapter interrogates the crisis concept anew by introducing the term 'slow crises'. 'Slow crises', in the plural, express the convergences, amplifications, and alternating and competing visibilities and temporalities of multiple crises in the South African context, for instance, the July 2021 riots in KwaZulu-Natal and Gauteng, and the TB and HIV/AIDS epidemics. The chapter also discusses South Africa's COVID-19 responses within the context of global lockdown models and pandemic preparedness strategies. By emphasising that crises cannot be singularised, the authors conclude that COVID-19 served to both surface and submerge the multiple, and nested, crises of our 'self-devouring' capitalist system.

In a variation on this focus on government and governance, Vinothan Naidoo in Chapter 6 problematises the public sector's response specifically. The chapter reviews how South Africa's public sector institutions responded to as well as sustained the effects of COVID-19. Firstly, the chapter unpacks the logic and consequences of the centralised disaster-managed approach adopted by the government to mobilise the public sector machinery to combat coronavirus. This approach reprised the government's historical tendency to employ overly complex and hierarchical co-ordination structures in government to respond to major policy problems, and in the process, generating sub-optimal results. Secondly, the chapter explains how the coronavirus amplified systemic governance challenges that public sector departments had been struggling with for years, namely, financial sustainability, the capacity to deliver, and ethical integrity. COVID-19 heightened these stresses at a time when the country's appetite for improved governance could not have been higher, and where the discourse around shifting to digital modes of public sector delivery appeared more aspirational than practically attainable.

In Chapter 7, Keymanthri Moodley considers the hugely political issue of vaccines. The COVID-19 pandemic, precariously situated at the intersection of science, ethics, the law, public health, the economy, and politics, unmasked deep-seated inequities. It stimulated profound reflection on a range of conflicts that were present in pre-COVID-19 times, but which re-surfaced in the context of this public health crisis. Central to bringing the pandemic under control was a toolbox of preventative measures that were developed and implemented – hygiene practices were intensified, physical distancing was advised, quarantine and isolation were implemented, mandatory masking became the norm, and vaccine development was accelerated. From a public health perspective, the tide of this pandemic turned after the development and administration of carefully tested vaccines. Previous natural infection in the first three waves of infection, in those who survived, also mitigated the mortality in later waves. This medical triumph of hybrid immunity was lauded in scientific and non-scientific circles alike but, sadly, against a backdrop of global inequity in access and supply. The world was split apart at its social and moral seams. As vaccine access improved, the conflict between myth and fact emerged as social media (both a blessing and a curse) fuelled the spread of misinformation with consequent vaccine hesitancy and refusal. Chapter 7 explores the bright and dark sides of vaccine development and implementation and how it impacted the pandemic in South Africa.

In Chapter 8, Guy Lamb analyses the relationship between the actions of the South African Police Service (SAPS) and police legitimacy during the height of the COVID-19 pandemic in 2020 and 2021. Select aspects of the 'trust-diminishing' police behaviours framework devised by Goldsmith (2005) are used to analyse the SAPS's approach to policing during the pandemic. The chapter demonstrates that South African communities, especially in poorer areas, regularly experienced indifference, low levels of police professionalism, and incompetence from the police. Moreover, trust in the police, and subsequently police legitimacy, was also undermined by the National Coronavirus Command Council's requirement that the police enforce several unpopular regulations, especially the prohibition on the sale of tobacco products and alcohol. Police legitimacy was further diminished by pervasive corruption within the SAPS and militarised approaches to police work which resulted in numerous incidents of excessive use of force by police officials.

In Chapter 9, Eldridge Moses and Ingrid Woolard consider the important role of temporary social grants in mitigating the poverty impact of COVID-19 in South Africa. The pandemic and associated lockdown responses revealed structural inequalities in the South African economy and subjected already vulnerable households to large negative and unexpected economic shocks. South Africa's well-developed cash transfer and social insurance systems facilitated swift and substantial interventions to ensure that economically vulnerable households were able to survive the economic impacts of the pandemic. The interventions were in the forms of existing grant top-ups, temporary relief to employers and employees, and a new special Social Relief of Distress grant aimed at the previously excluded unemployed population. The chapter finds that these interventions were relatively well targeted, although there is some evidence of non-poor households also benefiting from grants intended for the poor. Nevertheless, the temporary extension of the social assistance net to unemployed individuals assisted many vulnerable households in staving off the worst of the economic impacts of the pandemic. However, given South Africa's fragile fiscal outlook, it is important that the continuation of additional support to unemployed individuals works in tandem with focused labour market interventions to ensure that South Africa achieves its employment, economic growth, and longer-term fiscal sustainability objectives.

In Chapter 10, André Janse van Rensburg, Irvin Bhana, and Inge Petersen consider mental health in the context of the South African epidemic. As COVID-19 unfolded during 2020, there was growing cognizance of the short-, medium-, and long-term impacts of the event on individuals and communities globally. In South Africa, the mental health burden of the pandemic was identified relatively early, where a substantial mental health burden was identified under stages 3 and 4 of the country's lockdown measures. Collective trauma and psychological distress were experienced by many communities, in tandem with widespread uncertainty and socio-economic pressures, and severe restrictions in personal freedoms. Importantly, the contexts of infection prevention and control catalysed virtual support platforms, and this was exemplified by provincial health departments who worked with academic and technical partners to develop psychoeducational materials (audio-visual and print materials promoting COVID-19-related mental health literacy and help-seeking among healthcare workers and in communities) as well as a wellness training course for healthcare workers. The South African Federation for Mental Health, the South African Depression and Anxiety Group, and several others offered free telephonic counselling, while grassroots mobilisation like the development of Community Action Networks helped to rally community resources to support the basic needs of the vulnerable, which included looking after their mental health needs. While promising, many of these responses were at best reactive, emergency procedures, and not illustrative of a quality, people-centred health system. Time will tell how well the South African health system dealt with the multilevel, increasingly complex mental health challenges presented by COVID-19. While the pandemic exposed deep and persistent health system challenges, the chapter does identify promising, if isolated, partnerships that focus on comprehensive health system strengthening.

In Chapter 11, Gabrielle Wills and Jesal Kika-Mistry investigate the critical area of early childhood care and education provisioning in South Africa after COVID-19. Events surrounding the COVID-19 pandemic threatened to undo 20 years of sustained expansion in access to early childhood care and education in South Africa. The chapter explores the underlying structural weaknesses in non-grade R early childhood care and education provisioning that was exposed through the pandemic, and the strengths that have surfaced. Through a lens of sustainability, capacity, and accountability, the chapter also reviews the policy and civil society responses (and in some cases, non-responses) that emerged following the pandemic-induced early childhood care and education crisis. The chapter considers what these policy responses and events reveal about how the sector is viewed and prioritised by the government. Despite the challenges experienced through the pandemic, the lessons gathered are useful in preparing for structural reforms in the early childhood care and education system.

In the final chapter of this volume, Cindy Steenekamp considers the impact of the epidemic on South Africans' support for democracy. Democracy relies on the attitudes and acceptance of its citizens. When democratic governments are unable to secure or maintain popular support, they are vulnerable to political, economic, or social crises. Chapter 12 tracks popular support for democracy in South Africa during the global COVID-19 pandemic in 2020 and 2021. The chapter utilises micro-level data to measure citizen support for and evaluations of democracy and prominent political actors since the onset of the global pandemic as well as public opinion relating to the South African government's response to COVID-19 by means of a fivefold analytical framework. The findings suggest that South Africa is at increased risk of democratic breakdown given the low and declining levels of diffuse support (political community, regime principles, and regime performance) and specific support (regime institutions and political actors) for democracy.

Factors including political governance, policy regulations and enforcement, the national socio-economic context and impact of COVID-19 on the economy, as well as irregular expenditure relating to COVID-19 measures by various government agencies and public officials are used to illustrate the intrinsic and instrumental nature of support for democracy in South Africa.

Notes

1 The ideas in this section were first developed in Fourie and Follér (2012).
2 The philosopher Thomas Hobbes (1588–1679) famously argued in his book *Leviathan* that, without strong government, life would be 'solitary, poor, nasty, brutish, and short'.
3 For instance, see Altman (1986); Treichler (1999); Sontag (2002); Barnes (2005); Crawford (2007).

References

Altman, D. (1986). *AIDS in the Mind of America.* Garden City, NY: Anchor Press/ Doubleday.
Baker, R. (2007). *Epidemic: The Past, Present and Future of the Diseases That Made Us.* London: Vision.
Barnes, E. (2005). *Diseases and Human Evolution.* Albuquerque: University of New Mexico Press.
Carter, R. & Mendis, K. (2002). Evolutionary and historical aspects of the burden of malaria. *Clinical Microbiology Reviews, 15*(4), 564–594, doi.org/10.1128/CMR.15.4.564–594.2002.
Cartwright, F. & Biddiss, M. (2006). *Disease & History.* Stroud: Sutton Publishing Ltd.
Cohn, S. (2007). After the black death: Labour legislation and attitudes towards labour in late-medieval western Europe. *Economic History Review, 60*(3), 457–485, http://www.jstor.org/stable/4502106.
Cooper, A. & Kirton, J. (eds) (2008). *Innovation in Global Health Governance: Critical Cases.* Aldershot: Ashgate.
Crawford, D. (2007). *Deadly Companions: How Microbes Shaped Our History.* Oxford: Oxford University Press.
De Waal, A. (2021). *New Pandemics, Old Politics: Two Hundred Years of War on Disease and Its Alternatives.* Cambridge, UK: Polity Press.
Evans, R. (1988). Epidemics and revolutions: Cholera in nineteenth-century Europe. *Past & Present, 120*, 123–146, http://www.jstor.org/stable/650924.
Fourie, P. & Follér, M-L. (2012). AIDS hyper-epidemics and social resilience: Theorising the political. *Contemporary Politics, 18*(2), 254–268, doi.org/10.1080/13569775.2012.674342.
Fukuyama, F. (2003). *Our Posthuman Future: Consequences of the Biotechnology Revolution.* London: Profile Books.
Hays, J. (2009). *The Burdens of Disease: Epidemics and Human Response in Western History.* New Brunswick: Rutgers University Press.
McMichael, A. (2004). Environmental and social influences on emerging infectious diseases: Past, present and future. *Philosophical Transactions of the Royal Society of*

London. *Series B, Biological Sciences, 359*(1447), 1049–1058, https://doi.org/10.1098/rstb.2004.1480.

Sontag, S. (2002). *Illness as Metaphor and AIDS and Its Metaphors.* London: Penguin Books.

Sontag, S. (2003). *Regarding the Pain of Others.* New York: Picador/Farrar, Straus and Giroux.

Treichler, P. (1999). *How to Have Theory in an Epidemic.* Durham: Duke University Press.

UNAIDS (2022). *AIDS Fact Sheet 2022.* Available at: https://www.unaids.org/sites/default/files/media_asset/UNAIDS_FactSheet_en.pdf [Accessed 15 October 2022].

WHO (2022a). *Malaria Fact Sheet 2022.* Available at: https://www.who.int/news-room/fact-sheets/detail/malaria [Accessed 15 October 2022].

WHO (2022b). *Cholera Fact Sheet 2022.* Available at: https://www.who.int/news-room/fact-sheets/detail/cholera [Accessed 15 October 2022].

WHO (2022c). *International Health Regulations.* Available at: https://www.who.int/health-topics/international-health-regulations#tab=tab_1 [Accessed 15 October 2022].

Wilson, M. (1995). Infectious diseases: An ecological perspective. *BMJ (Clinical Research ed.), 311*(7021), 1681–1684, https://doi.org/10.1136/bmj.311.7021.1681.

2 COVID-19 in South Africa

History, impact, and government response – An overview

Christiane Struckmann

Introduction

In late 2019, a cluster of novel human coronavirus cases broke out in the Chinese city of Wuhan and subsequently spread like wildfire across the world. COVID-19 reached South African shores in early March 2020. President Ramaphosa declared a National State of Disaster on 15 March 2020, and the national lockdown began on 27 March 2020. As of October 2022, South Africa reported the highest number of COVID-19 cases in Africa, the 36th highest number in the world (WHO, 2022a). While 102 246 COVID-19-related deaths have been recorded in South Africa to date, the 18th highest number in the world (WHO, 2022b), some would argue that far more livelihoods were lost as a consequence of the economic impact of the pandemic (Schotte & Zizzima, 2022). Within the first month of the lockdown, 3 million South Africans had lost their jobs, leading to an increase in poverty and food insecurity (Haffajee, 2020). In response, the government announced a R500-billion stimulus package, and took out a R70-billion loan from the International Monetary Fund (IMF), accelerating South Africa's deficit spending to 83% of GDP for the 2020/2021 financial year (Felix, 2020). Unfortunately, large-scale corruption in the distribution of the R500-billion stimulus package as well as in the procurement of personal protective equipment (PPE) and health infrastructure had a significant negative impact on South Africa's efforts to fight the COVID-19 pandemic (Corruption Watch, 2020b). Corruption, police brutality, and an increase in gender-based violence during the lockdown led to a further loss of lives. This chapter provides a timeline of how the COVID-19 pandemic unfolded in South Africa and discusses a number of selected themes: the economic impact, corruption, law enforcement, and the gendered implications of the pandemic.

Background

The first human coronavirus was discovered by scientists in 1965. Coronaviruses, named after the crown-like appearance of their surfaces, are common human pathogens that are responsible for a large proportion of upper

DOI: 10.4324/9781003294931-2

and lower respiratory tract infections (Kahn & McIntosh, 2005:S223). Since their discovery in the 1960s, seven human coronaviruses have been identified. The most common of these are two alpha (229E and NL63) and two beta (OC43 and HKU1) coronaviruses (CDC, 2020). Zoonotic coronaviruses are also known to spread to humans. Severe acute respiratory syndrome (SARS), which emerged in China in February 2003 and subsequently spread to many other countries, led to the death of 774 people, and consequently put zoonotic transmission in the spotlight (CDC, 2017). Virological studies also point toward dromedary camels as the source of Middle East respiratory syndrome (MERS), which was first reported in Saudi Arabia in 2012 (ECDC, 2021). The World Health Organisation's (WHO) investigation into the origin of COVID-19, which is closely related to bat and pangolin coronaviruses, found that it first emerged in the Chinese city of Wuhan in December 2019 and suggested that the selling of animal products at Huanan Seafood Wholesale Market was the probable source of this coronavirus pandemic (Maxmen, 2021).

COVID-19 is an airborne disease. The virus can spread from an infected person's mouth or nose in small liquid particles when they cough, sneeze, speak, or breathe. Even though most people infected by the novel coronavirus experience only mild to moderate respiratory illness, and recover without requiring special treatment, older people, and those with underlying conditions, including cardiovascular disease, diabetes, chronic respiratory disease, or cancer, can experience severe respiratory disease, including pneumonia. Once humans contract the disease, they can remain contagious for up to 20 days, even if they are asymptomatic (WHO, n.d.). Recent studies are demonstrating that COVID-19 may lead to long-term acute health problems for certain populations (Johns Hopkins Medicine, 2022).

Once the novel coronavirus was identified in Wuhan city, others in Hubei province imposed lockdowns. This, however, failed to contain the outbreak of the disease, which spread to other parts of mainland China, and from there, around the globe. On 24 January 2020, a *Lancet* report recognised the virus's 'pandemic potential' and recommended testing as well as PPE for healthcare workers (Huang *et al.*, 2020). The first modelling study, which was published at the end of January 2020, called for 'large scale public health interventions' (Wu, Leung & Leung, 2020). On 30 January 2020, with almost 8,000 confirmed cases across 19 countries, the WHO declared the COVID-19 outbreak a public health emergency of international concern (WHO, 2020a). The organisation declared a pandemic on 11 March 2020. At this point, infection rates were rising significantly in specifically Italy, Iran, South Korea, and Japan.

WHO Director General, Tedros Adhanom Ghebreyesus, recommended that states 'detect, test, treat, isolate, trace, and mobilise their people' in response to the pandemic. He further emphasised that hospitals needed to be readied, and health workers trained and protected (WHO, 2020b). In January 2020, the WHO published a comprehensive package of guidance documents for countries, covering topics related to the management of an outbreak of a new disease. Early efforts to curb the transmission of the disease by, for example, restricting public gatherings, tracing close contacts, and self-isolation failed (Sanyaolu, Okoriem, Hosein *et al.*, 2020). Countries then began to establish stricter control measures for transportation facilities, workplace environments, schools, and civil aviation. These attempts, however, also proved inadequate, which led to states implementing emergency shutdowns as well as curfews to prevent hospital systems from being completely overwhelmed (Sanyaolu, Okoriem, Hosein *et al.*, 2020). By the end of March 2020, the United States had overtaken China and Italy as the country with the highest number of confirmed cases in the world. To date, the United States has consistently reported the highest number of COVID-19-related deaths, followed by India and Brazil (WHO, 2022a).

As of 18 October 2022, the WHO has reported around 622 million confirmed COVID-19 cases worldwide, and over 6.5 million deaths (WHO, 2022a). Mortality rates vary by region and demographics, but based on the aforementioned data, the global case-fatality ratio is currently at 1.05%. It may be important to note here that the principal determinant of the infection-fatality rate (IFR) is age. A study by Levin *et al.* (2020) showed that IFR increases exponentially with age, doubling every six years, and increasing by a factor of 7500 from those that are ten years old (0.002%) to those that are 85 years old (15%). An important consequence of this is that the IFR in Sub-Saharan Africa, where about 2% of the population is over the age of 65, is about ten times less than in Europe, where 20% of the population is over the age of 65. This may also explain why South Africa, where about 5% of the population is over the age of 65, has had a more severe epidemic impact than most other countries in Sub-Saharan Africa.

COVID-19 in South Africa

On 5 March 2020, the South African health minister at the time, Zweli Mkhize, confirmed that COVID-19 had spread to South Africa. The country's first known case was a 38-year-old man who tested positive upon his return from northern Italy (South African Government, 2020a). One week into the outbreak, South Africa reported 17 confirmed cases, 16 of which were individuals who had travelled to South Africa from high-risk countries. President Cyril Ramaphosa declared a national state of disaster on 15 March 2020. Schools were closed, and a travel ban was imposed with immediate effect. On 17 March 2020 the National Coronavirus Command Council, headed by the President, was established to come up with a national plan to contain the spread of the disease. The national lockdown, starting on alert-level 5, began on 27 March (BusinessTech, 2020a). On the same day, the country recorded its first COVID-19 death (South African Government, 2020b).

Under alert-level 5, only essential services were permitted to operate. Non-essential workers could only leave their homes to purchase essential goods or to seek medical care. The international and inter-provincial movement of people, as well as public gatherings, was prohibited. Restrictions were imposed on public transport, including limitations on vehicle capacity. All childcare facilities, schools, and institutions of higher learning were closed, but could continue with online teaching and learning. The sale of alcohol and tobacco was also banned (Department of Cooperative Governance and Traditional Affairs, 2021). On 10 April 2020, Minister Mkhize recommended that the general public use cloth facemasks when going out in public (Department of Health, 2020a). The country remained under the strictest alert-level lockdown until 31 April 2020.

While South Africa's initial lockdown measures were quite severe in comparison to those imposed in other countries, the hard lockdown appeared to have had a significant effect on reducing infections. The number of cases reported each day rose rapidly until the end of March and then fell by a factor of 10 in one week once lockdown alert-level 5 had been imposed (WHO, 2022b).

On 13 April, the chair of the Ministerial Advisory Committee on COVID-19, Prof. Salim Abdool Karim, South Africa's leading clinical infectious disease epidemiologist, who is widely recognised for his research contributions in HIV prevention and treatment, indicated that the lockdown had been effective in delaying transmission and easing the burden on South Africa's healthcare facilities. He nevertheless warned that the country could see an exponential increase in COVID-19 cases, were the lockdown to be lifted. He therefore recommended devising a plan to systematically ease the lockdown in stages to keep infection rates low (Basson, 2020). Abdool Karim described an eight-stage plan to combat the coronavirus. The first stage focused on preparing for COVID-19, including establishing testing capacity. Stage 2 involved primary prevention, including banning international travel, closing schools, restricting gatherings, and promoting social distancing and hand hygiene. Stage 3 consisted of the national lockdown. Stage 4 focused on the deployment of community health workers to engage in door-to-door screening and contact tracing. Abdool Karim emphasised Stage 5: surveillance to identify and intervene in hotspots, Stage 6: preparing a medical care response for the peak, including the construction of field hospitals, and Stage 8: vigilance and national surveillance, including administering vaccines, if available. Stage 7 involved expanding burial capacity and managing the psychological impact of bereavement (Abdool Karim, 2020).

On 1 May 2020, Ramaphosa announced that lockdown restrictions would gradually be eased, and the lockdown was phased down to alert-level 4.[1] At this point, the number of confirmed infections stood at approximately 5,600, with a reported 103 COVID-19 deaths (WHO, 2020:c5). Under the new alert-level regulations, the wearing of masks in public was made compulsory. On 1 June 2020, restrictions were lowered to alert-level 3, which also lifted the ban on alcohol sales (SAnews, 2020).

On 12 July 2020, in an address to the nation, the President announced that the anticipated surge in COVID-19 cases had arrived. With 86,695 new confirmed cases and 997 deaths, South Africa had reached its first COVID-19 peak (WHO, 2022b). The state of disaster was extended until 15 August 2020. Although the country remained on alert-level 3, the alcohol ban was reintroduced along with a new curfew from 9 pm to 4 am. The resumption of alcohol sales and distribution had led to increased pressure on hospitals, including trauma and ICU units, due to road traffic accidents, violence, and related trauma, which occurred mostly at night (Williams, 2020). A study by Moultrie *et al.* (2021) showed that the weekly number of unnatural deaths (motor vehicle accidents, suicides, and murders) was reduced by half while a full ban on alcohol was in place during the COVID-19 lockdown in South Africa.

On 23 July 2020, President Ramaphosa announced the reclosure of all public schools for four weeks from 27 July to 24 August 2020, and the extension of the academic year into 2021 (Fengu, 2020). During the month of July 2020, 341,947 new COVID-19 cases were recorded, raising the total number of confirmed cases to almost half a million. The death toll rose to 8,005 (WHO, 2020d:4). By mid-August, the first peak had, however, flattened, and on 17 August, restrictions were lowered to alert-level 2. The temporary ban on tobacco sales[2] was also lifted. Restrictions were further lowered to alert-level 1 on 21 September 2020. President Ramaphosa addressed the nation again on 11 November 2020, announcing the reopening of international travel to all countries, the relaxation of alcohol trading times, and the extension of COVID unemployment support (Nyathi, 2020).

In early December 2020, COVID-19 cases were again on the rise, particularly in the Eastern Cape and Western Cape, KwaZulu-Natal, and Gauteng. On 9 December 2020, Health Minster Zweli Mkhize announced that the country had entered its second wave of infections. Numbers rose from below 1,000 new cases a day at the end of September 2020 to over 6,000 new cases a day. The virus peaked particularly amongst those between the ages of 15 and 19. It was speculated that this was due to a growing number of social events, which involved young people drinking alcohol, and not adhering to social distancing and mask protocols (Evans, 2020). On 14 December 2020, the President addressed the nation, announcing a return to alert-level 3 restrictions for 14 days in order to flatten the second wave of infections during the festive season. A curfew was introduced from 9 pm to 6 am, the sale and distribution of alcohol was banned, and public amenities such as beaches, dams, rivers, and public parks were closed (Daniel, 2020). There were 267,157 new COVID cases in December 2020, raising the total number of confirmed cases to over a million. The COVID-19-related death toll rose to 28,469 (Department of Health, 2020b).

Enter vaccines

In December 2020, the United Kingdom was the first country to authorise the use of both the Pfizer-BioNTech as well as the Oxford-AstraZeneca COVID-19 vaccines. On 3 January 2021, Minister Mkhize announced South

Africa's vaccine rollout strategy. At this stage, the country had secured doses for 10% of its population, with more to follow. The country's target was to vaccinate 67% of the population by the end of 2021 to achieve herd immunity. It was announced that during the first phase of the vaccination rollout, 1.25 million frontline healthcare workers would be vaccinated (Department of Health, 2021a). On 27 January 2021, the Department of Health announced the approval of the AstraZeneca vaccine for emergency use, and that 1 million doses would be delivered to the country on 1 February 2021, with a further half a million doses said to arrive later in the month (BusinessTech, 2021a).

By mid-January, the COVID-19 beta variant had been found in all nine of South Africa's provinces. There were 396,600 new COVID cases in January 2021, raising the total number of confirmed cases to almost 1.5 million. The death toll rose to 44,164 (African Centre for Disease Control, 2021). A week after the 1 million doses of the AstraZeneca vaccine had been delivered to South Africa by the Serum Institute of India, Government suspended the use of the vaccine after evidence emerged that the vaccine did not protect clinical-trial participants from mild to moderate illness caused by the beta variant. Government sold the AstraZeneca doses to a number of other African states and decided to inoculate healthcare workers with the Johnson & Johnson (J&J) vaccine, which had proven effective in preventing severe cases and hospitalisations caused by the beta variant (Mueller, Robbins & Chutel, 2021; Ray, 2021). On 16 February 2021, the first consignment of 80,000 doses of the J&J vaccine arrived in South Africa (TimesLive, 2021a). A day after, South Africa's national COVID-19 vaccination programme was officially launched. Healthcare workers at Khayelitsha District Hospital received their J&J vaccine dose together with President Ramaphosa and Health Minister Mkhize[3] (Brandt, 2021). On 27 February, the country received its second consignment of 80,000 J&J vaccine doses (Mahlati, 2021).

By 5 March 2021, exactly a year after the first COVID-19 case was recorded in South Africa, 100 000 vaccines had been administered in the country (TimesLive, 2021b). The third consignment of 80 000 J&J vaccines arrived during the week of 15 March 2021. On 17 March 2021, the South African Health Products Regulatory Authority (SAHPRA) also approved the use of the Pfizer vaccine, of which the government ordered 20 million doses (eNCA, 2021a). More than 50 vaccine sites were operational nationwide at this point (Persens, 2021). Although the second wave of infections had been surpassed by the beginning of March 2021, the death toll had risen to over 50 000 (TimesLive, 2021b). On 29 March 2021, the Aspen Pharmacare manufacturing facility in Gqeberha (formerly Port Elizabeth) was given approval to manufacture 220 million doses of the J&J vaccine, of which 30 million were earmarked for South Africa (eNCA, 2021b).

Minister Mkhize announced the suspension of the J&J vaccine on 13 April 2021, after the United States Food and Drug Administration recommended a pause in the use of the vaccine, pending a review of a possible link between the vaccination and a rare type of blot clot in the brain, which had been reported in six women in the United States (Ellis, 2021). It was later established that the chances of developing a blood clot after receiving the J&J vaccine are one in a million. With such low probabilities, the continued use of the J&J vaccine was approved by SAHPRA. Vaccination was resumed on 28 April (McCain, 2021). The first consignment of 325,260 doses of the Pfizer vaccine arrived in South Africa on 3 May 2021 and began to be administered under phase two of South Africa's vaccine rollout plan on 17 May 2021. Under phase two, essential workers, those over the age of 60, and people living in congregate setting, such as prisoners, could be vaccinated. By 31 May 2021, over one million vaccine doses had been administered in South Africa (NICD, 2021). By 18 June 2021, this number had doubled, with over 2 million vaccine doses having been administered (Brandt, 2021b).

By the end of May 2021, the third wave of infections was well underway. On 30 May 2021, Cyril Ramaphosa addressed the nation, announcing the tightening of restrictions from alert-levels 1 to 2 (Omarjee, 2021a). On 15 and 27 June 2021, respectively, restrictions were adjusted to alert-levels 3 and 4. On 28 June 2021, the country recorded 132,450 new cases (with an almost 29,000 weekly increase), suggesting that the third wave had peaked (WHO, 2022b). On 26 July 2021 restrictions were lowered to alert-level 3.

The civil unrest and widespread looting that occurred in KwaZulu-Natal and Gauteng from 9 to 18 July 2021 – following the imprisonment of former President Jacob Zuma for contempt of court, and fuelled by increased job-lessness and inequality worsened by the pandemic – slowed down the vaccine rollout as many vaccines sites shut down during this period (Benghu, 2021). An estimated 120 private pharmacies were destroyed, which led to a loss of approximately 47,500 vaccine doses and lots of damage to infrastructure (Department of Health, 2021b). Nevertheless, from 15 July 2021 onwards, vaccinations could be administered to those between the ages of 50 and 59 (SAnews, 2021a). Vaccinations for those aged 35 to 49 opened on 1 August (Sanews, 2021b).

In mid-August 2021, the Department of Health announced that the challenge of reaching the target of vaccinating 70% of South Africa's adult population by December 2021 had shifted from a shortage of supply to a lack of demand. At this stage, about four million South Africans (about 7% of the population) had been vaccinated, but vaccination levels had dropped, particularly among men between the ages of 35 and 49 (Bloomberg, 2021). Vaccine hesitancy is a large problem in South Africa. A 2021 Afrobarometer study showed that 54% of South Africans were unlikely to get a COVID-19 vaccine and that almost half of the population believes that prayer provides more protection against contracting the disease than a vaccine (Moosa, Mpako & Felton, 2021).

In order to increase the demand for vaccines, Cabinet moved the start date of vaccinations for those over the age of 18 from 1 September to 20 August 2021. On 20 August 2021, 560,000 people aged 18 to 34 regis-tered on the Government's Electronic Vaccination Data System (EVDS). On

3 September 2021, new Health Minister Joe Phaahla[4] announced that South Africa had the capacity to vaccinate between 300,000 and 400,000 people a day. It was also reported that government was making progress in creating a system to vaccinate people without identity documents, such as undocumented migrants. Minister Phaahla further noted that the government was looking into 'soft incentives' (e.g., free entertainment, sports, and cultural events) to encourage vaccination. He called on the private sector and higher education institutions to implement policies within the law to mandate vaccination (Nkgadima, 2021).

On 17 September 2021, Phaahla announced that vaccination numbers were still falling short of the 300,000 daily target. At that point, 15.7 million vaccine doses had been administered, with 11.2 million people (28% of the adult population) having received one dose, and 7.7 million people (almost 20% of adults) being fully vaccinated. The daily rate of, vaccinations (around 184,000 at the time) would have to be sustained in order to reach the target of 70% of adult coverage by Christmas 2021 (Chambers, 2021).

On 29 September 2021, the Department of Health confirmed that digital vaccine certificates would be issued from early October 2021 to everyone whose vaccination data was on the EVDS platform. While certificates were not required to gain access to essential and emergency services, the private sector was free to use them to control access to businesses. The certificates could also be used for international travel; the UK confirming that it would accept them from 11 October 2021 (BusinessTech, 2021b).

On 1 October 2021, with under 6,000 new confirmed cases, restrictions were lowered to alert-level 1. A decision was made to allow for a maximum of 2,000 people to gather outdoors, and 750 people to gather indoors. While there was speculation that pressure from churches was behind this decision, municipal elections, scheduled to take place on 1 November 2021, were also a major factor. Experts claimed that President Ramaphosa was ignoring scientific advice, putting politics ahead of health and economic concerns. Experts warned that large public gatherings, together with low vaccination coverage and complacency around social distancing and mask protocols, could result in an early fourth wave of COVID-19 infections, thousands of avoidable deaths, and spending the festive season under hard lockdown. This, in turn, would limit economic recovery (Khoza, Farber & Ash, 2021).

Vaccinations for those between the ages of 12 and 17 opened on 20 October 2021. Minors could receive one Pfizer dose at any vaccination site in South Africa without their parents' consent. The second vaccine dose was, however, discouraged at this point due to concerns of myocarditis in teenage boys (Turner, 2021). In mid-October 2021, the Ministerial Advisory Committee on COVID-19 vaccines advised that booster shots could be administered to individuals with comprised immunity. They also recommended that healthcare workers who were vaccinated with the J&J vaccine receive a booster shot, pending SAHPRA approval (SA News, 2021c). The Health Department also confirmed that pilot programmes to vaccinate undocumented people were operational in eThekwini, Cape Town, and Tshwane, with more sites to be phased in (Malan, 2021a). On 15 October 2021, South Africa surpassed the 20 million mark of administered vaccine doses, with over 10 million people being fully vaccinated (Malan, 2021b). At this point, South Africa had recorded over 2.9 million confirmed COVID-19 cases and almost 90 000 deaths (WHO, 2022b). At the end of November 2021, South Africa was the first country to detect the new, heavily mutated, but milder symptom causing, coronavirus variant referred to as Omicron (Callaway, 2021). Despite the variant already being present in numerous countries around the world, several states imposed travel bans on South Africa. Scientists and international bodies, including the WHO, expressed their outrage about these selective restrictions, labelling them as racist, unscientific, and counterproductive (Malan, 2021c). President Ramaphosa again addressed the nation on 28 November 2021, announcing that no changes would be made to the country's coronavirus alert level. He pleaded to states that had imposed travel bans on South Africa to reverse their decisions – albeit to no effect (South African Government, 2021).

On 8 December 2021, 20,000 new COVID-19 cases were recorded in South Africa; a record since the start of the fourth wave (Reuters, 2021a). On the same day, SAHPRA approved the third dose of the Pfizer vaccine for those over the age of 18. This dose could be administered six months after the second dose (SAHPRA, 2021). Children between the ages of 12 and 17 could also now receive a second dose of the Pfizer vaccine, 42 days after their first dose (Department of Health, 2021c). By the end of 2021, 28 million vaccine doses had been administered in South Africa, with 66% of the target population being fully vaccinated (WHO, 2022b). Government had missed its target of vaccinating 70% of the population by the end of 2021 by only 4%.

On 30 December 2021, after surveillance indicators had suggested that the country had passed its peak of the fourth wave, the midnight to 4 am curfew was lifted (Reuters, 2021b). On 31 January 2022, the country's coronavirus alert-level 1 was adjusted so that those testing positive for the virus, but showing no symptoms, would not be required to self-isolate. Those who tested positive and who were symptomatic only had to isolate for seven days, instead of ten. All schools also returned to full daily attendance, with the requirement of a one-metre social distancing being removed (Department of Health, 2022).

At midnight on 4 April 2022, the National State of Disaster was lifted although some transitional provisions, such as the wearing of face masks indoors and restrictions on public gatherings, remained in place for another 30 days (South African Government, 2022b). On 22 June 2022, Health Minister Joe Phaahla repealed the country's COVID-19 regulations, including the mask mandate (BusinessTech, 2022). While the pandemic had not ceased, the number of new cases, especially those requiring hospitalisation, or leading to death, had decreased significantly. On 27 June 2022, only 2,842 new confirmed cases and 81 deaths were recorded (WHO, 2022b).

As of 18 October 2022, South Africa has recorded 4,023,358 confirmed COVID-19 cases and 102,246 deaths. By 9 October 2022, 37,679458 vaccine doses had been administered (WHO, 2022b).

Economic impact

At the end of 2019, before COVID-19 had reached South Africa, the country had slid into a technical recession. Economic growth was recorded at 0.2%. Formal unemployment stood at 29%, with youth unemployment (53%) being the biggest concern (StatsSA, 2020). Credit rating agencies such as Fitch and Standard and Poor had downgraded the country's sovereign debt from stable to negative. Due to revenue shortfalls, the budget deficit had widened to 4.5%. Household debt stood at 34% of GDP, meaning that more than one-third of families in South Africa relied on debt as part of their household income. Due to the volatility of the Rand, basic food costs rose and fuel and electricity prices increased, leading to a rise in inequality (Nyathi & Nicolaides, 2019). Therefore, once COVID-19 arrived in South Africa, the country was in a tenuous socio-economic position (Naidu, 2021). At the end of March 2020, when lockdown was imposed, economists predicted that the economy would shrink by 2.5%–10% as a consequence of the pandemic (Ryan, 2020).

While government received widespread support for immediately instituting a hard lockdown, it was widely criticised for putting lives ahead of livelihoods. Within the first month of lockdown, 3 million South Africans had lost their jobs, leading to an increase in poverty and food insecurity (Haffajee, 2020). In response, government announced a R500-billion stimulus package on 21 April 2020, accelerating South Africa's deficit spending to over 10% of GDP for the 2020 financial year (Tromp & Kings, 2020). The stimulus package included the adoption of the Temporary Employer/Employee Relief Scheme (TERS); debt relief for small to medium-sized enterprises affected by the pandemic; and Social Relief Distress measures, which extended child support and unemployment grants and provided food parcels to vulnerable households (Tromp & Kings, 2020). While these measures were deemed appropriate to lessen the socio-economic impact of the pandemic in the short term, government did not have the financial means to avert an economic crisis in the long term. In May 2020, it was estimated that the state would lose R285 billion in tax revenue during the 2020/21 financial year because of a near-total cessation of economic activity during the hard lockdown (Ajam & Davis, 2020).

In late July 2020 – for the first time in South Africa's democratic history – government took out a R70-billion loan from the IMF. Even though this loan is not subject to strict conditionalities, which would compromise South Africa's fiscal sovereignty, austerity measures continue to be implemented to appease international investors as well as to service the country's total debt-to-GDP ratio, which had now risen to 83% (Felix, 2020).

Small, medium, and micro enterprises were the worst affected by the lockdown. In total, 42.7% of small businesses were forced to shut down. Of these, less than 50% had applied for COVID-19 relief funding, however, 99.9% of those that had applied were rejected. Less than 10% of the potential R200 billion COVID-19 Loan Guarantee Scheme was dispersed (Buthelezi, 2022). Former finance minister, Tito Mboweni, blamed South Africa's banks for the scheme's failure. Even though the scheme was designed in such a way that the National Treasury and the South African Reserve Bank (SARB) would absorb 94% of the risk, should businesses not be able to repay their loans, banks insisted that the SARB instructed them not to lend irresponsibly (Buthelezi, 2022).

Large-scale unemployment was the result of almost half of South African businesses closing down (BusinessTech, 2020d). In the second quarter of 2021, South Africa's official unemployment rate was recorded at 34.4%, accounting for 7.8 million people. The youth continued to be worst affected with 64.4% of those between the ages of 15 and 24 being unemployed and 42.9% of those aged 25–34 being unemployed (Omarjee, 2021b). Despite a 4.9% rise in GDP in 2021, following −7% contraction in 2020, there was no recovery in employment levels (StatsSA, 2021). In the first quarter of 2022, South Africa's unemployment rate stood at 34.5% (StatsSA, 2022b).

Corruption

Corruption has had a significant negative impact on South Africa's efforts to fight the COVID-19 pandemic, putting increased lives at risk, and further eroding confidence in government institutions. According to Transparency International's (2020a) Corruption Perceptions Index, South Africa ranks 69th out of 180 countries with a score of 44 out of 100. During 2020, South African civil society group, Corruption Watch, received 4 780 reports of corruption, the second-highest number since the organisation's inception in 2012. On average, 11 complaints were received daily from across South Africa. In addition to incidents relating to procurement and the distribution of goods and services, 2020 was also the year that saw the highest number of reports implicating the police and health sector in corruption-related actions (Corruption Watch, 2020a).

Prior to the COVID-19 pandemic, South Africa was already mired in corruption. A special commission of inquiry, the Zondo Commission, was launched in 2018 to investigate allegations of state capture during the Jacob Zuma administration. The Zondo Commission found that some of the heads of state-owned enterprises, as well as a number of top law enforcement officials, Cabinet ministers, and Zuma himself, were paid off by corrupt businesses to secure large government contracts. After a motion of no confidence in Parliament, Zuma was forced to resign as president in February 2018. President Cyril Ramaphosa came to power, vowing to root out corruption, yet many government officials and business owners continued with the graft, viewing the pandemic as a further opportunity to enrich themselves (Imray, 2021). Many of government's emergency measures that were put in place to deal with the economic impact of COVID-19, such as the R500-billion relief package, the R70-billion IMF loan, as well as emergency procurement measures presented opportunities for further corruption (Corruption Watch, 2020b). Accountability measures to monitor the use of these large sums of money were relaxed to seemingly fast-track the procurement of essential goods and services needed to fight the pandemic. Given that most items were procured under the guise of emergency, public scrutiny, and accountability could be evaded. Simultaneously, temptations to personally benefit from these fortunes, in a culture where malfeasance tends to go unpunished, ran high (Aikins, 2022).

On 23 July 2020, in an address to the nation, Ramaphosa announced that there were various allegations of corruption, including fraudulent Unemployment Insurance Fund (UIF) claims; overpricing of goods and services; violations of emergency procurement regulations; collusion between government officials and service providers; abuse of food parcel distribution; and the creation of fake non-profit organisations to access relief funding (BusinessTech, 2020b). In order to hasten and strengthen corruption investigations, Cyril Ramaphosa signed a proclamation, authorising Government's Special Investigating Unit (SIU) to investigate any unlawful or improper conduct by state institutions in the procurement of goods, works, and services during or relating to the national state of disaster. The SIU investigated dozens of companies that were believed to have benefited from dubious COVID-19 tenders (BusinessTech, 2020b).

A large number of irregularities were found in terms of the procurement of PPE, needed to protect frontline healthcare workers and carers from the coronavirus. It was reported that Gauteng MEC for health, Bandile Masuku, and the health department's former chief financial officer, Kabelo Lehloenya, were behind the irregular awarding of PPE contracts. Two such contracts, to the value of R125 million were allocated to Thandisizwe Diko, the husband of the President's spokesperson, Khusela Diko (BusinessTech, 2020c). The SIU estimates that there was up to R2.2 billion in irregular expenditure on PPE in Gauteng alone. Millions of Rands in PPE tenders were also awarded to companies and individuals tied to African National Congress secretary general and former Free State premier, Ace Magashule (BusinessTech, 2020c). Frontline healthcare workers paid the price for this corruption. By the beginning of August 2020, 24 000 health workers had contracted COVID-19 and 181 had died, given that many of them were not properly protected (Aljazeera, 2020). This led WHO director-general, Tedros Adhanom Ghebreyesus, to state the following at a media briefing in Geneva in late August 2020:

> Any type of corruption is unacceptable, however, corruption related to personal protective equipment, for me it's actually murder. If health workers work without PPE, we're risking their lives and the lives of the people they serve. It is murder and it has to stop.
>
> (Nkanjeni, 2020)

Private companies were equally complicit in price gouging of PPE equipment, such as masks. Sicuro Safety and Hennox Supplies admitted guilt and were fined for inflating face mask priced by up to 900%. Even DisChem, a popular pharmacy chain, was fined for the excessive pricing of masks (Magome, 2020).

In the Eastern Cape, Health MEC Sindiswa Gomba and former head of the Department of Health, Dr Thobile Mbengashe, were responsible for a R10-million scandal involving the procurement of motorcycle clinics, which were intended to be used to access deep rural areas of the Eastern Cape where there are no proper roads. Instead of procuring much-needed ambulance scooters, motorcycles were ordered that were unable to withstand the conditions of the province's rural roads, which did not meet the basic criteria for patient transport (Ellis & Jubase, 2020). In July 2020, at the time of the scooter scandal, the Eastern Cape had become a COVID-19 hotspot, and many hospitals were facing a dire shortage of personnel, PPE, and basic equipment such as blood pressure cuffs and oxygen. As a result, deaths increased rapidly in Nelson Mandela Bay (Ellis, 2021). On 22 July, it was reported that 96 people had died in the metro since the start of the month – an average of almost five a day (Nkosi, 2020).

In late September 2020, investigations into allegations of corruption in the procurement of health infrastructure, particularly the building of four ICU COVID-19 field hospitals in Gauteng, began (Heywood, 2020b). Millions of Rands were spent on building 'barrack-style field hospitals' to increase ICU bed capacity in anticipation of the first COVID-19 surge. The field hospitals were, however, nowhere near completion when the first wave of infections peaked, and many medical professionals claimed the structures were not fit for purpose, and were not needed in Gauteng. Out of a total provincial allocation of R5.9-billion for the fight against COVID-19, R3 billion was allocated to hospital refurbishment and construction. The majority of this money was wasted on unneeded infrastructure (Heywood, 2020a). Unfortunately, this expenditure became impossible to track, given that the Gauteng government stopped publishing its monthly COVID-19 Expenditure Disclosure reports in January 2021 (Heywood, 2022). It is, however, very clear that there were irregularities in the tendering and construction of these hospitals. The construction sector in South Africa is known for accepting bribes and kickbacks, as well as for price fixing, and using substandard materials to increase profits (Gilili, 2022).

On 29 September 2021, the SIU released a report that found that several senior officials at the South African health ministry were engaged in corruption, fraud, and the misappropriation of billions of Rands meant to aid the fight against COVID-19. The report found that former health minister, Zweli Mkhize, who resigned in early August 2021, interfered in the procurement process of a COVID-19 communications contract worth R150 million, which he awarded to close associates. In return, he received payments to his and his family's benefit, which he used to renovate one of his homes and to buy his son a car (Magome, 2021).

The media and civil society organisations applied pressure on government to undertake measures to counteract corrupt practices. At the end of August 2020, government published a full list of contracts awarded under the emergency procurement regulations, opening them up for public scrutiny. On 2 September, the entire management of the UIF was suspended. Bandile Masuku was dismissed; Khusela Diko was suspended, although she will remain in the public service; and Zweli Mkhize resigned. South Africans and civil society remain hopeful that decisive action against deep-seated corruption will continue (Corruption Watch, 2020b; Heywood, 2020b).

Law enforcement

As mentioned above, Corruption Watch's 2020 annual report indicated that reports of police corruption increased during 2020, most likely due to the COVID-19 National State of Disaster and the subsequent hard lockdown which was imposed in late March 2020. Furthermore, Corruption Watch listed the South African Police Service as the most corrupt government institution in South Africa. Unfortunately, the country's apartheid-era culture of impunity, brutality, and abuse of power has found its way into democratic South Africa and has reduced the public's confidence in the police (Faull & Newman, 2011). On 18 March 2020, Transparency International (2020b) published an advisory, cautioning that 'corruption often thrives during times of crisis, particularly when institutions and oversight are weak, and public trust is low'. Lockdown conditions created an environment ripe for police corruption, with police officers having wide discretion to interpret whether members of the public were flouting regulations or not and extort bribes as a result (Knoetze, 2020).

While most types of violence decreased following the implementation of lockdown, incidents of police violence against civilians reportedly doubled after 26 March 2020, with security forces coercively enforcing quarantine measures (ACLED, 2020). Under lockdown level 5, nearly 3,000 soldiers were deployed mainly to townships across South Africa. The police set up hundreds of roadblocks and vehicle checkpoints across the country, and encouraged security forces to use force to enforce the liquor ban. During the first week of lockdown, 2,000 people had been arrested for flouting lockdown regulations. On 21 April 2020, additional soldiers were deployed to support the police (Trippe, 2020).

By 1 June 2020, 230 000 people had been arrested, mostly for minor violations such as being outdoors without a permit or possessing alcohol and/or cigarettes (Trippe, 2020). Amnesty International (2020) reports that at least 115 people died in police custody during lockdown in 2020 alone. By 24 June 2020, at least 10 South Africans (all of them Black) had died in police action. One such individual was Collins Khosa, who was assaulted by members of the SANDF (and subsequently died from his injuries) for allegedly having cups of alcohol in his front yard in Alexandra, a township north of

Johannesburg (Amnesty International, 2020). Further analysis on the policing of the COVID-19 lockdowns is provided in Chapter 8.

Gendered implications

As witnessed through previous pandemics such as the 2014–2016 Ebola outbreak in West Africa as well as the 2015–2016 Zika virus outbreak in South America, epidemics do have a disproportionate effect on women. Gendered norms result in women being more likely to be infected by a virus given their principal roles as family caregivers and frontline healthcare workers (WHO, 2019). Women are also more likely to be affected by the social and economic downturns that result from pandemics (Flor *et al.*, 2022). Nevertheless, given women's limited decision-making power, public health efforts and policies have not explicitly addressed the gendered effects of pandemics, including COVID-19 (Parry & Gordon, 2020:796). While women have been disproportionally affected by the COVID-19 crisis globally, women in South Africa were particularly hard hit (Casale & Shepherd, 2021).

The National Income Dynamics Study – Coronavirus Rapid Mobile Survey (NIDS-CRAM), a nationwide household survey conducted over five waves of the pandemic from May 2020 to July 2021, found that women were not only much more likely to lose their jobs and work fewer hours during the lockdown, but that they also endured a slower recovery relative to men when the economy started to reopen (Casale & Shepherd, 2021). As a result of school closures, women were also found to take on additional childcare responsibilities, which further limited their ability to engage in paid work, or to work as many hours as before. Despite these skewed labour market outcomes, women were less likely to benefit from COVID-specific government income support measures (Casale & Shepherd, 2021). A spike in gender-based violence during the lockdown further eroded gender equality gains.

Employment

Of the 2.9 million jobs that were lost during the first strict lockdown phase in April 2020, just under 2 million (or two-thirds) were accounted for by women (Casale & Shepherd, 2021:6). The agricultural, hospitality, and retail sectors, which typically employ large numbers of women, were hit hardest by the pandemic, and therefore laid off the most workers. Black women were particularly affected by job losses. Before the outbreak of the pandemic, 36.5% of black women in South Africa were unemployed. This number increased to 42.4% in the fourth quarter of 2021 (StatsSA, 2022a). Black women make up 47.6% of the informal sector and dominate the domestic work sphere (StatsSA, 2015). Given that they find themselves in more precarious employment relationships, often without formal employment contracts, it made it easier for employers to reduce their employment when lockdown restrictions were imposed (Casale & Shepherd, 2021:7).

In addition to experiencing greater job losses than men, employed women also saw much larger declines in mean hours worked once the hard lockdown was imposed. Between February and April 2020, mean hours worked fell by 35% for women compared to 26% for men (Casale & Shepherd, 2021:8). As mentioned above, women also experienced a slower recovery in employment levels than men when the economy reopened. By March 2021, the recovery for women was still 8% below pre-pandemic levels, while men's employment had fully recovered (Casale & Shepherd, 2021:1). Even in the case of women having returned to work, many were still working fewer hours on average compared to pre-pandemic times. This was not the case for men (Casale & Shepherd, 2021:24). One reason for the reduction in hours worked is that women had to take up increased care responsibilities under lockdown.

Unpaid labour

Women's 'double burden' of participating both in the labour market as well as in unpaid reproductive and care work was worsened by the pandemic. Women had to take on greater care responsibilities such as looking after ill and elderly family members as well as children. During lockdown, employed mothers were in many instances unable to call on support networks for childcare, given that childcare facilities and schools were closed, and grandparents were unable to fulfil their childcaring roles because of the higher mortality rate amongst the elderly (Alon *et al.*, 2020). When asked how much additional time was spent per day on childcare, 80% of women, compared to 65% of men, reported that they spent over four hours more per day on childcare during lockdown (Casale & Shepherd, 2021:19). This increased burden of unpaid labour has in many instances had a negative effect on women's careers and income. Additional caring responsibilities have reduced women's work productivity, which could make them less likely to be considered for promotions, and which may negatively affect their lifetime income and pension. In other instances, it has pressured women to leave their paid jobs for temporary employment (Power, 2020).

Income support

Even though women accounted for most job losses and reductions in mean hours worked during the lockdown, they were underrepresented in the COVID-19-specific government income support provided for unemployed and furloughed workers (those with employment, but unable to work because of lockdown restrictions). Only 35–39% of the UIF-TERS beneficiaries were women (Casale & Shepherd, 2021:11). Given that many women in South Africa do not have formal employment contracts, and few of them are registered by their employers for the UIF, they did not qualify for UIF-TERS assistance (Venter, 2020).

Women were also underrepresented in the disbursement of the COVID-19 Social Relief of Distress Grant (SRDG) of R350 a month. By March 2021, only 36% of the grant's recipients were women (Casale & Shepherd, 2021:13). A key reason for this underrepresentation is that the SRDG could not be held concurrently with other social grants. This deterred women, who make up the majority of Child Support Grant recipients, from applying. The eligibility criterion in fact penalised unemployed women for also caring for their children (Casale & Shepherd, 2021:14).

Domestic violence

Since the outbreak of the COVID-19 pandemic, gender-based violence, particularly intimate partner violence, has also increased as a consequence of mandatory lockdowns, quarantining, self-isolation as well as security, health, and income concerns worsened by confined living conditions (UN Women, 2020). A 2020 rapid gender assessment survey commissioned by UN Women and the United Nations Population Fund (UNFPA) showed that approximately one-third of participants know at least one person who was a victim of gender-based violence during the pandemic (UN Women & UNFPA, 2020). Before the pandemic, it was estimated that women in South Africa are five times more likely to be killed on account of their gender than elsewhere. Crowded homes, substance abuse, limited access to services, and reduced peer support were listed as aggravating circumstances (StatsSA, 2018). Within the first two weeks of lockdown, the Gender-Based Violence Command Centre had received 8 764 calls from women and children who experienced violence while confined to their homes. Domestic violence centres had at this point reached their capacity due to lockdown and social distancing measures and were therefore unable to take in many vulnerable women and children (van Dyk, 2020). Before the outbreak of the pandemic, some women were able to find refuge or seek support from their parents, friends, neighbours, or the community, but lockdown measures made it difficult for them to access this support (Nigam, 2020). This lack of access to regular social networks and sources of social and health support placed women in more vulnerable positions.

Conclusion

More than 100 000 lives have been lost in South Africa due to the COVID-19 virus. Were it not for the imposition of the national lockdown, many more individuals would likely have died. Nevertheless, containment measures had a substantial negative impact on South Africa's economy as well as on citizens' livelihoods and safety. Since August 2021, South Africa is the country with the highest unemployment rate in the world (Naidoo, 2021). More than half of the population live below the national poverty line, with women-headed households being worst affected by the COVID-19 economic slump. Government's R500-billion stimulus package was undermined by widespread corruption; food parcels and unemployment relief did not reach the truly destitute. During lockdown, some South Africans also died at the hands of the police and SANDF forces, and women and children became increasingly vulnerable to gender-based violence.

Professor Brian Gerard Williams, an eminent epidemiologist developed the first model to demonstrate that a policy of Test-and-Treat would make it possible to end the HIV epidemic in South Africa – a model which provided impetus for the development of the now widely accepted policy targets of '90-90-90' – argues the following: If only 10% of COVID-19 relief measures had been spent on putting in place a few basic measures: good monitoring and surveillance (i.e., contact tracing), developing test kits, treating and isolating those infected, and getting people vaccinated, South Africa could have contained the pandemic in its early stages, saved thousands of lives, livelihoods, and the economy (Williams, 2022). What this would, however, have demanded is good leadership – something South Africa (and many other countries who ineffectively responded to the pandemic) lacked. In preparation for the next inevitable pandemic, it would be worthwhile for government to invest in health systems, surveillance, data systems and epidemiological skills, as well as good leadership which results in strong government action.

Notes

1 The Ministerial Advisory Committee had the responsibility to advise the Minister of Health, regarding which Alert Level (level of restrictions to be applied during the national state of disaster) should be declared nationally, provincially, in a metropolitan area, or district. The Committee took into account the epidemiological trends of COVID-19 infections; the health system capacity to respond to the disease burden in a specified area; and any other factors that would influence the level of infection, hospitalization and mortality (South African Government, 2022a).
2 Evidence, in fact, strongly suggests that smoking reduces an individual's chances of developing COVID. The coronavirus attaches itself to the same cell membrane protein in the lungs which nicotine attaches itself to. It is therefore harder for the virus to attach itself to this cell membrane protein in smokers' lungs. While this should not be viewed as an incentive to start smoking, the ban in cigarette sales in South Africa was in fact unscientific and futile (Williamson *et al.*, 2020).
3 Government, and particularly the President and Health Minister's, urgency to respond to the COVID-19 pandemic contrasts markedly to the HIV/AIDS response under Thabo Mbeki and Manto Tshabalala-Msimang, which was characterised by denialism for almost a decade.
4 Zweli Mkhize resigned as health minister in early August amid corruption scandals (discussed in more detail below).

References

Abdool Karim, S.S. (2020). The South African response to the pandemic. *The New England Journal of Medicine*, 382, e95.
African Centre for Disease Control. (2021). *Outbreak Brief 55: Coronavirus Disease 2019 (COVID-19) Pandemic*. Retrieved from https://africacdc.org/download/

outbreak-brief-55-coronavirus-disease-2019-covid-19-pandemic/   [Accessed 22 September 2021].

Aikins, E.R. (2022). *Corruption in Africa Deepens the Wounds of COVID-19*. Pretoria: Institute for Security Studies.

Ajam, T. & Davis, D. (2020). Unprecedented tax collapse endangers post-Covid recovery. *The Daily Maverick*, 14 May. Retrieved from https://www.dailymaverick.co.za/article/2020-05-14-unprecedented-tax-collapse-endangers-post-covid-recovery/

Al Jazeera. (2020). South Africa sets up body to probe coronavirus corruption. *Al Jazeera*, 7 August.

Alon, T.M., Doepke, M., Olmstead-Rumsey, J. & Tertilt, M. (2020). *The Impact of COVID-19 on Gender Equality* (Working Paper No. 26947). Cambridge, MA: National Bureau of Economic Research.

Amnesty International. (2020). *South Africa 2020*. Retrieved from https://www.amnesty.org/en/location/africa/southern-africa/south-africa/report-south-africa/ [Accessed 1 November 2021].

Armed Conflict Location & Event Data Project (ACLED). (2020). *CDT Spotlight: South Africa*. Retrieved from https://acleddata.com/2020/06/04/cdt-spotlight-south-africa/ [Accessed 24 October 2021].

Basson, A. (2020). The difficult truth: Rise in cases expected after lockdown, says expert. *News24*, 13 April.

Benghu, L. (2021). #UnrestSA: Vaccine rollout halted in parts of KZN, Gauteng due to looting. *News24*, 13 July.

Bloomberg. (2021). South Africa's vaccine headache switches from supply to demand. *BusinessTech*, 13 August.

Brandt, K. (2021a). No tears: Ramaphosa gets his COVID-19 jab. *Eyewitness News*, 17 February.

Brandt, K. (2021b). SA vaccinates over 2 million people as authorities give J&J study thumbs up. *Eyewitness News*, 19 June.

BusinessTech. (2020a). Ramaphosa announces 21-day coronavirus lockdown for South Africa. *BusinessTech*, 23 March.

BusinessTech. (2020b). Billions of rands looted by South Africa's 'Covidpreneurs': Report. *BusinessTech*, 26 July.

BusinessTech. (2020c). Gauteng PPE tender corruption uncovered. *BusinessTech*, 9 August.

BusinessTech. (2020d). Lockdown forced nearly half of small businesses in South Africa to close: Study. *BusinessTech*, 9 August.

BusinessTech. (2021a). How South Africa's new Covid-19 vaccine 'ID system' will work – and the documents you will need. *BusinessTech*, 28 January.

BusinessTech. (2021b). Good news for South Africans travelling to the UK. *BusinessTech*, 15 October.

BusinessTech. (2022). South Africa ends Covid curbs including mask wearing. *BusinessTech*, 23 June.

Buthelezi, L. (2022). 'They wouldn't budge': Mboweni blames banks for failure of the Loan Guarantee Scheme. *Fin24*, 04 May.

Callaway, E. (2021). Heavily mutated Omicron variant puts scientists on alert. *Nature*, 600(21).

Casale, D. & Shepherd, D. (2021). 'The gendered effects of the COVID-19 crisis and ongoing lockdown in South Africa: Evidence from NIDS-CRAM Waves 1–5.'

National Income Dynamics (NIDS)-Coronavirus Rapid Mobile Survey (CRAM) Wave 5.

Centers for Disease Control and Prevention (CDC). (2017). *Severe Acute Respitory Syndrome (SARS)*. Retrieved from https://www.cdc.gov/sars/about/fs-sars.html [Accessed 16 July 2022].

Centers for Disease Control and Prevention (CDC). (2020). *Human Coronavirus Types*. Retrieved from https://www.cdc.gov/coronavirus/types.html [Accessed 20 September 2021].

Chambers, D. (2021). Vaccine passports and jabs for kids on the way, says Joe Phaahla. *TimesLive*, 17 September.

Corruption Watch. (2020a). *Annual Report 2020: From Crisis to Action*. Retrieved from https://www.corruptionwatch.org.za/wp-content/uploads/2021/05/Corruption-Watch-AR-2020-DBL-PG-20210324.pdf [Accessed 23 October 2021].

Corruption Watch. (2020b). *In South Africa, COVID-19 has Exposed Greed and Spurred Long-Needed Action Against Corruption*. Retrieved from https://www.transparency.org/en/blog/in-south-africa-covid-19-has-exposed-greed-and-spurred-long-needed-action-against-corruption# [Accessed 23 October 2021].

Daniel, L. (2020). SA back to 'adjusted' Level 3 – here are some of the new rules. *Business Insider*, 28 December.

Department of Cooperative Governance and Traditional Affairs (South Africa). (2020). Disaster Management Act, 2002 (Act No. 57 of 2002): Regulations made in terms of Section 27(2) by the Minister of Cooperative Governance and Traditional Affairs. (Notice 398). *Government Gazette*, 43148, 25 March.

Department of Health (South Africa). (2020a). Dr Zwele Mkhize recommends the widespread use of cloth masks. *COVID-19 Online Resource & News Portal*, 10 April. Retrieved from https://sacoronavirus.co.za/2020/04/10/dr-zweli-mkhize-recommends-the-widespread-use-of-cloth-masks/ [Accessed 21 September 2021].

Department of Health (South Africa). (2020b). Update on Covid-19 (31st December 2020). *COVID-19 Online Resource & News Portal*, 31 December. Retrieved from https://sacoronavirus.co.za/2020/12/31/update-on-covid-19-31st-december-2020/ [Accessed 22 September 2021].

Department of Health (South Africa). (2021a). Minister Zweli Mkhize public briefing statement South Africa's COVID-19 vaccine strategy 3 January 2021. *COVID-19 Online Resource & News Portal*, 3 January. Retrieved from https://sacoronavirus.co.za/2021/01/03/minister-zweli-mkhize-public-briefing-statement-south-africas-covid-19-vaccine-strategy-3-january-2021/ [Accessed 22 September 2021].

Department of Health (South Africa). (2021b). [Twitter] 23 July. Retrieved from https://twitter.com/healthza/status/1418537304113696768 [Accessed 16 October 2021].

Department of Health (South Africa). (2021c). Circular: Changes to vaccine roll-out eligibility criteria for adolescents (12–17 years). *COVID-19 Online Resource & News Portal*, 9 December. Retrieved from https://sacoronavirus.co.za/2021/12/09/circular-changes-to-vaccine-roll-out-eligibility-criteria-for-adolescents-12-17-years-09-dec-2021/ [Accessed 28 February 2022].

Department of Health (South Africa). (2022). Cabinet approved changes to adjusted alert level 1 COVID-19 regulations. *COVID-19 Online Resource & News Portal*, 9 December. Retrieved from https://sacoronavirus.co.za/2022/01/31/cabinet-approves-changes-to-adjusted-alert-level-1-covid-19-regulations/   [Accessed 28 February 2022].

Department of Statistics South Africa (StatsSA). (2018). *Quarterly Labour Force Survey – Quarter 2: 2018.* Pretoria, South Africa.

Department of Statistics South Africa (StatsSA). (2020). *Quarterly Labour Force Survey – Quarter 4: 2019.* Pretoria, South Africa.

Department of Statistics South Africa (StatsSA). (2021). *Gross Domestic Product: Second Quarter 2021.* Pretoria, South Africa.

Department of Statistics South Africa (StatsSA). (2022a). *Quarterly Labour Force Survey (QLFS) Q4: 2021.* Pretoria, South Africa.

Department of Statistics South Africa (StatsSA). (2022b). *Quarterly Labour Force Survey (QLFS) Q1: 2022.* Pretoria, South Africa.

Ellis, E. (2021). Eastern Cape Health MEC felled by medical scooters and Madiba funeral money. *The Daily Maverick*, 21 February.

Ellis, E. (2021). South Africa suspends use of J&J vaccine, 'hopefully for only a few days'. *The Daily Maverick*, 13 April.

Ellis, E. & Jubase, H. (2020). Ambulance scooters saga: 'We showed the minister the wrong vehicles'. *The Daily Maverick*, 15 July.

eNCA. (2021a). South Africa approves another COVID-19 vaccine. *eNCA*, 17 March.

eNCA. (2021b). COVID-19 vaccine: J&J commits 30 million doses for SA. *eNCA*, 29 March.

European Centre for Disease Prevention and Control (ECDC). (2021). *MERS-CoV Worldwide Overview.* Retrieved from https://www.ecdc.europa.eu/en/middle-east-respiratory-syndrome-coronavirus-mers-cov-situation-update   [Accessed 20 September 2021].

Evans, J. (2020). Covid-19: SA enters second wave as Mkhize warns of surge in infections among teens. *News 24*, 9 December.

Faull, A. & Newham, G. (2011). *Protector or Predator? Tackling Police Corruption in South Africa.* Pretoria: Institute for Security Studies Monograph, 182.

Felix, J. (2021). R70 billion IMF loan won't compromise SA's fiscal sovereignty, says Tito Mboweni. *Fin24*, 11 June.

Fengu, M. (2020). Public schools to close for 4 weeks, academic year will be extended. *City Press*, 23 July.

Flor, L.S., Friedman, J., Spencer, C.N., *et al.* (2022). Quantifying the effects of the COVID-19 pandemic on gender equality on health, social, and economic indicators: A comprehensive review of data from March, 2020, to September, 2021. *The Lancet*, 399(10344), P2381–2397.

Gilili, C. (2022). Public works, SIU declare war on infrastructure tender corruption. *Mail & Guardian*, 24 May.

Haffajee, F. (2020). The day the bottom fell out of South Africa – a triple pandemic has hit us. *The Daily Maverick*, 15 July.

Heywood, M. (2020a). Big questions loom over Gauteng's billion-rand ICU field hospitals. *The Daily Maverick*, 25 September.

Heywood, M. (2020b). Scandal of the Year: Covid-19 corruption. *The Daily Maverick*, 27 December.

Heywood, M. (2022). Gauteng's 'new' R1.2bn Covid-19 ICU hospitals still lie abandoned, unfinished or underused. *Daily Maverick*, 25 March.

Huang, C., Wang, Y., Li, X. *et al.* (2020). Clinical features of patients infected with 2019 novel coronavirus in Wuhan, China. *The Lancet*, 395(10223), 497–506.

Imray, G. (2021). Hope that South Africa's COVID-19 corruption inspires action. *Associated Press News*, 15 March.

Johns Hopkins Medicine. (2022). *Long COVID: Long-Term Effects of COVID-19.* Retrieved from https://www.hopkinsmedicine.org/health/conditions-and-diseases/coronavirus/covid-long-haulers-long-term-effects-of-covid19#:~:text=Breathing%20Issues%20after%20COVID%2D19,is%20possible%2C%20but%20takes%20time. [Accessed 18 October 2022].

Kahn, J.S. & McIntosh, K. (2005). History and recent advances in coronavirus discovery. *The Pediatric Infectious Disease Journal*, 24(11), S223–S227.

Khoza, A., Farber, T. & Ash, P. (2021). Cyril's Covid gamble. *Sunday Times*, 3 October: 1–2.

Knoetze, D. (2020). COVID-19: Lockdown creates ripe pickings for corrupt police. *GroundUp*, 15 April. Retrieved from https://www.groundup.org.za/article/covid-19-lockdown-creates-ripe-pickings-corrupt-police/ [Accessed 24 October 2021].

Levin, A.T., Hanage, W.P., Owusu-Boaitey, N., Cochran, K.B., Walsh, S.P. & Meyerowitz-Katz, G. (2020). Assessing the age specificity of infection fatality rates for COVID-19: Systemic review, meta-analysis, and public policy implications. *European Journal of Epidemiology*, 35, 1123–1138.

Magome, M. (2020). South Africa warns COVID-19 corruptions puts 'lives at risk'. *The Washington Post*, 26 July.

Magome, M. (2021). Report: Corruption at S Africa health ministry during COVID. *Associated Press News*, 29 September.

Mahlati, Z. (2021). Second batch of 80 000 doses of Johnson & Johnson vaccine arrives in SA. *Independent Online*, 27 February.

Malan, M. (2021a). [Twitter] 15 October. Retrieved from https://twitter.com/miamalan/status/1448906881234358277 [Accessed 16 October 2021].

Malan, M. (2021b). [Twitter] 15 October. Retrieved from https://twitter.com/miamalan/status/1449074521353375750 [Accessed 16 October 2021].

Malan, M. (2021c). Debunked: The cruel and racist logic of Omicron travel bans. *Mail & Guardian*, 8 December.

Maxmen, A. (2021). WHO report into COVID pandemic origins zeroes in on animal markets, not labs. *Nature*, 592, 173–174.

McCain, N. (2021). Johnson & Johnson vaccination drive to resume at more sites as jab safe to use – Zweli Mkhize. *News24*, 26 April.

Moosa, M., Mpako, A. & Felton, J. (2021). South Africans support government's COVID-19 response but are critical of corruption and sceptical of vaccines. *Afrobarometer*, Dispatch No. 467.

Moultrie, T.A., Dorrington, R.E., Laubscher, R., Groenewald, P., Harry, C.D.H., Matzopoulos, R. & Bradshaw, D. (2021). Unnatural deaths, alcohol bans and curfews: Evidence from quasi-natural experiment during COVID-19. *The South African Medical Journal*, 111(9), 834–837.

Mueller, B., Robbins, R. & Chutel, L. (2021). South Africa says AstraZeneca's vaccine doesn't work well against a new variant. *The New York Times*, 7 February.

Naidoo, P. (2021). South Africa's unemployment rate is now highest in the world. *Aljazeera*, 24 August.

Naidu, S. (2021). The impact of COVID-19: The conundrum of South Africa's socio-economic landscape. *Accord*, 3 March. Retrieved from https://www.accord.

org.za/analysis/the-impact-of-covid-19-the-conundrum-of-south-africas-socio-economic-landscape/ [Accessed 17 October 2021].

National Institute for Communicable Diseases (NICD). (2021). *Latest Confirmed Cases of COVID-19 in South Africa (1 June 2021).* Retrieved from https://www.nicd.ac.za/latest-confirmed-cases-of-covid-19-in-south-africa-1-june-2021/ [Accessed 25 September 2021].

Nigam, S. (2020). *COVID-19: Right to Life with Dignity and Violence in Homes.* Retrieved from https://papers.ssrn.com/sol3/papers.cfm?abstract_id=3631756 [Accessed 23 October 2021].

Nkanjeni, U. (2020). 'Any type of corruption is unacceptable': WHO boss scolds SA for Covid-19 corruption. *Sunday Times*, 24 August.

Nkgadima, R. (2021). Government looking into 'soft incentives' to encourage COVID-19 vaccinations, says Joe Phaahla. *Independent Online*, 3 September.

Nkosi, N. (2020). Report Eastern Cape Covid-19 deaths daily, Mkhize tells Gomba. *DispatchLive*, 22 July.

Nyathi, M. (2020). Ramaphosa extends UIF and TERS payment by a month, relaxes alcohol trade and international travel restrictions. *City Press*, 11 November.

Nyathi, A. & Nicolaides, G. (2019). Oil price spike and weakening rand feed massive fuel price hike. *Eyewitness News*, 31 March.

Omarjee, H. (2021a). Ramaphosa urges diligence as he tightens COVID-19 restrictions. *Business Day*, 30 May.

Omarjee, L. (2021b). SA's unemployment rate hits record 34.4%. *Fin24*, 24 August.

Parry, B.R. & Gordon, E. (2021). The shadow pandemic: Inequitable gendered impacts of COVID-19 in South Africa. *Gender Work Organ*, 28, 795–806.

Persens, L. (2021). SA to receive more tranches of J&J vaccine this week, authorities say. *Eyewitness News*, 15 March.

Power, K. (2020). The COVID-19 pandemic has increased the care burden of women and families. *Sustainability: Science, Practice and Policy*, 16(1), 67–73.

Probst, C., Parry, C.D.H., Wittchen, H. & Rehm, J. (2018). The socioeconomic profile of alcohol-attributable mortality in South Africa: A modelling study. *BMC Medicine*, 16(97).

Ray, S. (2021). Report: South Africa asks Indian maker of AstraZeneca vaccine to take back one million doses. *Forbes*, 16 February.

Reuters. (2021a). South Africa reports nearly 20,000 COVID-19 cases, an Omicron-wave record. *Reuters*, 9 December.

Reuters. (2021b). South Africa lifts curfew as it says COVID-19 fourth wave peaks. *Reuters*, 31 December.

Ryan, C. (2020). SA economy could crater up to 10% this year. *Moneyweb*, 25 March.

SA News. (2021). South Africa to look at first use of booster COVID-19 vaccines. *BusinessTech*, 15 October.

Sanyaolu, A., Okorie, C., Hosein, Z. *et al.* (2020). Global pandemicity of COVID-19: Situation Report as of June 9, 2020. *Infectious Diseases: Research and Treatment*, 14, 1–8.

Schotte, S. & Zizzamia, R. (2022). The livelihood impacts of COVID-19 in urban South Africa: A view from below. *Social Indicators Research*. https://doi.org/10.1007/s11205-022-02978-7.

South African Government. (2020a). *Minister Zweli Mkhize reports first case of Coronavirus COVID-19.* Retrieved from https://www.gov.za/speeches/health-reports-first-case-covid-19-coronavirus-5-mar-2020-0000 [Accessed 21 September 2021].

South African Government. (2020b). *Minister Zweli Mkhize Confirms Total of 1170 Cases of Coronavirus COVID-19.* Retrieved from https://www.gov.za/speeches/minister-zweli-mkhize-confirms-total-1170-cases-coronavirus-covid-19-27-mar-2020-0000 [Accessed 21 September 2021].

South African Government. (2021). *President Cyril Ramaphosa: Address on South Africa's Response to Coronavirus COVID-19 Pandemic – 28 Nov.* Retrieved from https://www.gov.za/speeches/president-cyril-ramaphosa-address-south-africas-response-coronavirus-covid-19-pandemic-28 [Accessed 28 February 2022].

South African Government. (2022a). *About Alert System.* Retrieved from https://www.gov.za/covid-19/about/about-alert-system [Accessed 17 July 2022].

South African Government. (2022b). *President Cyril Ramaphosa: South Africa's Response to Coronvirus COVID-19 pandemic.* Retrieved from https://www.gov.za/speeches/president-cyril-ramaphosa-south-africas-response-coronavirus-covid-19-pandemic-4-apr-2022 [Accessed 16 July 2022].

South African Government News Agency (Sanews). (2020). *SA Moves to Alert Level 3.* Retrieved from https://www.sanews.gov.za/south-africa/sa-moves-alert-level-3 [Accessed 21 September 2021].

South African Government News Agency (Sanews). (2021a). *COVID Vaccination for those Aged 50 and above to Start on 15 July.* Retrieved from https://www.sanews.gov.za/south-africa/covid-vaccination-those-aged-50-and-above-start-15-july [Accessed 25 September 2021].

South African Government News Agency (Sanews). (2021b). *35–49 Age Group to be Vaccinated from 1 August.* Retrieved from https://www.sanews.gov.za/south-africa/35-49-age-group-be-vaccinated-1-august [Accessed 25 September 2021].

South African Government News Agency (Sanews). (2021c). *SAHPRA Approves Protocol for J&J Vaccine Booster Trial for Health Workers.* Retrieved from https://www.sanews.gov.za/south-africa/sahpra-approves-protocol-jj-vaccine-booster-trial-health-workers [Accessed 25 September 2021].

South African Health Products Regulatory Authority (SAHPRA). (2021). *SAHPRA Approval of Booster Dosing with the Pfizer (Comirnaty) COVID-19 Vaccine.* Retrieved from https://www.sahpra.org.za/press-releases/sahpra-approval-of-booster-dosing-with-the-pfizer-comirnaty-covid-19-vaccine2/ [Accessed 28 February 2022].

TimesLive. (2021a). J&J vaccines arrive in SA on Tuesday night. *TimesLive*, 16 February.

TimesLive. (2021b). SA hits vaccine milestone as 100,000 shots have now been administered. *TimesLive*, 05 March.

Transparency International. (2020a). *Corruption Perceptions Index: South Africa.* Retrieved from https://www.transparency.org/en/cpi/2020/index/zaf [Accessed 23 October 2021].

Transparency International. (2020b). *Corruption and the Coronavirus.* Retrieved from https://www.transparency.org/en/news/corruption-and-the-coronavirus [Accessed 23 October 2021].

Trippe, K. (2020). Pandemic policing: South Africa's most vulnerable face a sharp increase in police-related brutality. *Atlantic Council*, 24 June. Retrieved from https://www.atlanticcouncil.org/blogs/africasource/pandemic-policing-south-africas-most-vulnerable-face-a-sharp-increase-in-police-related-brutality/ [Accessed 1 November 2021].

Tromp, B. & Kings, S. (2020). Ramaphosa announces R500-billion Covid-19 package for South Africa. *The Mail & Guardian*, 21 April.

Turner, K.J. (2021). Covid-19 vaccine roll-out expands to 12–17 age group from next week. *Independent Online*, 15 October.

United Nations Entity for Gender Equality and the Empowerment of Women (UN Women). (2020). *COVID-19 and Ending Violence against Women and Girls*. Retrieved from https://www.unwomen.org/en/digital-library/publications/2020/04/issue-brief-covid-19-and-ending-violence-against-women-and-girls [Accessed 23 October 2021].

United Nations Entity for Gender Equality and the Empowerment of Women (UN Women) & United Nations Population Fund (UNFPA). (2020a). *Rapid Gender Assessment (RGA) on the Impact of COVID-19 on Women and Men in South Africa*. Retrieved from https://data.unwomen.org/sites/default/files/documents/Publications/SA%20RGA%20report.pdf [Accessed 20 October 2022].

Van Dyk, J. (2020). Home sweet hell: Calls for help surge from women locked down with abusers. *Bhekisisa Centre for Health Journalism*. Retrieved from https://bhekisisa.org/health-news-south-africa/2020-04-14-home-sweet-hell-calls-for-help-surge-from-women-locked-down-with-abusers/ [Accessed 23 October 2021].

Venter, Z. (2020). Plight of domestic workers under lockdown. *Pretoria News*, 14 May.

Williams, M. (2020). 'This is a fight to save every life': Ramaphosa bans booze, enforces masks and announces curfew. *News 24*, 12 July.

Williams, B.G. (2022). Personal interview. 1 July, Geneva.

Williamson, E.J., Walker, A.J., Bhaskaran, K. *et al.* (2020). Factors associated with COVID-19-related death using OpenSAFELY. *Nature*, 584, 430–436.

World Health Organisation (WHO). (n.d.). *Coronavirus Disease (COVD-19)*. Retrieved from https://www.who.int/health-topics/coronavirus#tab=tab_1 [Accessed 18 July 2022].

World Health Organization (WHO). (2019). *Delivered by Women, Led by Men: A Gender and Equity Analysis of the Global Health and Social Workforce*. Geneva: WHO.

World Health Organisation (WHO). (2020a). *COVID-19 Public Health Emergency of International Concern (PHEIC) Global Research and Innovation Forum*. Retrieved from https://www.who.int/publications/m/item/covid-19-public-health-emergency-of-international-concern-(pheic)-global-research-and-innovation-forum [Accessed 18 October 2022].

World Health Organisation (WHO). (2020b). *WHO Director-General's Opening Remarks at the Media Briefing on COVID-19 – 11 March 2020*. Retrieved from https://www.who.int/director-general/speeches/detail/who-director-general-s-opening-remarks-at-the-media-briefing-on-covid-19---11-march-2020 [Accessed 21 September 2021].

World Health Organisation (WHO). (2020c). *Coronavirus Disease (COVID-19) Situation Report – 102*. Retrieved from https://web.archive.org/web/2020 0503174111/https://www.who.int/docs/default-source/coronaviruse/situation-reports/20200501-covid-19-sitrep.pdf?sfvrsn=742f4a18_4 [Accessed 21 September 2021].

World Health Organisation (WHO.) (2020d). *Coronavirus Disease (COVID-19) Situation Report – 194*. Retrieved from https://web.archive.org/web/20200809 061355/https://www.who.int/docs/default-source/coronaviruse/situation-reports/20200801-covid-19-sitrep-194.pdf?sfvrsn=401287f3_2 [Accessed 21 September 2021].

World Health Organisation (WHO). (2022a). *WHO Coronavirus (COVID-19) Dashboard*. Retrieved from https://covid19.who.int [Accessed 16 July 2022].

World Health Organisation (WHO). (2022b). *South Africa Situation*. Retrieved from https://covid19.who.int/region/afro/country/za [Accessed 28 February 2022].

Wu, J.T., Leung, K. & Leung, G.M. (2020). Nowcasting and forecasting the potential domestic and international spread of the 2019-nVoV outbreak originating in Wuhan, China: A modelling study. *The Lancet*, 395(10225), 689–697.

3 The rough and the smooth

South Africa's uneven response to COVID-19

Warren Parker

The making of pandemics

Pandemic preparedness is defined as a 'continuous process of planning, exercising, revising and translating into action, national and subnational pandemic preparedness and response plans' (ECDC, 2021). As such, it is an iterative process that draws on global, regional, and national data as new epidemics emerge, employing standardised and nuanced responses to ensure fit with local conditions.

While epidemics involve outbreaks of disease that spread over large geographic areas, pandemics involve outbreaks affecting many people that span country and regional boundaries and pose a global health threat. Influenza epidemics include widespread transmission, but are generally not considered pandemics unless they are highly infectious and occur within the same timeframe across regions. Epidemics with high fatality rates, such as Ebola Virus Disease, have tended to be confined to only a few countries and are thus not pandemics. Other considerations for defining a pandemic include a lack of population immunity, the novelty of infectious agents, the vulnerability of particular sub-populations, and the attack rates of infection that contribute to rapid spread. There is disagreement as to whether disease severity should also be included as part of the definition (Morens, Folkers & Fauci, 2009). The World Health Organisation (WHO) does not have a formal definition of a pandemic, and focuses instead on defined epidemic phases, including verification of human-to-human transmission and sustained community outbreaks, which translate into pandemics when there is multi-country and multi-region transmission (WHO, 2018).

Over the past two decades, pandemic preparedness exercises have been conducted to inform efficient and effective responses. These exercises have been carried out by donor organisations, universities, governments, and United Nations bodies and provide insights for strategic response. A pandemic preparedness exercise led by Johns Hopkins University in 2019 explored the possibility of a respiratory pathogen and touched on many considerations that are informative for COVID-19 response (Johns Hopkins Center for Health Security, 2019).

DOI: 10.4324/9781003294931-3

The track record of the WHO in response to pandemics is uneven. When the severe respiratory syndrome (SARS) epidemic emerged in the early 2000s, the WHO was said to have provided 'objective and neutral policy and technical advice' that mobilised effective response in the affected countries and regions (Mackenzie et al., 2004: 45). In this instance, the WHO was operating in a context of months-long suppression of information on the outbreak by China in late 2002 (Huang, 2004). It was only in February 2003, when a doctor who had treated SARS patients in China's Guangdong Province travelled to Hong Kong and transmitted SARS to 16 other guests at his hotel, that the disease became apparent. Soon after, SARS was observed to have spread to other countries, mostly via major airline routes (Oberholtzer et al., 2004).

The WHO response to the H1N1 pandemic of 2009 was roundly critiqued, including in relation to the imposition of the 'swine flu' descriptor, and over-elaboration of the extent of transmission and risks of severe outcomes. Additionally, guidelines that countries focus on vaccine manufacturing and stockpiling were made early on, which along with the removal of the guidelines from the WHO website, appeared to have been linked to concerns about links to pharmaceutical manufacturers within WHO decision-making structures (Kamradt-Scott, 2018).

In 2014, the WHO response to the Ebola epidemic in West Africa involved delays in declaring a Public Health Emergency of International Concern (PHEIC). The delays were attributed to analyses of the epidemic being omitted for some severely affected countries, which in turn, delayed international coordination. There was also a failure to address the immediate needs of infection control and direct patient care – with the WHO instead focusing on producing technical guidance documents and conducting meetings on vaccines, diagnostics, and laboratory services (Wenham, 2017).

In 2016, the WHO declared a PHEIC in response to Zika epidemics in Brazil and other countries in South America. Diagnostics and vaccines were made available, but emphasis on contraception and access to safe terminations of pregnancy for the most vulnerable poorer pregnant women were de-emphasised in the context of political and religious regimes in the most-affected countries (Wenham et al., 2019).

Clearly, providing leadership in response to global epidemics and pandemics is complex and challenging, but as these experiences show, there is a need for nuance that goes beyond what the WHO has to offer.

A novel respiratory pandemic

The COVID-19 pandemic arose following the emergence of a growing number of cases of 'pneumonia of unknown origin' that were identified in Wuhan, China, during December 2019. Doctors in the city shared their concerns via the *WeChat* social network using the phrase 'atypical pneumonia' – a common term for SARS. Reference to SARS and the implications of a severe coronavirus epidemic raised the ire of the Chinese government, who viewed such assertions as rumour-mongering, with doctors who had voiced them being roundly disciplined by local authorities (Mai, 2020). At the same time, the Taiwan Centre for Disease Control (TCDC), which was monitoring the situation, shared their concerns about the outbreak with the regional WHO focal point on 31 December 2019. Their communication emphasised that Taiwan's public health professionals could discern from the wording of communication on the disease and that human-to-human transmission was occurring (TCDC, 2020).

While the WHO did not acknowledge Taiwan's warning, the country remained steadfast in implementing its own epidemic response. For example, on 1 January 2020, border controls and health checks on travellers from Wuhan were instituted, as were quarantines and other measures. A number of other East Asian countries followed suit in the same early timeframe (Parker & Barclay, 2020).

On 1 January 2020, the WHO mobilised an Incident Management Support Team and immediately rolled out a well-defined protocol that included investigative enquiries and meetings, reports in Disease Outbreak News, day-to-day assessments, and press briefings. Although much attention was given to suspected animal-to-human transmission at the Huanan Seafood Market, there were also known cases of transmission between family members, and by 13 January 2020, a traveller from China had been diagnosed with the coronavirus in Thailand (Allam, 2020).

On 14 January 2020, a briefing that included an announcement by WHO official, Dr Maria van Kerkhove, stated that limited human-to-human transmission was occurring and that there were risks of super-spreading events in health care settings (Reuters, 2020). Her suggestion was, however, immediately quashed via an official tweet from WHO stating that there was 'no clear evidence' for such concerns and that investigations were ongoing (WHO, 2020b). The WHO took until 22 January 2020 to acknowledge human-to-human transmission, ten more days to declare a PHEIC, and nearly six weeks to declare a pandemic on 11 March 2020 (Maxmen, 2021). Clearly, the possibility for an urgent response was on the back foot.

Stringency measures

In Taiwan, Hong Kong SAR, and South Korea, epidemic stringency measures in January and February 2020 included restrictions on international travel, COVID-19 screening, testing, quarantines, and contact tracing. Supplies of face masks were fortified by halting exports and scaling up local production. Mandatory mask mandates were implemented in public spaces, and social distancing measures included closing schools, restricting gatherings, and implementing work-from-home arrangements (Ma, Wang & Wu, 2021).

China's response intensified in late January 2020, with strict lockdowns in Wuhan and Hubei Province, shutdowns of public transport, bans on outbound travel, closures of shops, schools and other public facilities, face mask mandates, case detection, quarantines and contact tracing, disinfection campaigns, and rapid construction of emergency hospitals (Liu, Yue & Tchounwou, 2020). In the remainder of the country, a travel health code was implemented in conjunction with intensive community testing to stifle outbreaks. As a result of these measures, the first-wave epidemics in China, Taiwan, Hong Kong SAR, and South Korea remained very low per capita in the following period (Yu, Li & Dong, 2021).

The United States imposed a travel ban on travellers from China on 31 January 2020, and a number of other countries restricted international travel in February. The WHO opposed travel and trade restrictions during this time, with WHO Director, Tedros Adhanom Ghebreyesus, stating that there was no need for measures that 'unnecessarily interfere with international travel and trade', praising China's proactive response to their epidemic, and observing that the virus' spread was 'minimal and slow' (Nebahay, 2020). Reinforcing this position, the WHO required that countries imposing travel restrictions that 'significantly interfere with international traffic' to explain their rationale and scientific basis to the WHO within 48 hours (WHO, 2020b).

Apart from travel restrictions, social distancing and personal protective measures were immediate options for countries to prevent the spread of COVID-19, and these were gradually scaled up over February and March. However, by the time WHO declared the pandemic, only a few countries had implemented diversified prevention measures – notably Italy, Spain, Denmark, Iran, Albania, Czechia, Slovakia, Kosovo, and Macedonia – which met the criteria for stronger responses identified in a 'stringency index' developed by Oxford University (Oxford, 2021). In Italy, Spain, and Iran, stringency measures corresponded with rapidly growing numbers of cases and were essentially too late, while in other countries, they served the purpose of slowing new infections. 'Think different' approaches were also in play. Sweden and the United Kingdom were strongly opposed to implementing comprehensive prevention measures, and instead aligning with the concept of herd immunity through natural infection and letting the epidemic 'run', which meant focusing on managing people who were ill (The Guardian, 2020; Vanttinen & Lawton, 2020).

Other WHO guidance remained off-track. The organisation was adamant that the route of SARS-COV-2 was via respiratory droplets that spread only at a short range in conjunction with fomite transmission (surface spread). These assumptions translated into recommendations for hand washing, respiratory hygiene (coughing or sneezing into a tissue or elbow), avoiding touching one's face, disinfecting surfaces, avoiding people with obvious symptoms, and maintaining a distance of at least 1 metre between people. Face masks were advised only for people who were ill or their carers and were not recommended for 'healthy persons' in wider community settings. This guidance included assertions – without evidence – that 'masks in the community may create a false sense of security', 'result in unnecessary costs', and 'take masks away from health care workers who need them most' (WHO, 2020d). These spurious notions ran counter to the prioritisation of face masks by East Asian countries where epidemics were already declining. It also ran counter to the growing evidence of asymptomatic infection and risks of transmission. Asian researchers were baffled, voicing their concerns in an article in *The Lancet* on 20 March 2020, observing that face masks were a demonstrably effective and a vital complementary COVID-19 prevention measure (Feng et al., 2020).

The WHO was also opposed to the understanding that viral transmission of COVID-19 included airborne modes – i.e. transmission via particles that were smaller than respiratory droplets that could linger in the air and travel longer distances. A study had shown that the SARS coronavirus had been transmitted from a single source to multiple passengers on an aircraft and there was extensive research on the airborne transmission characteristics of many respiratory viruses that there was a very strong likelihood that SARS-CoV-2, the virus that causes COVID-19, could spread in this way (Olsen et al., 2003; Kutter et al., 2018; Molteni, 2021). The WHO's attachment to droplet spread specifically reduced the possibilities of emphasising the benefits of ventilating of indoor spaces to disperse viral particles and implementing mask mandates (Shiu, Leung & Cowling, 2019; Tellier, Cowling & Tang, 2019).

It was against this background that the WHO set countries up for failure. But there was also the opportunity to nuance prevention approaches at the country level.

South Africa's response

The WHO's insistence on not curtailing air travel had severe implications for countries in the global South where COVID-19 had not yet taken route – South Africa and many African countries among these. There was a high risk that early infections would be seeded through international air travel – a risk that was immediately apparent when, on 5 March 2020, South Africa's first case was confirmed to be a traveller returning from Italy. The next 16 cases were also linked to international travel, and an invisible spread was well underway.

In South Africa, the decades-long response to HIV provided a point of reference for COVID-19 response that could potentially be mobilised. An urgent response was also needed. On 15 March 2020, President Cyril Ramaphosa declared a National State of Disaster, closing land ports of entry, curtailing international air travel, limiting public gatherings, closing schools, and introducing a package of economic measures. This was followed by a strict national 'hard' lockdown imposed on 27 March 2020 (SAHO, 2021). Guidance for the response included the establishment of a National Command Council (NCC) comprising cabinet ministers and senior officials, and an opaquely constituted Ministerial Advisory Council (MAC) that was comprised almost entirely of biomedical experts to the exclusion of other fields of expertise.

President Ramaphosa's initial pronouncements reiterated WHO guidance on individual-level prevention measures while also introducing two novel approaches – a ban on alcohol and a ban on tobacco products. The alcohol ban was linked to concerns that hospital trauma cases were often alcohol-related – including injuries from violence and vehicle accidents. There was a need to ensure sufficient hospital capacity by removing this risk, as well as reducing the risks of respiratory transmission through social drinking (Oosthuizen, 2021). The tobacco ban was premised on the assumption that SARS-CoV-2 would be spread through sharing of 'cigarettes' in conjunction with the likelihood that smokers were more likely to develop severe symptoms, thereby impacting on health system resources (Vardavas & Nikitara, 2020). Another key measure was the relaxation of procurement requirements to fast-track the emergency response – in particular to increase the availability of personal protective equipment (PPE) for health care workers and other essential supplies.

There was no epidemiological evidence to back the alcohol ban, nor was there scientific evidence to inform the risks of sharing cigarettes. Cessation of current smoking would also not make any difference to the risks of severe illness, and instantly curtailing access to a known addictive requires a programme of treatment – a core principle in overcoming addiction. Of all other countries around this time, only Greenland had implemented an alcohol ban. And for all the red flags already waving regarding government tenders, there was not a hint of concern at the relaxation of procurement measures.

Understanding the longer-term trajectory of COVID-19 in South Africa was necessary. And while the cases among international travellers were readily identified, as were isolated outbreaks, more epidemiological data was needed. To improve understanding of the extent of infections, a door-to-door community screening programme via community health workers (CHWs) was instituted to identify cases. The approach, which included training and deployment of 28 000 CHWs, was implemented through the Department of Health's primary care approach. It was intended to understand COVID-19 epidemiology as well as slowing down transmission through diagnosis and contract tracing and provide an opportunity to prepare for hospitalisations (David & Mash, 2020).

The 'hard' lockdown

South Africa's response to COVID-19 was conveyed to the public through government pronouncements supported by advisories led by the Chair of the MAC, Professor Salim Abdool Karim. The approach was substantially top-down. Directives were issued and supported through cabinet ministers and government departments supported via the government communication system. Edicts included reassurances that the government's strategy was being guided by 'top class scientists and doctors' (Muller, 2020). Membership of the MAC group, which was only officially announced on 21 April 2020, clarifying the lack of multidisciplinary representation. It was unclear why this was the case. Singh (2020) describes the absence of experts from the humanities and social sciences as unfathomable. The biomedical bias over-rode key lessons in the HIV response which emphasised multidisciplinary and multisectoral approaches (Dell & Paterson, 2020; Singh, 2020).

The first nationwide 'hard' lockdown involved severe restrictions on movement that were to be enforced by the South African Police Services (SAPS) in conjunction with the deployment of the South African Defence Force (SANDF) in various communities. This included restrictions on outdoor movement and curfews, business closures, border closures, and restrictions on public transport and vehicle movements.

Over-reach and brutality by soldiers and police immediately followed – a response particularly evident in impoverished township settings where frustrations included loss of informal sector income and food insecurity. Protests took place in poorer communities in response to uneven access to food parcels and inadequacies in service delivery (Open Democracy, 2020). Liquor stores were looted, and cases of domestic violence increased (AP News, 2020). By 1 June 2020, there had been more than 230 000 arrests – most of which were for minor infringements of COVID-19 regulations (Trippe, 2020). Little had been done to understand the contexts of poverty within which many South Africans live, nor was there any demonstrable attempt to engage with the public at this level (Parker & Hlatshwayo, 2020). Public communication devolved primarily to key messages via political announcements, and message-based communication through conventional channels in combination with seeding social media (Moonasar et al., 2020). In the context of communication diversity and misinformation, public trust was not established (Koch et al., 2020).

Epidemiological modelling and community screening

Epidemiological data that underpinned the lockdown followed epidemiological modelling exercises that were initially kept out of the public domain – ostensibly to avoid increasing public fear. Various models released were not sufficiently informative regarding underlying assumptions and also did not adequately factor in the potential effects of prevention measures (Cowan, 2020). For example, in mid-May 2020, predictions by the South African COVID-19 Modelling Consortium predicted 1-million active cases, with over 90 000 non-ICU and 30 000 ICU beds needed, and 20 000 deaths by mid-August 2020 (South African COVID-19 Modelling Consortium, 2020; National Institute for Communicable Diseases, 2020). The predictions for cases and deaths were roughly twice as high as what actually transpired (Muller, 2020).

While some data were emerging through South Africa's novel national-level community screening initiative, a particular challenge was the large-scale deployment of screening teams. Each team needed access to PPE, testing materials, rapid turnaround of laboratory results, and logistical support to conduct extensive contact tracing. In low-incidence provinces, a great deal of groundwork elicited very few cases, whereas in high-incidence areas, laboratory results were delayed and contact tracing could not be effectively conducted. In epidemiological terms, given the rapid spread of COVID-19 from any index case, near-immediate case identification, and follow-up would be needed to contain outbreaks. Any epidemiological insights were also immediately skewed by delays in test results. Laboratory turn-around times were of the order of five to 14 days, and there were soon shortages of test kits. Test kits, PPE, and laboratory resources were urgently also needed beyond the community screening initiative, notably at hospitals and clinics responding to symptomatic cases, outbreak tracking, contact tracing, and follow-up (Mendelson & Mahdi, 2020). And other approaches were likely to be more informative – for example, the DATCOV hospital-based surveillance system that at least provided real-time data on cases on a national basis (Jassat et al., 2021).

Contradicting WHO recommendations on face masks

The fundamental assumptions of the WHO in preventing SARS-CoV-2 transmission were not questioned by the biomedically weighty MAC, who simply pushed the standard guidance including recommendations that face masks were not needed by all. During March and April 2020, major retailers also fell in line, prominently displaying signs that read *'In line with the WHO, we have been advised against using face masks as they do not prove to be effective in preventing infection for the wearer'*. Hospitals did not require universal masking of patients or staff, except in wards dedicated to COVID-19 treatment, and little was done to counter the hazards of asymptomatic and airborne transmission. Indeed, many cases were likely to have been seeded in crowded minibus taxis conveying essential workers from distant townships to worksites in city centres during the initial lockdown period in the absence of adequate protection measures.

The most frequent outbreaks during this period occurred in retail outlets, shops, and hospitals, many of which shut down partially or entirely for days for 'deep cleaning' – a requirement that also lacked underpinning science. Outbreak analyses were also poorly conceived. For example, an analysis of infections of 119 patients and staff at St Augustines Hospital in Durban rejected the possibility of aerosol transmission and focused attention largely on surface hygiene with deference to mask wearing in line with droplet spread (Lessels, Moosa, & de Oliveira).

The scientific evidence for universal mask wearing in the context of a respiratory pandemic was sound, albeit not framed in the randomised controlled trial (RCT) evidence format that many in the medical research fraternity consider to be a 'gold standard'. Obviously, evidence specific to COVID-19 did not exist, since it is a novel virus, but there were many small-scale studies and meta-analyses that provided a sound basis for prevention guidance, including for using cloth masks in pandemic circumstances (MacIntyre & Chuhtai, 2015). In the context of shortages of medical face masks, civic-minded groups globally and in South Africa had already identified cloth face masks as a protective measure, and by late March 2020, an initiative entitled Masks4All led by a group of South African doctors and predominantly Muslim community organisations, had already initiated home-based manufacture of cloth face masks. Separately, an ad hoc scientific advisory group was established to guide strategy on cloth face masks to inform response for the Department of Health, duly gathering sufficient evidence to support nationwide uptake. Nonetheless, it did take some persuading to get senior MAC members to agree that face masks including cloth face masks were a viable option, and mandatory guidance was issued on 1 May 2020 (Parker, 2021). Cloth masks were increasingly being used in other countries, and there was a gradual implementation of mandatory guidelines for use by all people in public settings. The WHO, however, continued to malign mask mandates, only shifting their guidance in June 2020. And the WHO remained intransigent on airborne transmission. This blocked the urgent emphasis needed on ventilating indoor spaces. It took on open letter by 239 experts to effectively argue the case in July 2020, although it still took months for the WHO to issue an acknowledgement of this mode of transmission in October 2020 (Molteni, 2021).

Alcohol and tobacco bans

Although there was a disinclination by country authorities to flout the WHO guidance, even though the underlying science to support alternate guidance was widely available, South Africa did not hesitate to follow hybrid approaches that were scientifically tenuous at best – the alcohol and tobacco bans.

The sale of alcohol and tobacco was prohibited on 27 March, with limited reintroduction of sales during shifting 'risk adjusted' phases of response throughout 2020 (Myers et al., 2021). Whether or not banning alcohol would have led to decline in the need for hospital beds could not be predicted in a context where the movement was already highly restricted through the lockdown. Policing this ad hoc arrangement would not necessarily address the likely underground markets that are inevitable when products such as alcohol or tobacco are not available through ordinary commercial channels (Theron et al., 2022).

Indeed, the bans negatively impacted the alcohol and tobacco industries quite rapidly, with an estimated 117 000 jobs lost in 2020. Some R9.5 billion was estimated to have been lost in forfeited tax revenue, and criminal networks profited from illegal distribution. Investment deals by companies such as Consol Glass (R1.5 billion), South African Breweries (R2.5 billion), and Heineken (R6 billion) fell through. Illicit cigarette sales increased, and an estimated 93% of consumers were buying from illegal sellers, raising an estimated R2 billion in profits for organised crime. Prices of illicit alcohol and tobacco to consumers far exceeded legal pricing structures. At the same time, tax shortfalls due to the bans were estimated at R12–R15 billion by the end of 2020 (Holmes, 2020; PMI, 2020).

The blight of corruption

The South African government has been blighted by corruption since the arms deal, with later corrupt practices morphing into the capture of key parastatals and widespread looting enabled through government tenders and cronyism. Billions of rands have been removed from the fiscus, and key service providers such as Eskom, Transnet, and South African Airways remain severely fractured (Gottschalk, 2022).

It did not take long for the fast-tracked COVID-19 procurement arrangements to fall into unscrupulous hands. Deals worth more than R2.2 billion for PPE in Gauteng were soon suspect, and in July 2020, spokesperson to the President, Khusela Diko, took a leave of absence following her links to a R125-million PPE tender (Chabalala, 2020; Sunday Independent, 2020). In the Eastern Cape, PPE for schools included procurements of R2.4 billion and R2.8 billion, respectively (McCain, 2022). Food parcels, social grants, and temporary employer/employee relief funds were also corruptly redirected, and by 27 August 2020, South Africa's Special Investigations Unit was reviewing contracts in excess of R5 billion – mostly in Gauteng and the Eastern Cape (Gerber, 2020).

Taking stock of the early response in South Africa

Many countries took bold steps to counter the impending threat of the COVID-19 pandemic, and countries in Africa at least had some lead time, albeit undermined by the WHO's open-skies guidance.

Like all countries responding to COVID-19, South Africa followed a mix of global guidance and indigenous adaptations to prevent infections and mitigate impacts. The epidemic pattern in South Africa followed the global trends over time, with a series of waves characterised by high rates of infection and mortality which subside and re-occur. By late 2021, a study in Gauteng determined that 85% of residents had been infected with SARS-COV-2 at least once, and in the context of relatively low rates of vaccination, underlying immunity and the decreased severity of the Omicron variant, the epidemic had subsided to low levels by March 2022 (Ellis, 2022). Through to 30 June 2022, there were an estimated 93 186 COVID-19 deaths and 295 135 excess deaths in South Africa during the COVID-19 period.

While COVID-19 is complex to contain, and emerging virus variants are capable of overcoming immunity from previous infections or vaccines, South Africa could have done better. While the MAC was ostensibly grounded in the wisdom of the country's elite scientists, it was untransparent and constituted without consultation. It is unclear how much the MAC shaped the understanding of the science underpinning COVID-19 or defining the public health measures relevant to slowing its spread. But there is no doubt that whatever was done did not meet the moment. The inclusion of a wider diversity of experts and thought leaders alongside multisectoral and community representation in decision-making structures would have had a unifying effect in the context of a common challenge. Perhaps even a foundation for new ways of solving other crises by drawing on the power of national unity.

Instead, it was business as usual through various expressions of top-down power, and deference to the habit of corruption. Lives were lost unnecessarily as a result, and the economy remains overburdened with just another crisis.

There is seldom accountability for decision-making regarding public health decision-making. Yet we cannot escape the bald fact that lives were lost to COVID-19 in South Africa due to shoddy science and poor strategic thinking. This was not helped by uncritical deference to slew of slow, obstructive, and ill-conceived guidance emanating from the WHO.

There is talk of pandemic preparedness for future pathogens, but it is important to also consider the possibility that COVID-19 might drag along intractably, even though, with considered analysis drawing on diverse insights, it might well be overcome.

Clearly, nearly every step taken in the early response to COVID-19 was significantly flawed. And this view does not depend on hindsight. The human-to-human transmission was clearly evident well before it was acknowledged: COVID-19 had already spread across regions well in advance of the declaration of a pandemic, the science of respiratory viral transmission was more than sufficient to guide preventive measures such as ubiquitous use of cloth and medical face masks, and to acknowledge airborne transmission and measures to address this mode of transmission. Clearly, international air travel represented a severe risk for seeding country epidemics, especially in countries with lower exposure such as South Africa. Indeed, the early East Asia examples demonstrated how effective controls on international travel could be, and stand in sharp contrast to the WHO's haughty demands for an explanation from countries that deigned to consider such restrictions.

While the South African government can be admired for its prompt response, albeit a heavy-handed 'hard' lockdown, the potential to strategise while marking time was quickly lost. The community screening programme was wholly unsuited to informing the epidemiological dimensions of a disease with a short infectious period that was already known to reveal itself through symptomatic cases. Vital supplies of COVID-19 tests, PPE, and laboratory resources were misdirected as a result, at the same time hampering outbreak and case detection following more conventional approaches. Epidemiological modelling was imprecise, with overestimates feeding into justifications for harsher measures and less nuance.

The alcohol and tobacco bans had spurious foundations, and on balance, did more harm than good. The whimsy of the latter is well exposed in the song 'When people zol', which directly quotes Co-operative Governance and Traditional Affairs Minister Nkosazana Dlamini-Zuma: *'When people zol, they put saliva on the paper, and then they share that zol'* (Pitjeng, 2020). The alcohol ban, which indeed contributed to some reductions in trauma cases, involved considerable negative macroeconomic impacts and had no long-term impact on the hazardous context of alcohol use that prevails in the country (Matzopoulos et al., 2020; Chu et al., 2022).

Top-down edicts were unhelpful as the epidemic progressed, and the biomedical overrepresentation within the MAC, excluded sectors and communities that had historically been important actors in the country's HIV response. Public trust was an immediate casualty, creating space for burgeoning and divisive discourses on social media, and undermining any possible broader civic leadership (Schmidt et al., 2020).

There was an absence of introspection attached to the laissez-faire approach that led to the adoption of COVID-19 procurement guidance – a convenient myopia in the face of a glaring and unresolved fault line. Corruption ensued.

While COVID-19 is not over, there has not been an adequate critical appraisal of South Africa's response. There is no shortage of lessons to be learned, and it is unfortunate that the country's early response was underscored by naiveté in a context where humble deference to the full extent of leaders embedded across disciplines, in sectoral networks and communities. Many are well-schooled in HIV response among other health and social issues and had much to contribute. On the longer term, the challenges of COVID-19 remain, and there are many more touchstones to explore in the post-2020 response to the epidemic. Will the response to another public health crisis be any different?

References

Allam, Z. (2020). The first 50 days of COVID-19: A detailed chronological timeline and extensive literature documenting the pandemic. Surveying the Covid-19 Pandemic and its Implications. *Elsevier Public Health Emergency Collection*, 1–7. doi: 10.1016/B978-0-12-824313-8.00001-2

AP News. (13 April 2020). South Africa's lockdown effective, but problems emerge. *AP News*. Retrieved from https://apnews.com/article/africa-johannesburg-crime-photography-international-news-d61d033687711d56f0d37790b3bd38ea [Accessed 22 July, 2022]

Chabalala, J. (19 August 2020). Gauteng PPE scandal: David Makhura 'displayed recklessness' in awarding contract, tribunal hears. *News 24*. Retrieved from https://www.news24.com/news24/southafrica/news/gauteng-ppe-scandal-david-makhura-displayed-recklessness-in-awarding-contract-tribunal-hears-20210819 [Accessed 22 July, 2022]

Chu, K. M., Marco, J. L., Owolabi, E. O., Duvenage, R., Londani, M., Lombard, C., & Parry, C. D. (2022). Trauma trends during COVID-19 alcohol prohibition at a South African regional hospital. *Drug and Alcohol Review*, 41(1), 13–19.

Cowan, K. (20 May 2020). One million Covid-19 cases, 40 000 deaths and a dire shortage of ICU beds - SA's shocking projections. *News24*. Retrieved from https://www.news24.com/news24/SouthAfrica/News/one-million-covid-19-cases-40-000-deaths-and-a-dire-shortage-of-icu-beds-sas-shocking-projections-20200520 [Accessed 22 July, 2022]

David, N., & Mash, R. (2020). Community-based screening and testing for Coronavirus in Cape Town, South Africa. *African Journal of Primary Health Care and Family Medicine*, 12(1), 1–3.

Dell, S., & Paterson, M. (19 May 2020). COVID-19 – Academy joins calls for multidisciplinary approach. *University World News*. Retrieved from https://www.universityworldnews.com/post.php?story=20200519162236692 [Accessed 22 July, 2022]

ECDC. (2021). Why is pandemic preparedness planning so important. Retrieved from https://www.ecdc.europa.eu/en/seasonal-influenza/preparedness/why-pandemic-preparedness. Accessed 1 July 2022. [Accessed 22 July, 2022]

Ellis, E. (25 February 2022). 'Measures to prevent infection failed' – study finds 85% of Gauteng residents were likely infected in first three Covid-19 waves. *The Daily Maverick*. Retrieved from https://www.dailymaverick.co.za/article/2022-02-25-measures-to-prevent-infection-failed-study-finds-85-of-gauteng-residents-were-likely-infected-in-first-three-covid-19-waves/ [Accessed 22 July, 2022]

Feng, S., Shen, C., Xia, N., Song, W., Fan, M., & Cowling, B. J. (2020). Rational use of face masks in the COVID-19 pandemic. *The Lancet Respiratory Medicine*, 8(5), 434–436.

Gerber, J. (2020). SIU probes PPE contracts worth R5bn, Eastern Cape tops alleged irregular cases. *News 24*. Retrieved from https://www.news24.com/news24/southafrica/news/siu-probes-ppe-contracts-worth-r5bn-eastern-cape-tops-alleged-irregular-cases-20200819 [Accessed 22 July, 2022]

Gottschalk, K. (8 February 2022). State capture in South Africa: How the rot set in and how the project was rumbled. *The Conversation*. Retrieved from https://theconversation.com/state-capture-in-south-africa-how-the-rot-set-in-and-how-the-project-was-rumbled-176481. [Accessed 22 July, 2022]

Holmes, T. (26 August 2020). Fraud and corruption in the COVID-19 era. *Mail & Guardian*. Retrieved from https://mg.co.za/special-reports/2020-08-26-fraud-and-corruption-in-the-covid-19-era [Accessed 22 July, 2022]

Huang, Y. (2004). The SARS epidemic and its aftermath in China: A political perspective. In S. Knobler, Mahmoud, A., Lemon, S., et al. (Eds). *Learning from SARS: Preparing for the next disease outbreak*, pp. 116–36. Washington, DC: National Academies Press.

Jassat, W., Cohen, C., Masha, M., Parker, W., DATCOV Team, & Blumberg, L. (2021). COVID-19 in South Africa: Lessons from implementing a new national hospital surveillance platform. In A. Dhai, D. Ballot, & M. Veller (Eds). *Pandemics in health care,* pp. 288–297. Cape Town: Juta.

Johns Hopkins Center for Health Security (2019). *Preparedness for a High-impact Respiratory Pathogen Pandemic*. Retrieved from https://www.centerforhealthsecurity.org/our-work/pubs_archive/pubs-pdfs/2019/190918-GMPBreport-respiratorypathogen.pdf [Accessed 1 July, 2022]

Kamradt-Scott, A. (2018). What went wrong? The World Health Organization from swine flu to Ebola. In A. Kruck, K. Opperman, & A. Spencer (Eds). *Political mistakes and policy failures in international relations*, pp. 193–215. London: Palgrave Macmillan.

Koch, A., Masuku, B., Young, E., & Warner, D. (24 June 2020). Messaging during Covid-19: What can we learn from previous crises of infectious disease. *Daily Maverick*. Retrieved from https://www.dailymaverick.co.za/article/2020-06-24-messaging-during-covid-19-what-can-we-learn-from-previous-crises-of-infectious-disease/ [Accessed 22 July, 2022]

Kutter, J. S., Spronken, M. I., Fraaij, P. L., Fouchier, R. A., & Herfst, S. (2018). Transmission routes of respiratory viruses among humans. *Current Opinion in Virology*, 28, 142–151.

Lessels, R., Moosa, Y., & de Oliveira, T. (2020). *Report into a Nosocomial Outbreak of Coronavirus Disease 2019 at Netcare St. Augustine's Hospital*. University of KwaZulu-Natal. Retrieved from https://www.krisp.org.za/manuscripts/StAugustinesHospitalOutbreakInvestigation_FinalReport_15may2020_comp.pdf. [Accessed 22 July, 2020]

Levitt, J. (18 May 2020). Nkosazana Dlamini-Zuma slid into 'Zol' song producer's DMs: 'Well done on entertaining the nation. *Times Live*. Retrieved from https://www.timeslive.co.za/news/south-africa/2020-05-18-nkosazana-dlamini-zuma-slid-into-zol-song-producers-dms-well-done-on-entertaining-the-nation/ [Accessed 22 July, 2022]

Liu, W., Yue, X. G., & Tchounwou, P. B. (2020). Response to the COVID-19 epidemic: The Chinese experience and implications for other countries. *International Journal of Environmental Research and Public Health*, 17(7), 2304. doi: 10.3390/ijerph17072304

Ma, M., Wang, S., & Wu. F. (2021). COVID-19 prevalence and wellbeing: Lessons from East Asia. In F. Helliwell, R. Layard, J. Sachs, J. de Neve, L. Aknin, & S. Wang (Eds). *World Happiness Report*. Sustainable Solutions Network. https://happiness-report.s3.amazonaws.com/2021/WHR+21.pdf

MacIntyre, C., & Chughtai, A. (2015). Facemasks for the prevention of infection in healthcare and community settings. *British Medical Journal*, 9, 350.

Mackenzie, J. S., Drury, P., Ellis, A., Grein, T., Leitmeyer, K. C., Mardel, S., & Ryan, M. (2004). The WHO response to SARS, and preparations for the future. In K. Oberholtzer, L. Sivitz, A. Mack, S. Lemon, A. Mahmoud, & S. Knobler (Eds). *Learning from SARS: Preparing for the next disease outbreak: Workshop summary*. Washington DC: National Academies Press.

Mai, J. (29 January 2020). Coronavirus 'rumour' crackdown by Wuhan police slammed by China's top court. *South China Morning Post*. Retrieved from https://www.scmp.com/news/china/society/article/3048042/chinas-top-court-hits-out-wuhan-police-over-coronavirus-rumour [Accessed 22 July, 2022]

Matzopoulos, R., Walls, H., Cook, S., & London, L. (2020). South Africa's COVID-19 alcohol sales ban: The potential for better policy-making. *International Journal of Health Policy and Management*, 9(11), 486.

Maxmen, A. (23 January 2021). Why did the world's pandemic warning system fail when COVID hit? *Nature*. Retrieved from https://www.nature.com/articles/d41586-021-00162-4 [Accessed 22 July, 2022]

McCain, N. (28 January 2022). How COVID-19 contracts were used to steal millions from Eastern Cape education department. *News 24*. Retrieved from https://www.news24.com/news24/southafrica/news/how-covid-19-contracts-were-used-to-steal-millions-from-eastern-cape-education-dept-20220128 [Accessed 22 July, 2022]

Mendelson, M., & Madhi, S. (2020). South Africa's coronavirus testing strategy is broken and not fit for purpose: It's time for a change. *South African Medical Journal*, 110(6), 429–431.

Molteni, M. (13 May 2021). The 60-year-old scientific screwup that helped COVID kill. *Wired*. Retrieved from https://www.wired.com/story/the-teeny-tiny-scientific-screwup-that-helped-covid-kill/ [Accessed 22 July, 2022]

Moonasar, D., Pillay, A., Leonard, E., Naidoo, R., Mngemane, S., Ramkrishna, W.,...&
Pillay, Y. (2021). COVID-19: Lessons and experiences from South Africa's first
surge. *BMJ Global Health*, 6(2), e004393.

Morens, D. M., Folkers, G. K., & Fauci, A. S. (2009). What is a pandemic?. *The
Journal of Infectious Diseases*, 200(7), 1018–1021.

Muller, S. (8 June 2020). South Africa's use of COVID-19modelling has been deeply
flawed. Here's why. *The Conversation*. Retrieved from https://theconversation.
com/south-africas-use-of-covid-19-modelling-has-been-deeply-flawed-heres-
why-140002 [Accessed 22 July, 2022]

Muller, S. (4 June 2020). A 'scientific' approach to pandemic lacking transparency.
University World News. Retrieved from https://www.universityworldnews.com/
post.php?story=20200604074841475 [Accessed 22 July, 2022]

Myers, B., Carney, T., Rooney, J., Malatesta, S., White, L. F., Parry, C. D.,... &
Jacobson, K. R. (2021). Alcohol and tobacco use in a tuberculosis treatment cohort
during South Africa's COVID-19 sales bans: A case series. *International Journal of
Environmental Research and Public Health*, 18(10), 5449.

National Institute for Communicable Diseases. (2020). *Latest Confirmed Cases of
COVID-19 in South Africa*. 8 August 2020. Retrieved from https://www.nicd.
ac.za/latest-confirmed-cases-of-covid-19-in-south-africa-8-aug-2020/ [Accessed
22 July, 2022]

Nebahay, S. (3 February 2020). WHO chief says widespread travel bans not needed
to beat China virus. *Reuters*. Retrieved from https://www.reuters.com/article/
us-china-health-who/who-chief-says-widespread-travel-bans-not-needed-to-
beat-china-virus-idUKKBN1ZX1H3 [Accessed 22 July, 2022]

Oberholtzer, K., Sivitz, L., Mack, A., Lemon, S., Mahmoud, A., & Knobler, S.
(Eds.). (2004). SARS: Emergence, detection, and response. In K. Oberholtzer,
L. Sivitz, A. Mack, S. Lemon, A. Mahmoud, & S. Knobler (Eds). *Learning from
SARS: Preparing for the next disease outbreak: Workshop summary*. Washington, DC:
The National Academies Press.

Olsen, S. J., Chang, H. L., Cheung, T. Y. Y., Tang, A. F. Y., Fisk, T. L., Ooi, S. P. L.,... &
Dowell, S. F. (2003). Transmission of the severe acute respiratory syndrome on
aircraft. *New England Journal of Medicine*, 349(25), 2416–2422.

Oosthuizen, A. (2020). Banning alcohol during lockdown: It is not just about the virus
or economics. Retrieved from http://www.hsrc.ac.za/en/review/hsrc-review-
covid19-april-2020/banning-alcohol-during-lockdown [Accessed 22 July, 2022]

Open Democracy (24 April 2020). "We are still waiting" – protesting under
lockdown in South Africa. Retrieved from https://www.opendemocracy.net/
en/beyond-trafficking-and-slavery/we-are-still-waiting-protesting-under-
lockdown-in-south-africa/ [Accessed 22 July, 2022]

Oxford COVID-19 response tracker. Oxford University. Retrieved from https://
ourworldindata.org/grapher/covid-stringency-index?time=2020-03-14 [Accessed
22 July, 2022]

Parker, W. (2021). Disentangling science and ideology in a rapidly evolving pandemic:
Moments in the COVID-19 maelstrom. In M. Lewis, E. Govender, & K. Holland
(Eds). *Communicating COVID-19. Interdisciplinary perspectives*. London: Palgrave.

Parker, W., & Barclay, J. (2020). *COVID-19 arising: Lessons learned in proactive response
in East Asia*. Balsillie Papers 01. Balsillie School of International Affairs. Retrieved
from https://balsilliepapers.ca/bsia-paper/covid-19-arising-lessons-in-proactive-
response-in-east-asia/ [Accessed 22 July, 2022]

Parker, W., & Hlatshwayo, M. (14 May 2020). The voices we should be listening to: Informal settlement residents on Covid-19. *Daily Maverick*. Retrieved from https://www.dailymaverick.co.za/article/2020-05-14-the-voices-we-should-be-listening-to-informal-settlement-residents-on-covid-19/ [Accessed 22 July, 2022]

Reuters. (14 January 2020). WHO says new China virus could spread, it's warning all hospitals. *Reuters*. Retrieved from https://www.reuters.com/article/china-health-pneumonia-who/who-says-new-china-virus-could-spread-its-warning-all-hospitals-idUSL8N29F48F [Accessed 22 July, 2022]

SAHO. (2021). COVID-19 timeline 2019–2020. Retrieved from https://www.sahistory.org.za/article/covid-19-timeline-2019-2020 [Accessed 22 July, 2022]

Schmidt, T., Cloete, A., Davids, A., Makola, L., Zondi, N., & Jantjies, M. (2020). Myths, misconceptions, othering and stigmatizing responses to Covid-19 in South Africa: A rapid qualitative assessment. *PloS One*, 15(12), e0244420.

Shiu, E. Y., Leung, N. H., & Cowling, B. J. (2019). Controversy around airborne versus droplet transmission of respiratory viruses: Implication for infection prevention. *Current Opinion in Infectious Diseases*, 32(4), 372–379.

Silal, S., Pulliam, J., Meyer-Rath, G., Nichols, B., Jamieson, L., Kimmie, Z., & Moultrie, H. (2020). *Estimating Cases for COVID-19 in South Africa Update: 19 May 2020*. Retrieved from https://www.nicd.ac.za/wp-content/uploads/2020/05/SACMC_19052020_slides-for-MoH-media-briefing.pdf [Accessed 22 July, 2022].

Singh, J. A. (2020). How South Africa's ministerial advisory committee on COVID-19 can be optimised. *South African Medical Journal*, 110(6), 439–442.

Sunday Independent. (26 July 2020). Under the spotlight: The MEC's wife, Diko and a R125m PPE contract. *Sunday Independent*. Retrieved from https://www.iol.co.za/sundayindependent/news/under-the-spotlight-the-mecs-wife-diko-and-a-r125m-ppe-contract-06eb0951-4b22-402e-9110-cdd247e29102 [Accessed 22 July, 2022]

TCDC. (11 April 2020). *The Facts Regarding Taiwan's Email to Alert WHO to Possible Danger of COVID-19*. Retrieved from https://www.cdc.gov.tw/En/Bulletin/Detail/PAD-lbwDHeN_bLa-viBOuw?typeid=158 [Accessed 22 July, 2022]

Tellier, R., Li, Y., Cowling, B. J., & Tang, J. W. (2019). Recognition of aerosol transmission of infectious agents: A commentary. *BMC Infectious Diseases*, 19(1), 1–9.

The Guardian. (13 March 2020). Herd immunity: Will the UK's coronavirus strategy work? *The Guardian*. Retrieved from https://www.theguardian.com/world/2020/mar/13/herd-immunity-will-the-uks-coronavirus-strategy-work [Accessed 22 July, 2022]

Theron, M., Swart, R., Londani, M., Parry, C., Petersen Williams, P., & Harker-Burnams, N. (2022). Did COVID-19-related alcohol sales restrictions reduce alcohol consumption? Findings from a national online survey in South Africa. *International Journal of Environmental Research and Public Health*, 19(4), 2422.

Trippe, K. (24 June 2020). Pandemic policing: South Africa's most vulnerable face a sharp increase in police-related brutality. *Atlantic Council*. Retrieved from https://www.atlanticcouncil.org/blogs/africasource/pandemic-policing-south-africas-most-vulnerable-face-a-sharp-increase-in-police-related-brutality/ [Accessed 22 July, 2022]

Vanttinen, P., & Lawton, S. (13 March 2020). Sweden tops EU rate of new daily COVID-19 cases. *Euractiv*. Retrieved from https://www.euractiv.com/section/health-consumers/short_news/sweden-update-covid-19/ [Accessed 22 July, 2022]

Wenham, C. (2017). What we have learnt about the World Health Organization from the Ebola outbreak. *Philosophical Transactions of the Royal Society B: Biological Sciences*, 372(1721), 20160307.

Wenham, C., Arevalo, A., Coast, E., Corrêa, S., Cuellar, K., Leone, T., & Valongueiro, S. (2019). Zika, abortion and health emergencies: A review of contemporary debates. *Globalization and Health*, 15(1), 1–7.

WHO. (20 June 2020). *Listing of WHO's response to COVID-19*. Retrieved from https://www.who.int/news/item/29-06-2020-covidtimeline. [Accessed 22 July, 2022]

WHO. (2018). WHO pandemic phase descriptions and main actions by phase. Retrieved from https://www.who.int/influenza/resources/documents/pandemic_phase_descriptions_and_actions.pdf [Accessed 22 July, 2022]

WHO. (2020b). (14 January 2020). Retrieved from https://twitter.com/who/status/1217043229427761152?lang=en [Accessed 22 July, 2022]

WHO. (2020c). (29 February, 2020). Updated WHO recommendations for international traffic in relation to COVID-19 outbreak. Retrieved from https://www.who.int/news-room/articles-detail/updated-who-recommendations-for-international-traffic-in-relation-to-covid-19-outbreak [Accessed 22 July, 2022]

WHO. (2020e). Advice on the use of masks in the community, during home care, and in health care settings in the context of COVID-19. 19 March 2020. Retrieved from https://apps.who.int/iris/bitstream/handle/10665/331493/WHO-2019-nCoV-IPC_Masks-2020.2-eng.pdf?sequence=14&isAllowed=y [Accessed 22 July, 2022]

Yu, X., Li, N., & Dong, Y. (2021). Observation on China's strategies to prevent the resurgence of the COVID-19 epidemic. *Risk Management and Healthcare Policy*, 14, 2011.

4 Placing the South African COVID-19 epidemic in a global context

Alan Whiteside

Introduction: Disease threats to human health

A standard measure of human well-being is life expectancy, and it is one of the four key metrics of the United Nations (UN) Human Development Index. The others are: expected years of schooling; average years of schooling; and gross national income (GNI) per capita.[1] In Europe and the America's life expectancy at birth (LEB), the number of years a person could expect to live on average stood at about 35 years up to about the 1860s. This is a somewhat misleading statistic since rates of infant and child mortality were high. Provided an individual survived to their fifth birthday, they could expect to live well beyond 35. Today, globally, life expectancy is 73 years. In Organisation for Economic Co-operation and Development (OECD) countries, it is 80 years and in Sub-Saharan Africa 62 years.[2]

Life expectancy began rising from the mid-1800s in the west and in the rest of the world from the beginning of the 1900s. From about 1995 to about 2010, Acquired Immune Deficiency Syndrome (AIDS) mortality was high enough to halt the growth in this indicator in a number of countries, primarily in Africa (Whiteside and Zebryk, 2017: 305). There was a small decrease in life expectancy in the United States (US), between 2014 and 2016, variously ascribed to the opioid crisis, suicide, and alcohol: 'deaths of despair' (Harper, Riddell, and King, 2021). Within a year of its emergence, the number of deaths from COVID-19 was already affecting life expectancy in South Africa (Aburto et al., 2022). According to Statistics South Africa, 'Life expectancy at birth for males declined from 62.4 in 2020 to 59.3 in 2021 (3.1 year drop) and from 68.4 in 2020 to 64.6 for females (3.8 year drop)' (Statistics SA, 2021). In the USA, males lost 2.2 years of life expectancy in 2020 (Aburto et al., 2022). The full effect of COVID-19 will take time to be seen in this indicator as increased poverty, unemployment, and educational disruptions work through economies and societies.

The increase in life expectancy and concomitant decrease in mortality were primarily due to public health advances (Davies et al., 2014). In her masterly assessment of the drivers of increased health and well-being, Sally Davies identified five waves of public health development. From about 1830 to 1900,

DOI: 10.4324/9781003294931-4

there were structural improvements addressing physical and environmental conditions: water and sewerage, food safety, and working conditions. The second wave (approximately 1890–1950) was characterised by biomedical and scientific advances. The third (approximately 1940–1980) was clinical and scientific, with understanding of the causes of communicable diseases, and development of treatments. The fourth, from approximately 1960 to the present, looked at social determinants of health. She speculated we may be entering a fifth wave: 'a culture for health', with healthy choices incentivised, and unhealthy ones discouraged.

Infectious diseases were on the retreat. The rapid development, adoption, and administration of vaccinations lead to greatly reduced morbidity and mortality from many childhood diseases, from measles to whooping cough. The eradication of smallpox, in 1980, marked a moment when it appeared infectious diseases could be conquered. This was short-lived. Within a year, in 1981, the first cases of a new disease, AIDS were reported. The cause, a virus, the Human Immunodeficiency Virus (HIV) was identified in 1983. HIV-1 crossed into humans from chimpanzees, HIV-2, a less virulent variety, originated in Sooty Mangabey monkeys, both were zoonotic (animal to human) infections.

HIV spread from human to human mainly through unprotected sex, through sharing needles, and receiving contaminated blood, although it can also be passed from mother to infant. Once a person is infected, they will, after a period of about eight years, in the absence of treatment, experience episodes of illness that increase in severity, duration, and frequency until they die. Despite the best efforts of scientists working internationally, effective treatments were not available until 1996. Treatment with the appropriate antiretroviral drugs will lead to recovery for most patients, but they must remain adherent to the drugs for the rest of their lives. There is no cure yet.

Until COVID-19 appeared, HIV had been the most serious pandemic humans had faced. In the early years, it was unclear as to where, and how much, it would spread, but, in the absence of treatment, an infection was a death sentence. Over time, it became apparent the pandemic would be unevenly distributed. Today, the epicentre is Sub-Saharan Africa and particularly Southern Africa. HIV infections and AIDS are found in certain 'key populations': men who have sex with men; intravenous drug users; and sex workers in much of the world. An additional vulnerable population are the infants of infected mothers, but this transmission can be largely prevented with drugs. In 2020, 85% of pregnant women living with HIV had access to antiretroviral medicines.

From 1981 to 2020, there had been 79 300 000 AIDS cases worldwide, of whom 36 300 000 had died. HIV is preventable, and AIDS is treatable if not curable.[3] New HIV infections have been reduced by 52% since the peak in 1997. However, the HIV and AIDS epidemic is not over. In 2020, an estimated 1.5 million people were newly infected with HIV and 680 000 people died from AIDS-related illnesses. By June 2021, 28.2 million people were accessing antiretroviral therapy. It is estimated 74% of adults (aged 15+ years) and 54% of children (aged 0–14 years) had access to treatment.[4] AIDS has not gone away, but COVID-19 has arrived.

From the beginning of the new century, there seemed to be a potential pandemic every few years. First, Severe Acute Respiratory Syndrome (SARS) began in China in 2002. It is a zoonotic disease, caused by the SARS Coronavirus (SARS-CoV-1). By the end of the outbreak in June 2003, 8,422 cases and 774 deaths had been recorded, a case-fatality rate (CFR) of 11% (Chan-Yeung and Xu, 2003). The worst affected countries, those with more than 100 cases, were China 5,327 cases, Hong Kong 1,755 cases, Taiwan 346 cases, Canada 251, and Singapore 238.

The 'Swine Flu' or H1N1/09 pandemic started in Mexico in April of 2009 and spread rapidly, reaching pandemic proportions within weeks. It began to taper off toward the end of the year and by May of 2010, it was declared over. It is estimated between 700 million and 1.4 billion people were infected, but only 18,449 lab-confirmed deaths were reported to the World Health Organization (WHO).[5] The event caused panic. Unfortunately, when the feared levels of mortality did not emerge, confidence in public health services and messages was eroded.

Middle East Respiratory Syndrome (MERS) is a viral respiratory infection caused by MERS-related Coronavirus (MERS-CoV). First reported from Saudi Arabia in 2012, it is a zoonotic disease that spread from camels to humans. The infected numbers are small, fewer than 3,000, since it was first identified. It rarely spreads from human to human, but has a high CFR, about 35%.

The next potential pandemic was different. The Ebola virus is endemic in Central and West Africa. It is zoonotic and its reservoir is probably fruit bats. The outbreak of 2014–2016 began in Guinea in December 2013, then spread to Sierra Leone and Liberia with small numbers of cases recorded in Nigeria and Mali. One person travelled to Texas and died in September of 2014, after infecting two nurses. The west and particularly the US mobilised to contain the outbreak. On 8 August 2014, WHO declared the epidemic an international public health emergency. In this outbreak, up to May 2016, 28,646 suspected cases and 11,323 deaths were reported. Ebola is a nasty, viral haemorrhagic fever. Symptoms can include fever, sore throat, muscle pain, headaches, vomiting, diarrhoea, rash, decreased liver and kidney function, and internal and external bleeding. The CFR is between 25% and 90%, but generally accepted to be about 50%.[6] There have been reports of sporadic new mini outbreaks, but these have been contained.

The Zika virus outbreak began in Brazil in 2015. It is a mosquito-borne disease and is generally mild. It caught global headlines because it can cause Guillain–Barré syndrome in adults, and severe microcephaly (skull deformity) in children of infected mothers, and because it was seen as a threat to the west in particular parts of the USA. Borders do not keep out mosquitoes, and it was reported in the southern US states. In February 2016, WHO declared the outbreak a Public Health Emergency of International Concern (PHEIC).

The public health community knew there would be new diseases and were braced for the next pandemic (Garrett, 1994). The WHO has been tracking diseases for decades beginning with the Global Influenza Surveillance and Response System set up in 1952 (Maxmen, 2021). Following the outbreaks described above, in February 2018 WHO adopted the place holder name 'Disease X' and began preparing for it (Tahir et al., 2021). This was not 'an actual disease caused by a known agent, but a speculated source of the next pandemic that could have devastating effects on humanity' (Huremović, 2019). This is done through a research and development (R&D) blueprint, and its global strategy and preparedness plan for rapid activation of R&D activities. There was a list of 'priority' diseases. At the same time, most OECD governments commissioned studies and developed plans to help prepare for the inevitable (Brownlie et al., 2006). However, there was a degree of complacency in the west, and in the USA, Trump's administration decided to end a project called Predict, run by the US Agency for International Development since 2009. This had been designed to warn of potential pandemics (Milman, 2020).

Disease X is COVID-19

Of the six coronaviruses known to science at the end of 2019, two were sources of concern, SARS and MERS, but both had been contained. The other four caused only mild disease, and two are sources of the common cold (Horton, 2020: 2). In December 2019, a new disease, presenting as pneumonia, was reported from Wuhan in Hubei province in China. Beijing authorities informed the WHO on 31 December 2019 and they set up an incident management team. Over the next weeks, as case numbers climbed, the WHO made a more formal notification of the disease and issued guidance on how to detect, test, and manage cases (2020: 2). In a truly remarkable feat, Chinese scientists were able to isolate the virus, sequence the genome, and make this public by 12 January 2020 (2020: 2).

The first reports to reach the west came through ProMED-Mail. This is produced by The Program for Monitoring Emerging Diseases (ProMED), set up by the International Society for Infectious Diseases (ISID) in 1994 'to identify unusual health events related to emerging and re-emerging infectious diseases and toxins affecting humans, animals and plants'.[7] It is funded by a range of donors and provides publicly available, global reporting of infectious disease outbreaks. ProMED operates 24 hours a day and, for many, the first news of the new pandemic came from this network. 'ProMED is an essential source of information for clinicians and laboratorians around the globe, providing timely reporting of important emerging pathogens and their vectors'.[8] Sarah Gilbert, one of the developers of the Oxford AstraZeneca vaccine, wrote in her book *Vaxxers: The Inside Story of the Oxford AstraZeneca Vaccine and the Race Against the Virus*:

> I checked in with ProMED-Mail … and something caught my eye. There
> were reports of "pneumonia of unknown cause" in Wuhan, China. Four
> cases with high fever and pneumonia not responding to antibiotics. First
> patient worked at a seafood market. Interesting.
>
> (Gilbert and Green, 2021: 29)

The race to develop a vaccine, aided by the release of the genetic sequence, was on. It was not so much a competition between developers, as a race against the virus itself, which was rapidly spreading around the world. At the WHO, the Director General Dr Tedros Adhanom Ghebreyesus and his senior staff deliberated over declaring a PHEIC. Doing this would indicate the disease could spread internationally and threaten other nations, and a coordinated response was needed to address it. This was not done by Tedros until 30 January 2020, by which time there was evidence that the disease could spread between people. It was also evident that COVID-19 had features that made it a unique disease, and an unprecedented threat to health and wellbeing, although as is discussed, the response to the pandemic magnified this. The delay was politically motivated, China did not want to be blamed for the outbreak, and Tedros bowed to this pressure. An additional challenge was the inevitable under-reporting of the disease. Many people had no or only mild symptoms and so are not identified by disease surveillance. This has been well-documented by a number of scholars (Chisale et al., 2021; Lewis et al., 2022).

Disease infectivity, progression, and prevention

COVID-19 is mainly transmitted via the airborne routes and usually attacks the respiratory system. Most people are infected through inhaling the virus particles that others breathe out. Less common are infections from larger airborne particles, uncommon, but possible, are infections from surfaces (fomites).[9] The small airborne particles are known as aerosols and infected people expel these out as they breathe, talk, cough, sneeze, or sing. The greatest risk is when people are close to infected people, who are expelling aerosols, especially if they are facing each other. The chance of infection will depend on the level and length of exposure, in other word the longer someone is exposed and the more virus they inhale, the greater the likelihood of them being infected.

What is unusual and concerning with COVID-19 is people are infectious for up to three days before symptoms appear and are most infectious just before they show symptoms. However, an additional issue is that up to 30% of those infected may not develop any symptoms – but they can still infect others. The majority, up to 55%, will only experience mild to moderate symptoms. The worry is with the balance of infections, 10% will develop severe symptoms, most requiring hospitalisation and some form of supplementary oxygen, five percent will be critically ill and will need oxygen and possibly ventilation and a proportion of these will die. It is this last cohort that puts pressure on health care systems, from Prague to Pofadder, Durban to Delhi.

The mortality rate varies over time and by population. One standard measure, as already mentioned, is the CFR. This is calculated by taking the number of people who have died from COVID-19 and dividing it by the number of people diagnosed with the disease. Obviously, there are many issues with the robustness of the data: how many people died of COVID-19; how do we know how many COVID-19 cases there are? In the United Kingdom (UK), the COVID-19 deaths reported in the daily briefings were people who died within 28 days of a positive COVID-19 test. The highest CFR in the world, to date, was in the UK on 20 April 2020, at 15.24%, next was Italy on 22 June 2020 at 14.53%. Globally, the peak was on 29 April 2020, at 7.32%. The CFRs have fallen dramatically in most countries, but not in South Africa. On 1 July 2022, the rates were 0.79% in the UK, 0.92% in Italy, 2.55% in South Africa, and 1.16% globally.[10] The South Africa rate peaked at 3.44% in at the end of April 2021 and has remained between 2.5 and 3% since. This may be because of underlying population health conditions (comorbidities), including high HIV prevalence, or because new variants seem to develop in the region.

Early in the epidemic, the most vulnerable were the elderly (over 65 years old) and those with comorbidities (Whiteside and Clement, 2020). This was seen on television screens around the world as, especially in the west, the virus ripped through care homes. The older and the more comorbidities people had, the more likely they were to fall ill and die, and as with the early HIV epidemic there were few proven treatments. The main comorbidities associated with poor prognosis are cancers, diabetes and hypertension, as well as respiratory, cardiac, and renal diseases (Pana et al., 2021).

The virus evolved and new variants appeared, some more infectious or deadly than others. Initially, they were named for the countries where they were first identified, which led to stigma. The South African variants seemed particularly infectious and resulted in the extension of restrictions on travellers from South Africa to the UK. WHO established a new naming system for COVID-19 variants, using letters of the Greek alphabet. The current (July 2022) main variants are Alpha, the B.1.1.7 variant, first documented in the UK; Beta the B.1.351 variant, first seen in South Africa; Gamma from Brazil; Delta found in India; and Omicron.

Omicron was first identified in Botswana and South Africa in November 2021. It quickly became the dominant strain globally, spreading faster than any previous strain. It should be noted that there are relatively few laboratories with the equipment and expertise to identify specific varieties, and one is South African. This is a two-edged sword since it can result in stigma against a nation. The evidence to date seems to show that Omicron is more infectious but less deadly than previous variants. There is some hope that COVID-19 may be evolving as a less serious endemic disease, but the high

CFA rate in South Africa suggests baseline health in a population may be significant as to how deadly it will be.

The spread of COVID-19 across the world

The global spread of COVID-19 was rapid. The crucial number is the reproductive number R_0, the number of new infections from each case. If it is greater than one (1) the epidemic is spreading, the higher the number the faster the spread. Lower than one and the epidemic is diminishing.

The Chinese authorities responded rapidly to the virus. On 23 January 2020, Wuhan was locked down completely with schools and shops closed and most citizens not allowed to leave their homes. These measures were extended as the cases spread. Cases were soon reported from Japan, South Korea, Nepal, Hong Kong, Malaysia, and Taiwan. By the end of January, cases had been reported from France, Germany, and the UK. Italy experienced a traumatic outbreak in the Lombardy region and on 9 March 2020 the entire country was placed in lockdown. Spain followed on 14 March, France on the 17th, and the UK on 24 March. The only OECD country not to have imposed a draconian lockdown was Sweden.

South Africa was one of the first African countries to report COVID-19 cases. On 5 March 2020, the Minister of Health Zweli Mkhize reported the first case, a male South African who had been infected in Italy. On 15 March, President Cyril Ramaphosa declared a national state of disaster, with travel restrictions and the closure of schools. A National Coronavirus Command Council was established, 'to lead the nation's plan to contain the spread and mitigate the negative impact of the coronavirus'.[11] A national lockdown was announced from 27 March 2020. This was extremely strict and included the banning of cigarette and alcohol sales. The levels of restrictions and draconian enforcement meant that much South African public was, initially at least, compliant.

There are a number of websites that track the progress of the epidemic. The one that I have used the most is the Johns Hopkins Coronavirus Resource Centre.[12] This gives a good overview, and it is possible to look at individual countries. Others include the outstanding Our World in Data and the SDG-Tracker, which

> are collaborative efforts between researchers at the University of Oxford, who are the scientific editors of the website content; and the non-profit organization Global Change Data Lab, who publishes and maintains the website and the data tools that make our work possible.

The sources of support are: 'the Quadrature Climate Foundation, the Bill and Melinda Gates Foundation, and a grant from the German entrepreneur, businesswoman and philanthropist Susanne Klatten'.[13] Most countries have their own publicly available websites, the South African Online Resource &

News Portal is managed by the Department of Health,[14] and in the UK there is a Coronavirus dashboard.[15]

The Financial Times has a brilliant graphic that illustrates the application and easing of restrictions around the world.

> This page provides an ongoing visual representation of the worldwide imposition and relaxation of lockdown measures. It uses the COVID-19 government response stringency index, a composite score developed by researchers at Oxford university, to compare countries' policy responses to the coronavirus pandemic.
>
> (*Financial Times*, 2022)

Globally, there have been waves of the epidemic. The first peak in December 2020 had 5,209,000 million cases per week, the second was in April 2021 with 5,780,000 cases, the third in August 2021 with 4,590,000 cases and the fourth peak came at the end of January 2022, with 23,226,000 cases. Deaths have followed a similar pattern with peaks in April 2020, January, May, and July 2021, and February 2022. Numbers fell consistently in the first half of 2022.[16] Since vaccines became available the number of people vaccinated has risen rapidly, but Africa lags behind the rest of the world.

Prevention

The first public health response to COVID-19 was to use the tried and tested infectious disease prevention activities: quarantine of infected cases and their contacts. There was, of course, frantic work going on in laboratories across the world to understand the virus, how it worked and what could be done about it. With extensive experience from HIV, my colleagues and I wrote: …

> it is clear from our long experience with HIV that this will change the world as we know it … While more complex understandings of the current pandemic will certainly emerge, we can immediately offer some lessons from our experiences in HIV: don't overlook what works; don't allow political imperatives to undermine rational action; and be open to the possibility that directives from esteemed bodies may not be entirely adequate … Practicable and effective prevention and containment measures rest on information that is underpinned by good data, sound analysis and appropriate conclusions.
>
> (Whiteside, Parker and Schramm, 2020: v–vi)

The nature of COVID-19, with the period of asymptomatic infection, created specific problems for containment. It should also be noted that early in the pandemic there were no proven medical control measures. South Korea was one of the first countries outside China to see COVID-19 and instituted a series of public health measures. In late January 2020, quarantine and isolation of infected individuals and their contacts were imposed. This required active and efficient diagnosis and tracing. It also demanded the ability to impose these restrictions. In addition, the authorities imposed school closures and social distancing, all to reduce contact and therefore transmission (Lee, Kwon and Lee, 2021). These were successful up to August 2020 when there was a small spike, followed by a second in December 2020. At the time of writing (July 2022) the number of cases had shot up reaching 2,717,000 per week at the end of March 2022, with deaths peaking at 2,429 in the week of 27 March.[17] This shows the price of epidemic control is sustained vigilance, but as telling, the lack of media coverage suggests that COVID-19 no longer reaches the front pages.

> School closure is considered one of the most effective ways to mediate disease transmission because it is well known that the contact rate is much higher in the school-age group than in others. Most educational institutes in South Korea including elementary, middle, and high schools and colleges delayed resumption of classes and have meanwhile started on-line classes. This imposes a burden on society, triggering various issues … several studies have reported that the rate of contact decreases by 25% – 75% during the school break.
>
> (Lee, Kwon and Lee, 2021: 8)

However, school closures bring their own challenges: children missing education, socialisation and, in some countries, school feeding programmes no longer reach children in need. These will have long-term consequences.

The lockdowns introduced across the world caused economies to contract, unemployment to rise, and resulted in increased poverty and hunger. The OECD countries were able to put mitigation measures in place, an example being the furlough schemes where governments ensured workers were paid a portion of their wages. In the UK, this was 80% of normal pay up to a maximum of £2,500 a month. The scheme ended at the end of September 2021. In most of the developing world, the ability of governments to provide social support was limited and the suffering was immense. This was illustrated by pictures of millions of unemployed and destitute Indian workers desperately walking to their rural homes.

The effect of COVID-19 on the global and national economies was as if an iron bar had been pushed into the spokes of the back wheel of a bicycle, a crashing halt. My personal metric concerns air traffic. My home in the UK is located near a small regional airport. At the peak in 2020, there were over 25 aircraft, from a range of carriers, parked in storage, on the apron, in one corner of the airport. Prior to the pandemic, there were four flights per day to Amsterdam, our hub to the world. In September 2021, there were just four flights per week!

The pandemic brought renewed nationalism in parts of the world as nations and, in some cases regions, closed their borders, imposed pre- and post-travel testing, quarantine for travellers, and generally turned inward. The actions were indicated, but the way they were generally imposed was not. It spoke of panic.

One of the major changes was the imposition of wearing of face masks. On 20 September 2020, the UK government introduced the 'Hands Face Space' public information campaign, which urged 'the public to continue to wash their hands, cover their face and make space to control infection rates and avoid a second peak'.[18] Continuing use of facemasks in crowds and on public transport is still advised by many governments and health authorities, although it may no longer be mandatory or enforced.

Science, treatment, and vaccines

Initial responses were to control transmission, and support people who were infected and had the misfortune to become seriously ill. There were no known effective drugs available at the start of the pandemic. The main medical intervention was to provide oxygen to patients. It was discovered that 'proning' (placing them face down) helped. COVID-19 cases were placed in isolation, and staff wore personal protective equipment to reduce the risk of infection. The most serious cases were put into medically induced comas and on ventilators, although the chances of recovery for these individuals were low. Of course, all of this was labour intensive and there were few ventilators available in many health services, especially in the developing world.

A very visible effect of the response was the scramble to increase capacity. In the UK, sports arenas were commandeered and adapted as emergency hospitals; in China, new facilities were built in a matter of days; in the USA, Navy hospital ships were docked in Los Angeles and New York City.[19] The expected deluge of patients did not materialise, the facilities were underutilised, and, without fanfare, they were decommissioned. However, the hospitals were under huge pressure due to the infection control measures, staff absences, and death. Many routine procedures and appointments were cancelled, adding to the burden of excess deaths recorded around the world.

There are still relatively few proven treatments against COVID-19. It was briefly thought that a drug, Ivermectin, used for the treatment of people and animals for parasitic diseases could help. The Scientific American noted:

> several groups of doctors are encouraging and enabling people to take the drug off-label to treat or prevent COVID-19—despite a lack of solid evidence that it works against the disease and the fact that high doses can be harmful.
>
> (Szalinski, 2021)

Hydroxychloroquine was proposed as a possible treatment (and taken by some high-profile patients), it is used to treat malaria, lupus erythematosus, and rheumatoid arthritis. It is not recommended for COVID-19. The drug Remdesivir, administered intravenously, was the first antiviral treatment 'approved by the US Food and Drug Administration (FDA)—despite its uncertain benefit to patients. The World Health Organization said the drug had "no meaningful effect" on mortality or the need for ventilation' (Neville and Asgari, 2021).

Obviously, treatments are essential and governments, research institutes, and drug companies around the world are working to develop them. In August 2021, the UK's Medicines and Healthcare products Regulatory Agency (MHRA) approved a monoclonal antibody treatment against COVID-19.

> The decision to authorise Ronapreve, Regeneron and Roche's casirivimab and imdevimab cocktail, was made after a review of clinical trial data showed the drug that may be used to prevent and treat acute COVID-19 infection and reduce hospital admissions due to coronavirus.
>
> Phase III studies of the treatment found it reduced the risk of hospitalisation or death in high-risk, non-hospitalised patients by 70% compared with placebo. Ronapreve also reduced the duration of coronavirus symptoms from 14 to ten days in those with the virus.
>
> (Jimenez, 2021)

A number of drugs have been developed and are being used. They include Merck's Molnupiravir and Paxlovid and Ritonavir tablets, made by Pfizer. Remdesivir, developed to treat people with the Ebola and hepatitis C, has been repurposed.[20] In the UK, an inhaled interferon treatment is being developed by Synairgen. The Swiss company Roche is developing an oral antiviral with Atea Pharmaceuticals with dual potential: to treat patients and prevent illness in people exposed to the virus.

Many treatments are in the pipeline; they will take time to gain approval. As with the early antiretrovirals for HIV and AIDS, there are questions around the accessibility and price, although unlike AIDS these drugs will not be needed for life. It is quite possible that treatment will be out of the reach of poorer nations unless there are interventions by the wealthy nations, the United Nations and especially the WHO and Unitaid.[21] The latter is a global health initiative working with partners on innovations to prevent, diagnose, and treat major diseases in the less developed world.

The global health community recognised that the best way forward was to develop a vaccine as rapidly as possible. Bill Gates said:

> One of the questions I get asked the most these days is when the world will be able to go back to the way things were in December before the coronavirus pandemic. My answer is always the same: when we have an almost perfect drug to treat COVID-19, or when almost every person on the planet has been vaccinated against coronavirus. The former is unlikely to happen anytime soon … Which leaves us with a vaccine.
>
> (Gates, 2020)

I produced a blog from 4 March 2020 up to 11 August 2021 to try to keep friends and colleagues informed on developments related to COVID-19. The information on vaccines is primarily drawn from this (Whiteside, 2021).

In June 2020, there were 125 vaccines in the preclinical phase; eight in Phase I trials where the safety and dosage are tested; eight in Phase II, expanded safety trials; and two in Phase III trials which meant large-scale efficacy tests. All these phases must be completed before a vaccine can be approved for use. Only in Phase III do we know if they actually work. The research was primarily in Europe (including the UK), North America, and China. The US government established 'Operation Warp Speed' to develop a vaccine, this started with five projects that received billions of dollars in federal funding and support. *New York Times* (2021) noted:

> The first vaccine safety trials in humans started in March, but the road ahead remains uncertain. Some trials will fail, and others may end without a clear result. But a few may succeed in stimulating the immune system to produce effective antibodies against the virus.

The news of potential vaccines came towards the end of 2020. First off the blocks were US-based pharmaceutical company Pfizer Inc. and BioNTech SE, a German biotechnology company. Reports on 9 November 2020 stated their vaccine was 90% effective (Hopkins, 2020). By the end of November, Moderna, a company based in Cambridge, Massachusetts, reported they had 94.5% effective vaccine. Shortly after this, the launch of the Oxford AstraZeneca vaccine was announced (Whiteside, 2021). The story of the Oxford AstraZeneca vaccine is comprehensively covered by scientists Sarah Gilbert and Catherine Green (2021). An overview of the epidemic and vaccines is provided by Jeremy Farrar, Director of the Wellcome Trust in *Spike: The Virus versus the People. The Inside Story* (Farrar, 2021).

Outside the OECD countries, by the end of 2020, there were three candidate vaccines from China and one from Russia. The Chinese company CanSino Biologics developed a vaccine in partnership with the Institute of Biology of the Academy of Military Medical Sciences. The Wuhan Institute of Biological Products developed and tested a vaccine with the state-owned company Sinopharm. Phase III trials were run in the United Arab Emirates, Morocco, and Peru. The Russian Gamaleya Research Institute, part of the Ministry of Health, developed Sputnik V which was approved in August 2020, even before Phase III trials had begun.

In September, there was an announcement of a new Chinese-developed vaccine produced by Clover Biopharmaceuticals (Cohen, 2021). Two doses of this vaccine protect against five variants of the virus, including the highly infectious Delta strain. The vaccine reduces the risk of disease among people who have not been infected and those who have.

There is no shortage of vaccines if all manufacturers are considered. However, Africa, including South Africa, lags in delivering vaccines. Initially, South Africa appeared to be doing reasonably well. It

> led major African economies by fully vaccinating 17.5% of its population, or 7 million people, with either the Johnson & Johnson single-dose vaccine or Pfizer's two-dose jab. This compares with under 3% of Africans overall, on a continent that risks falling further behind as richer countries chase limited global supplies.
>
> (Cotterill, Schipani and Pilling, 2021)

In addition, there is COVAX defined as 'the vaccines pillar of the Access to COVID-19 Tools (ACT) Accelerator'. This is

> a ground-breaking global collaboration to accelerate the development, production, and equitable access to COVID-19 tests, treatments, and vaccines. COVAX is co-led by Gavi [the Vaccine Alliance], the Coalition for Epidemic Preparedness Innovations (CEPI) and WHO. Its aim is to accelerate the development and manufacture of COVID-19 vaccines, and to guarantee fair and equitable access for every country in the world.[22]

An oft-repeated mantra is that until everyone is vaccinated no one will be safe and the epidemic will not be under control. This is informed by the view that variants will develop and spread in populations that are only partially vaccinated or unvaccinated. There is no evidence yet to suggest whether this is likely or unlikely. However, in July 2022 globally 60.99% of the population had received the initial doses. In South Africa, this figure was 31.76%. In the USA, it was 66.95% and in the UK, 73.49%.[23] It is not clear how long protection lasts from the different vaccines and protocols. This is under intense scrutiny. Uptake rather than supply seems to be the problem.

Conclusion and ways forward

In October 2021, I published an editorial in the African Journal of AIDS Research based on six new books on COVID-19 I had read over the previous two months (Whiteside, 2021). These were by the Editor of *The Lancet*, Richard Horton, *The COVID-19 Catastrophe: What's Gone Wand How to Stop It Happening Again* (Horton, 2020); an epidemiologist friend and colleague Daniel Halperin *Facing COVID Without Panic: 12 Common Myths and 12 Lesser Known Facts about the Pandemic: Clearly Explained by an Epidemiologist* (Halperin, 2020); investigative journalist Michael Lewis' *The Premonition: A Pandemic Story* (Lewis, 2021); Jeremy Farrar's *Spike The Virus vs the People The Inside Story*; Gilbert and Green's *Vaxxers*; and Adam Tooze's *Shutdown: How*

COVID-19 Shook the World's Economy (Tooze, 2021). All were well written, informed, and deeply interesting. A common theme was COVID-19 should not have been a surprise, and humankind has been exceptionally fortunate in that it was not a more virulent disease.

The quality and speed of the science, including epidemiology, was extraordinary. It was soon clear, in the absence of a vaccine, how to react to slow and, hopefully, stop the pandemic. We had examples of where these interventions worked: China, Taiwan, Hong Kong, Japan, and other east Asian nations. These non-medical interventions (NMIs) included social distancing, wearing face masks, and practising good hygiene. The most effective way to do this was through draconian lockdowns, confining all but the essential workers to their homes, suspending schools and universities, and banning gatherings of all kinds – from sporting events to church services. These effectively brought economies and societies to a grinding halt. In the OECD, social safety nets either existed or were put in place to ensure people could survive. Many countries set up scientific advisory groups or expanded the mandate of existing ones (Colman et al., 2021). These were able to advise on the science and suggest responses, although it should be remembered that this was sometimes contested.[24]

We can track infections, hospitalisations, and deaths from COVID-19 with varying degrees of accuracy in different countries (Troeger, 2021). At the moment, this virus is the leading cause of death in many countries. Vaccination uptake is urgently needed, but in the absence of this NMIs are critical. Unfortunately, societies have not yet adapted to living with the pandemic. The economic, educational, social, and cultural harms that come from stringent controls are increasingly seen to outweigh the benefits. The middle ground and trade-offs have not yet been established or communicated.

It is hard to predict what the future looks like. A binary one would be that new variants of COVID-19 become less deadly, but perhaps more infectious, as has been the case with Omicron. It is also possible they could become more deadly. The second option will lead to an isolated, suspicious world. There has already been increased inequality in all societies and the importance of social safety nets is clear.

The rest of this book digs into some of the big issues we face in South Africa. This is a time of great challenge, but it can also be one of opportunity. South Africa is a resilient society. The relatively peaceful transition from Apartheid to a democratic society was a miracle, albeit an imperfect one. The country faced one of the worst HIV/AIDS epidemics in the world. It has managed to keep millions of infected people alive with anti-retroviral therapy. The COVID-19 epidemic is the greatest challenge of the new century to date. We can learn how to respond to infectious diseases from this, and maybe, just maybe, we will learn how to respond to and mitigate the environmental catastrophes we are facing.

Notes

1 See https://ourworldindata.org/human-development-index (Accessed: 2 July 2022).
2 See https://data.worldbank.org/indicator/SP.DYN.LE00.IN (Accessed: 2 July 2022).
3 See https://www.unaids.org/en/resources/fact-sheet (Accessed: 2 July 2022).
4 See https://www.unaids.org/en/resources/fact-sheet (Accessed: 2 July 2022).
5 See https://www.who.int/emergencies/disease-outbreak-news/item/2010_08_ 06-en (Accessed: 8 April 2020).
6 See https://ourworldindata.org/mortality-risk-COVID-19 (Accessed: 2 July 2022).
7 See https://promedmail.org/about-promed/ (Accessed: 2 July 2022).
8 See https://promedmail.org/about-promed/ (Accessed: 2 July 2022).
9 Effectively touching a contaminated surface and transferring the viremia to a mucous membrane such as the eyes or nose, giving it entry to the body.
10 See https://ourworldindata.org/mortality-risk-COVID-19. It should be noted that raw data are sourced from the COVID-19 Data Repository by the Center for Systems Science and Engineering (CSSE) at Johns Hopkins University. (Accessed: 27 September 2021 and 3 July 2022).
11 See   https://www.gov.za/speeches/president-cyril-ramaphosa-meets-political- parties-combat-coronavirus-covid-19-18-mar-18-mar#:~:text=On%20 Tuesday%2C%2017%20March%202020,negative%20impact%20of%20 the%20 coronavirus (Accessed: 7 July 2022).
12 See https://coronavirus.jhu.edu/map.html (Accessed: 29 September 2021).
13 See https://ourworldindata.org/funding (Accessed: 29 September 2021).
14 See https://sacoronavirus.co.za/ (Accessed: 29 September 2021 and 2 July 2022).
15 See https://coronavirus.data.gov.uk/ (Accessed: 29 September 2021).
16 See https://coronavirus.jhu.edu/map.html (Accessed: 2 July 2022).
17 See https://coronavirus.jhu.edu/map.html (Accessed 2 July 2022).
18 See https://www.gov.uk/government/news/new-campaign-to-prevent-spread- of-coronavirus-indoors-this-winter. The campaign was launched on 9 September 2020. (Accessed: 29 September 2021).
19 See https://news.usni.org/2020/05/25/beyond-mercy-navys-COVID-19-hospital- ship-missions-and-the-future-of-medicine-at-sea (Accessed: 30 September 2021).
20 See https://www.hopkinsmedicine.org/health/conditions-and-diseases/corona- virus/coronavirus-treatment-whats-in-development (Accessed: 2 July 2022).
21 See https://unitaid.org/#en (Accessed: 2 July 2022).
22 See https://www.who.int/initiatives/act-accelerator/covax (Accessed: 2 July 2022).
23 See https://ourworldindata.org/covid-vaccinations (Accessed: 2 July 2022).
24 In the UK the British government's Scientific Advisory Group for Emergencies (SAGE) was quick to respond but it took pressure to make the SAGE minutes public. It is not widely known that a group of independent scientists and thinkers set up an alternative group, Independent SAGE. See https://www.gov.uk/gov- ernment/organisations/scientific-advisory-group-for-emergencies and https:// www.independentsage.org/.

References

Aburto, J. M., Schöley, J., Kashnitsky, I., Zhang, L., Rahal, C., Missov, T. I., Mills, M. C., Dowd, J. B., & Kashyap, R. (2022). Quantifying impacts of the COVID-19 pandemic through life-expectancy losses: A population-level study of 29 countries. *International Journal of Epidemiology*, *51*(1), 63–74, doi.org/10.1093/ije/dyab207.

Brownlie, J., Peckham, C., Waage, J., Woolhouse, M., Lyall, C., Meagher, L., Tait, J., Baylis, M., & Nicoll, A. (2006). *Infectious Diseases: Preparing for the Future – Future Threats. Foresight.* London: Office of Science and Innovation.

Chan-Yeung, M., & Xu, R. H. (2003). SARS: Epidemiology. *Respirology, 8*(s1), S9–14, doi:10.1046/j.1440–1843.2003.00518.x.

Chisale, M. R. O., Ramazanu, S., Mwale, S. E., Kumwenda, P., Chipeta, M., Kaminga, A. C., Nkhata, O., Nyambalo, B., Chavura, E., & Mbakaya, B. C. (2022). Seroprevalence of anti-SARS-CoV-2 antibodies in Africa: A systematic review and meta-analysis. *Reviews in Medical Virology, 32*(2), e2271, doi:10.1002/rmv.2271.

Cohen, J. (2021). New Chinese vaccine could bolster global arsenal: Protein-based shots developed by Clover shown to protect against five variants. *Science, 374*(6563), 12–13.

Colman, E., Wanat, M., Goossens, H., Tonkin-Crine, S., & Anthierens, S. (2021). Following the science? Views from scientists on government advisory boards during the COVID-19 pandemic: A qualitative interview study in five European countries. *BMJ Global Health, 6*(9), e006928, doi:10.1136/bmjgh-2021–006928.

Coronavirus Resource Centre. (n.d.). Johns Hopkins University of Medicine. *Global Map.* Available at: https://coronavirus.jhu.edu/map.html. [Accessed: 29 September 2021 & 2 July 2022]

Cotterill, J., Schipani, A., & Pilling, D. (2021). South Africa battles to boost take-up of COVID-19 vaccines Supplies are growing but the poor struggle to reach clinics or get time off work. *Financial Times*, 12 September. Available at: https://www.ft.com/content/b6a964fc-69c7-4247-9d06-0c7d3de11420. [Accessed: 2 July 2022]

Davies, S. C., Winpenny, E., Ball, S., Fowler, T., Rubin, J., & Nolte, E. (2014). For debate: A new wave in public health improvement. *The Lancet, 384*(9957), 1889–1895, doi.org/10.1016/S0140–6736(13)62341-7.

Farrar, J., & Ahuja, A. (2021). *Spike: The Virus versus the People – The Inside Story.* London, UK: Profile Books.

Financial Times (2022). *Lockdowns Compared: Tracking Governments' Coronavirus Responses.* Available at: https://ig.ft.com/coronavirus-lockdowns/. [Accessed: 29 September 2021 & 2 July 2022]

Garrett, L. (1994). *The Coming Plague: Newley Emergent Diseases in a World out of Balance.* New York, NY: Penguin.

Gates, B. (2020). What you need to know about the COVID-19 vaccine. *Gates Notes – The Blog of Bill Gates*, 30 April. Available at: https://www.gatesnotes.com/health/what-you-need-to-know-about-the-covid-19-vaccine. [Accessed: 2 July 2022]

Gilbert, S., & Green, C. (2021). *Vaxxers: The Inside Story of the Oxford AstraZeneca Vaccine the Race Against the Virus.* London, UK: Hodder and Stoughton.

Halperin, D. T. (2020). *Facing COVID Without Panic: 12 Common Myths and 12 Lesser Known Facts about the Pandemic: Clearly Explained by and Epidemiologist* [Online]. Available from: http://www.amazon.com/dp/B08D25GQX6 and https://davisny.edu/wp-content/uploads/2021/09/ABHE-Facing-COVID-Without-Panic.pdf. [Accessed: 2 July 2022]

Harper, S., Riddell, C. A., & King, N. B. (2021). Declining life expectancy in the United States: Missing the trees for the forest. *Annual Review of Public Health*, (April) 42, 381–403, doi.org/10.1146/annurev-publhealth-082619–104231.

Hopkins, J. S. (2020). Pfizer's COVID-19 vaccine proves 90% effective in latest trials: Drugmaker and partner BioNTech could seek FDA authorisation by end of November. *Wall Street Journal*, 9 November. Available at: https://archive.is/www.

wsj.com/articles/covid-19-vaccine-from-pfizer-and-biontech-works-better-than-expected-11604922300. [Accessed: 2 July 2022]

Horton, R. (2020). *The COVID-19 Catastrophe: What's Gone Wrong and How to Stop It Happening Again.* Cambridge, UK: Polity.

Huremović, D. (2019). Brief history of pandemics (pandemics throughout history). *Psychiatry of Pandemics*, (May) 16, 7–35, doi:10.1007/978-3-030-15346-5_2.

Jimenez, D. (2021). Ronapreve: UK approves first-of-its-kind antibody cocktail to treat COVID-19. *Pharmaceutical Technology*, 20 August. Available at: https://www.pharmaceutical-technology.com/news/ronapreve-uk-approves-antibody-cocktail-COVID-19/. [Accessed: 2 July 2022]

Lee, T., Kwon, H-D., & Lee, J. (2021). The effect of control measures on COVID-19 transmission in South Korea. *PLOS One*, *16*(3): e0249262, doi.org/10.1371/journal.pone.0249262.

Lewis, H., Ware, H., Whelan, M., Subissi, L., Li, Z., Ma, X., Nardone, A., Valenciano, M., et al. (2022). SARS-CoV-2 infection in Africa: A systematic review and meta-analysis of standardised seroprevalence studies, from January 2020 to December 2021. *medRxiv* [Online], 15 February. doi:10.1101/2022.02.14.22270934.

Lewis, M. (2021). *The Premonition: A Pandemic Story.* London, UK: Allen Lane.

Maxmen, A. (2021). Has COVID taught us anything about pandemic preparedness? Researchers warn that plans to prevent the next global outbreak don't consider the failures that have fuelled our current predicament. *Nature*, (August) Volume 596. Available at: https://www.nature.com/articles/d41586-021-02217-y. [Accessed: 2 July 2022]

Milman, O. (2020). Trump administration cut pandemic early warning program in September. *The Guardian*, 3 April. Available at: https://www.theguardian.com/world/2020/apr/03/trump-scrapped-pandemic-early-warning-program-system-before-coronavirus. [Accessed: 2 July 2022]

Neville, S., & Asgari, N. (2021). Antiviral pill: How close are we to a drug to treat COVID-19? *Financial Times*, 27 September. Available at: https://www.ft.com/content/48cf11f5-9588-4487-b262-f6f26e901ec2. [Accessed: 2 July 2022]

Pana, T. A., Bhattacharya, S., Gamble, D. T., Pasdar, Z., Szlachetka, W. A., Perdomo-Lampignano, J. A., Ewers, K. D., McLernon, D. J., et al (2021). Country-level determinants of the severity of the first global wave of the COVID-19 pandemic: An ecological study. *BMJ Open*, *11*(2), e042034, doi:10.1136/bmjopen-2020–042034.

Statistics South Africa (2021). COVID-19 Epidemic Reduces Life Expectancy in 2021. Available at: https://www.statssa.gov.za/?p=14519#:~:text=This%20resulted%20in%20a%20significant,at%20birth%20for%20South%20Africa. [Accessed: 2 July 2022]

Szalinski, C. (2021). Fringe Doctors' Groups Promote Ivermectin for COVID despite a Lack of Evidence. *Scientific American*, 29 September. Available at: https://www.scientificamerican.com/article/fringe-doctors-groups-promote-ivermectin-for-covid-despite-a-lack-of-evidence/. [Accessed: 2 July 2022]

Tahir, M. J., Sawal, I., Essar, M. Y., Jabbar, A., Ullah, I., & Ahmed, A. (2021). Disease X: A hidden but inevitable creeping danger. *Infection Control & Hospital Epidemiology*, (July) 26, 1–2, doi:10.1017/ice.2021.342.

Tooze, A. (2021). *Shutdown: How COVID-19 Shook the World's Economy.* London, UK: Alan Lane.

Troeger, C. (2022). Just How Do Deaths Due to COVID-19 Stack Up? Despite a likely undercount in many places, COVID-19 is the leading killer in most of Latin America and Western Europe. *Think Global Health*, 12 May. Available at: https://www.thinkglobalhealth.org/article/just-how-do-deaths-due-COVID-19-stack.

UNAIDS. (n.d.). *Global HIV & AIDS Statistics – Fact Sheet*. Available from: https://www.unaids.org/en/resources/fact-sheet. [Accessed: 2 July 2022]

Wang, H., Paulson, K. R., Pease, S. A., Watson, S., Comfort, H., Zheng, P., Aravkin, A. Y., Bisignano, C., et al. – COVID-19 Excess Mortality Collaborators (2022). Estimating excess mortality due to the COVID-19 pandemic: A systematic analysis of COVID-19-related mortality, 2020–21. *The Lancet*, *399*(10334), 1513–1536, doi:10.1016/S0140–6736(21)02796-3.

Whiteside, A. (2020a). Covid-19 watch: A different background. *Alan Whiteside: Covid-19 Watch*, 17 June. Available at: https://alan-whiteside.com/2020/06/17/COVID-19-watch-a-different-background/#more-3440.

Whiteside, A. (2020b). Covid-19 watch: Vaccines, vaccines, vaccines! *Alan Whiteside: Covid-19 Watch*, 25 November. Available at: https://alan-whiteside.com/?s=Vaccines%2C+vaccines%2C+vaccines&submit=Search.

Whiteside, A. (2021). Reflecting on pandemic publishing, now and then: COVID-19 and HIV. *African Journal of AIDS Research*, *20*(3), 189–191, doi:10.2989/16085906.2021.1984039.

Whiteside, A., & Clement, F. (2020). COVID-19, age and mortality: Implications for public policy. *Balsillie Papers*, (2 June) *2*(1), doi:10.51644/bap21.

Whiteside, A., Parker, W., & Schramm, M. (2020). Editorial: Managing the march of COVID-19: Lessons from the HIV and AIDS epidemic. *African Journal of AIDS Research*, *19*(2), iii–vi, doi.org/10.2989/16085906.2020.1749792.

Whiteside, A., & Zebryk, N. (2017). New and re-emerging infectious diseases in Sub-Saharan Africa. In: H. Groth & J. F. May (Eds.). *Africa's Population: In Search of a Demographic Dividend*, pp. 299–313. Switzerland & Washington, DC: Springer.

5 Slow crises

South Africa's governmental responses to COVID-19 in times of 'crisis within crisis'

Laurin Baumgardt and Steven Robins

Introduction

Throughout the world, COVID-19 triggered drastic public health interventions, including dramatic hard lockdowns in countries such as South Africa. Unlike so many other crises in the past, it would seem, governments prioritised the health of their citizens above the economic health of countries. In South Africa, like elsewhere in the world, COVID-19 triggered rapid, extensive, and drastic responses from the South African government in terms of the implementation of a hard lockdown and other public health measures. It would appear that the urgency, scale, and intensity of these COVID responses have not been replicated when it comes to other crises, not even the devastating HIV/AIDS pandemic that exploded in South Africa in the early 2000s – a crisis that came into national visibility largely as a result of the concerted actions and social mobilisation undertaken by AIDS activists and public health professionals. Why did the COVID-19 crisis produce such immediate responses from government? Furthermore, what was, and remains, the relationship between this crisis and many other 'slow crises' such as the structural conditions underpinning racialised inequality and chronic poverty, gender-based violence, violent crime, massive unemployment, climate-related drought, and water scarcity, and problems in housing, sanitation, service delivery, and so on? What is it about the latter kinds of 'slow crises' that do not appear to generate the kind of urgent government responses as COVID-19 did? What we seek to highlight is how and why 'crises' are rendered visible and invisible in particular historical conjunctures, and what this can tell us about governmental responses and policies in relation to the various temporalities of crisis.

By exploring how convergences of crises open or foreclose change, and how crises can leave positive traces, we will complement scholarly debates of crisis, which often either focus too narrowly on a singular 'crisis' or overemphasise an understanding of 'crisis talk' as a stabilising force. More specifically, we will use this analysis of 'crisis' to understand how the South African government, like many other governments throughout the world, came to respond to COVID-19 by means of hard lockdowns and other drastic public

DOI: 10.4324/9781003294931-5

health measures. We aim to not only understand how multiple crises are interlinked or nested within each other – what Joseph Masco termed 'crisis in crisis' (Masco, 2019) – but also how various crises surface with various levels of gravity, speed, and visibility. We are curious about how some crises can be hyper-transient, quickly vanish, and come in and out of focus, while they continue to exist endemically.

Thinking through the concept of crisis

To capture the current climate of political instability, uncertainty, precarity, structural violence, and enduring, chronic suffering, we draw on the term 'slow crises'. By using 'crises' in the plural, we also signal that those crises cannot be singularised and are not slow per se. Rather, crises always work in conjunction with alternate and competing temporalities and visibilities. Living in South Africa's highly stratified and racialised, unequal and violent society can mean, for the majority of citizens, to live with unemployment, insecure housing conditions, daily violence, constant threats of murder, rape, and theft, without modern infrastructures, and rendered vulnerable to air pollution, and other ecological dangers like floods, droughts and fires, to name but a few of the slow, everyday crises. These crises are slow not only in the sense that they are here to stay, permanently, chronically, and endemically. Rather, 'slow crises' are expressions of both ongoing slow violence (Nixon, 2011) and possibilities of 'slow activism' (Robins, 2014) and 'slow justice' (Neville & Martin, 2022), namely, collective responses that work against the continuous violence of infrastructural exclusions and toxic exposures (Ahmann, 2018).

In light of the ongoing pandemic, we thus aim to interrogate the crisis concept anew, especially in regard to how the South African government has responded to these multiple and interlocking crises in the time of COVID. Across the globe, COVID-19 has become a new, ordinary, and enduring endemic crisis, but not without still being hyper-visible across the media, political discussions, and human perceptions. The COVID-19 crisis started as a spectacularly horrifying and paralysing event but continues to get normalised and backgrounded with time. However, as the emergence of the Omicron variant in late 2021 revealed, COVID-19 globally shifting and alternating 'waves' in different countries secure continuous returns of attention in the media and among state officials and the wider citizenry.

As Janet Roitman argued in her book *Anti-Crisis* (2013), crisis is not so much a singular historical event, rather than an enduring existential condition and self-referential system. It is a 'blind spot', a 'placeholder' for the production of narratives and knowledge (Roitman, 2013). Following Roitman and others, we thus aim to understand the South African crises as enduring conditions and not singular events. Unlike in the Global North, where COVID-19 crisis talk continued to dominate and permeate all public discourse, in South Africa, these other crisis phenomena cannot be ignored.

Whether it is police or gender-based violence, crime, state capture, systemic problems with electricity supply, or the July 2021 'riots' in KwaZulu-Natal and Gauteng Provinces, these multiple eruptions of crisis periodically push themselves to the centre of public discussion. Crises in South Africa are not aberrations, they are endemic rather than episodic. For Henrik Vigh, crisis is the common background, 'the context', that is the terrain of action and meaning (Vigh, 2008). As a mediatic and governmental management tool and homeostatic device, 'crisis' seems to rarely offer new horizons or address structural changes. According to Chloe Ahmann, 'crisis' is a 'privileged designation' that is not 'necessarily transformative' and often 'reinscribes existing forms of inequality by diverting attention' (Ahmann, 2018: 147).

In his article 'Crisis in Crisis', Joseph Masco (2019: 236) shares these sentiments and asks, 'how and why crisis has come to be so dominant in our media cultures?' While examining what he terms the 'narrative saturation' and the 'radical presentism of crisis talk' in American media cultures, he shows how crisis, as 'an ever-present, near-permanent negative "surround" … [and] is thus a predominantly conservative modality, seeking to stabilize an existing structure within a radically contingent world' (Masco, 2019: 237). If the climate crisis was nested within the nuclear crisis during the 20th century, as Joseph Masco has pointed out, how are the above-mentioned slow crises, including the climate crisis, nested within the COVID-19 crisis today?[1] The nuclear crisis and climate crisis were based on and originated in a particular type of post-World War II securitisation and consumerist- and industrial-complex. Although it is beyond the scope of this chapter, it would seem that the structural underpinnings of South Africa's multiple and endemic slow crises are part of a racial capitalist system that shapes the broad contours of these crises. It would also appear that these crises are the product of underlying political-economic conditions and dynamics of what Nancy Fraser understands as the self-devouring, cannibalistic tendencies of capitalism, with 'the system's built-in tendency to ecological crisis' (Fraser, 2021: 95). According to Fraser, the world is not only facing 'a crisis of ecology, to be sure, but also one of economy, society, politics and public health – that is, a *general crisis* whose effects metastasize everywhere, shaking confidence in established worldviews and ruling elites' (Fraser, 2021: 95).

In the following sections, we will provide a commentary on South Africa's most recent pandemic history based primarily on our readings of investigative journalism, which continues to help us understand these intersecting crises in 'real-time'. First, we will start with a general elaboration on some specificities of this new crisis and its global emergence. Whilst maintaining a clear focus on how draconian public health measures like the lockdown model were adopted by the South African government, we also examine how this newly emergent crisis, and its governmental responses, reshape, and reconfigure multiple other already-existing 'slow crises'. Second, we exemplify these crisis relationships by pointing to the emerging public health 'blind spots' of other recent epidemics like TB and HIV/AIDS which, perhaps due to their normalisation and 'slower' or less spectacular framing, were not receiving the same public and national attention. Third, we take a closer look at how other wider societal crises such as gender-based violence, land dispossessions, and security force brutality are directly related to and become re-enforced in the wake of the COVID-19 crisis. By reading through three of South Africa's highly mediatised violent events in 2020, we highlight how the COVID-19 crisis and draconian lockdown responses have come to function as amplifiers, as well as portals, of slow violence, or what Lauren Berlant terms the 'crisis ordinary' (2011), that is an everyday condition of layered and extended crises. Fourth, we shed light on the July 2021 unrest as another spectacular instantiation of the convergence of crises. Unlike other crisis scholars (Roitman, 2013; Masco, 2016; Ahmann, 2018; Anderson, 2021), we propose a rather more balanced outlook on 'crisis', one which not only highlights governmental responses that reproduce and stabilise social hierarchies and inequalities through 'crisis talk', but one which also considers the converging crisis conditions that demand government actions and reconsiderations of earlier South African activist ideas such as the Basic Income Grant (BIG), a proposal which was first put forward by the labour union federation, the Congress of South African Trade Unions (COSATU) in the late 1990s and gained more traction in the early 2000s (Ferguson, 2009: 175ff).

Urban geographer Matthew Gandy has observed that the COVID-19 pandemic occupies an ambiguous zone between two biopolitical modes of intervention: a 'disciplinary nexus of control' as manifest in lockdown, testing, and quarantine measures, as well as an 'inoculation model' which is based on large-scale vaccination productions and campaigns (Gandy, 2021: 9). As a result of the 'real-time' media coverage and chronological writing process of this paper, we have put more emphasis throughout the chapter on the former, although we briefly discuss the latter in the conclusion. We will thus end our discussion with some concluding thoughts on the intersecting crises dynamics between the global South and Global North in light of the unequal vaccine rollouts and the international travel bans that were implemented in response to the detection of the Omicron variant.

Global lockdown models and South Africa's 'hard' response

It would seem that there were many factors responsible for the swift uptake by governments of the COVID-19 lockdown model and other drastic public health measures. Governments and international health agencies such as the WHO needed to come up with clear, coherent, and replicable containment strategies that could be rapidly rolled out and trigger drastic behavioural change of an unprecedented scale. In light of the uncertainties around the reproduction and mortality rates, lockdown came to be seen as the safest and most radical form of virus containment and suppression. Implementing nation-wide lockdowns, and Stay-at-Home or Shelter-in-Place orders, were quickly taken up as a replicable blueprint solution, a travelling public health model. Of course, not all people were, and are, impacted in the same way, but this intervention model seemed capable of producing dramatic and instant behavioural change. Considering the rapid chain of events, it seemed that the lockdown model allowed governments throughout the world to act in ways that appeared to be decisive and effective from both a public health and governance perspective. Being seen to be acting decisively seemed to override the 'collateral damage' of lockdown measures, and national lockdowns were quickly accepted by governments as necessary for saving lives, notwithstanding these unavoidable side effects in terms of adverse economic, social, and political consequences.[2] Afterall, many lives were expected to be saved by these drastic lockdown measures (Beaubien, 2020): the COVID-19 crisis was understood as a special type of global crisis that required unprecedented, radical governmental responses.

Lockdown became the default global health response even though, prior to the Covid-19 outbreak, it had not been part of global pandemic prevention and containment planning (Caduff, 2020). 'Pandemic prophecies' had, however, been circulating for a number of years already (Caduff, 2014). Pandemic preparedness plans (Lakoff, 2008) and pandemic bond speculation (Erikson, 2019) had been simulating and calculating the likelihood of potential pandemic outbreaks. Preparedness plans entailed the establishment of early warning and outbreak detection systems through disease surveillance technologies, antiviral drug stockpiling, international emergency operations centres, and potential vaccine distribution systems (Lakoff, 2010; Samimian-Darash, 2013). The pandemic preparedness plans in place are intended to safeguard vital security and critical urban infrastructures rather than protect the security of populations directly (Collier & Lakoff, 2015; Wolf, 2012). In an interview in late May 2020, medical anthropologist and pandemic expert Carlo Caduff lamented that 'a model-based policy brackets out the social and economic consequences of the pandemic response' (Caduff & Bonilla, 2020; Mostowlansky & Caduff, 2020). Caduff highlighted that national lockdowns were never part of pandemic preparedness plans. Rather, lockdowns were a theoretical option in mathematical disease models in which modellers stated that lockdowns needed to stay in place between 12 and 18 months until a vaccine became available. Caduff also pondered about how China's locked-city approach became the global norm; in other words, how a locked-city approach was turned into a locked-country approach (Caduff, 2020). Considering the extraordinary responses from governments, Caduff in fact argued that the coronavirus crisis demanded a more moderate response from governments, as well as a new perspective that 'looks beyond the virus' and 'beyond the crisis' (Caduff, 2020: 10). For him, the pandemic response, collective panic, and fantasies of control are what makes this public health crisis unprecedented, not the virus itself. He concluded that 'this pandemic will haunt us for decades in ways we can barely imagine at this point' (Caduff, 2020: 6).

The 'hard' lockdown, for which President Cyril Ramaphosa was initially widely lauded, was supposed to only last 21 days, starting 26 March 2020, but continued for about three months and was then substituted with a phased reopening of the South African economy and the society. According to the Oxford COVID-19 Government Response Stringency Index, South Africans were subjected to one of the world's most stringent lockdowns which included stay-at-home orders, curfews, bans on alcohol sales, and national and international travel, as well as the closure of schools, universities, transport systems, and entire industries (New Frame, 2020). Between February and April 2020, there were almost 3 million net job losses and the informal economy contracted, with women being the most negatively affected (Haffajee, 2020). According to the South African National Income Dynamics Study Coronavirus Rapid Mobile Survey (NIDS-CRAM) data, 37% of those self-employed reported zero earnings in April 2020, and women's typical earnings in informal sector jobs decreased by nearly 70% between February and April 2020 (Rogan & Skinner, 2020). Journalist and Daily Maverick associate editor, Ferial Haffajee went so far as to speak of a 'triple pandemic' that was hitting South Africa: COVID-19 deaths, unemployment (significantly higher for women), and hunger (Haffajee, 2020).

While the top-down imposition of the South African lockdown attempted to tackle the pressing epidemic crisis, it simultaneously exacerbated and unleashed ongoing structurally embedded crises. The lockdown could be seen as having been less successful at mitigating or suppressing this newly emergent health crisis, rather than reconfiguring and redistributing it. The emergence of COVID-19, together with a lockdown suppression approach, allowed for a convergence of multiple crises – crises such as chronic poverty and inequality, HIV and TB, structural violence and massive unemployment that overlap, intensify, and worsen, each other. Moreover, in the global South, large-scale institutional responses such as lockdowns have largely misrecognised the existing and emerging modes of 'collective life' and thus under/mined everyday urban practices and local economies (Bhan et al., 2020).

The blind spots of South Africa's governmental lockdown

The South African government's response to the COVID-19 crisis by means of national lockdowns both suspended politics in the name of public health and signalled that this crisis was of a qualitatively different order to the many other crises facing the country. This served to produce 'blind spots' that obscured the everyday realities of those experiencing the chronic crises of slow violence and structural poverty referred to above. As technical machinery, the lockdown attempted to 'buy time' and mobilise essential health resources and ramp up the intensive care unit (ICU) capacity and the production of ventilators and protective gear. Along with the virus, the dramatic lockdown model travelled rapidly across the globe to more than

100 countries, which partially or fully initiated nation-wide lockdowns. This extraordinary crisis also created new conditions for the economically privileged who were able to stay at home, while others made 'sacrifices' and risked their lives as essential frontline workers, also sometimes referred to as the 'corona warriors'. In the midst of the COVID-19 crisis, governments assumed powers to 'make live and let die' in dramatic responses that claimed to defend the capacity of public health systems and secure the lives of the most vulnerable, feeble, and old. For a moment, COVID-19 sidelined all other global crises and centred all attention on the production of pandemic-related equipment, expertise, media rhetoric, visualisation, and narrativisation. Differently put, the lockdown staged the 'spectacular' deaths through COVID-19, while it obscured the 'slow deaths' in places like South Africa through, for example, TB, malaria, HIV/AIDS, homicide, traffic fatalities and injuries, malnutrition, gender-based violence, or cancer. In short, COVID-19 and its lockdown response produced a number of blind spots for other societal ailments and chronic health issues. In many parts of the world, pre-existing and ongoing crises have come to impede and complicate government responses to COVID-19, for instance in terms of emergency food distribution demands, and sanitation and social distancing requirements. The ongoing war in Ukraine is similarly producing its own 'crises within a crisis', along with the emergence of crisis convergences and blind spots in many parts of the world, including South Africa.

Many of the very same South Africans, who were and are facing the lethal threats of coronavirus exposure and lockdown consequences, continue to live through the everyday realities of racial inequalities that were historically produced by apartheid, an especially extreme form of racial capitalism that has its roots in the colonial era in South Africa (Robinson, 2005; Ralph & Singhal, 2019). Many of them will also have lived through one of the most devastating recent epidemics, HIV/AIDS. In 2018, UNAIDS produced the following AIDS statistics for South Africa: 7.7 million people were living with HIV; and there were 240,000 new HIV infections and 71,000 AIDS-related deaths (Avert, 2020). It is with these statistics in mind that the journalist Janet Giddy wrote that

> the South African government's overreaction, overinvolvement and overfunctioning with regard to COVID-19, relative to many other health, societal and economic issues (all of which are, arguably, equally or more important and urgent), has been striking. It is in stark contrast with past responses to TB and HIV.
>
> (Giddy, 2020)

When it comes to TB in South Africa, the situation is especially grim – in 2018 an estimated 301,000 South Africans became ill with TB and 63,000 people died from the disease (WHO, 2019). Even though TB deaths in 2017 were four times greater than the 21,022 murders between April 2018 and

March 2019, and South Africa has the fifth-highest burden of TB in the world, this disease has become normalised and is not seen as a national crisis (Tswanya, 2019). Sidelined during the lockdown, TB was also described by journalist Dennis Webster as 'South Africa's forgotten killer' (Webster, 2022). With the implementation of the first series of lockdowns, there was growing evidence that many citizens were not coming to clinics and hospitals for vaccinations or for TB and HIV treatment. Based on estimates from UNAIDS in August 2020, it was reported that about 80% of TB, HIV, and malaria programs worldwide experienced disruptions in services and that one in four people living with HIV had problems with gaining access to medications (Mandavilli, 2020; The Global Fund, 2020; Msomi et al., 2020). HIV testing also sharply decreased in the first month of lockdown in South Africa, especially in KwaZulu-Natal (Dorward et al., 2021).

So why are TB and HIV/AIDS not seen to be national crises and emergencies? Could this be attributed to the 'unspectacular', slow-moving nature of these diseases, or what Rob Nixon refers to as the 'slow dyings' of unspectacular and slow violence? As Nixon has observed, writers, journalists, and activists often face difficulties and dilemmas in drawing attention to crises that are not spectacular, but are instead about 'ordinary suffering' and structural violence that unfold slowly, and without much public and media attention and visibility (Nixon, 2011; Shepherd, 2019). Chloe Ahmann shows how activists in Baltimore in the United States go about 'working time' – speeding up or slowing down events – in ways that seek to optimise the obstacles *and* opportunities presented by the 'slow violence' of environmental pollution and ecological damage (Ahmann, 2018: 147). Examples of the latter include the long-term health consequences of human disasters such as the Chernobyl and Fukushima Daiichi nuclear meltdowns, the Bhopal gas explosion, HIV/AIDS, TB, climate change, and countless other forms of 'slow violence' that do not conform to the graphic imagery of instant media spectacles. While the spectacular explosions at Chernobyl, Fukushima and Bhopal initially drew international television crews, this media attention was short-lived as international journalists and NGOs were quickly redeployed to other crises elsewhere. Similarly, the 'slow dyings' from diseases such as HIV and TB do not draw the same kind of media and public attention as the dramatic imagery of trucks being used as temporary mortuaries during the COVID-19 crisis in New York City.

In the midst of the COVID-19 crisis, top South African scientists such as Professors Glenda Gray and Shabir Mahdi warned government that the lockdown measures were causing 'collateral damage' in relation to other serious health conditions (Schimke, 2020; Davis, 2020). Professor Gray caused a political storm when she claimed that malnutrition was becoming a problem in the country because of the hard lockdown and the exclusive focus on responding to the COVID-19 crisis. Regardless of whether Janet Giddy's wholesale indictment of the South African government's 'overreaction' to the new coronavirus is valid or not, what seems clear is that the COVID-19 crisis produced unprecedented public health responses all over the world. The most dramatic and draconian of these responses were the country-wide lockdowns that were introduced in so many parts of the world, including South Africa. It is perhaps not surprising that citizens and human rights activists became alarmed that the government of a vibrant constitutional democracy such as South Africa's was able to introduce draconian lockdown measures so seamlessly. This was done by declaring a national disaster in the name of fighting the pandemic.

'Crisis ordinary': The intensification of slow violence in South Africa

A crisis occurs when the ordinary, without one's influence and control, starts to overwhelm. A crisis amplifies and multiplies the predicaments, impasses, and hardships that were already there, just below the surface. In an interview about her article 'The Pandemic is a Portal', Arundhati Roy remarked that 'COVID-19 is like an X-Ray. It exposes the bare bones of existence. It amplifies the terrible things that are happening, the inequalities, and puts them on display' (Hasan & Roy, 2020). COVID-19 reveals the underlying crisis hot spots and blind spots – as mentioned earlier, these can include the lack of decent housing, services and infrastructure, security, financial stability, health care, and women's safety. The lockdowns also generally exacerbated South Africa's ongoing crisis of gender-based violence (Udo, 2020; Warah, 2021) and sidelined other health problems such as access to TB, cancer, and HIV treatment (Healy, 2021; Webster, 2022).

In the wake of declaration of South Africa's lockdown, which followed an early announcement by President Cyril Ramaphosa on 23 March 2020, three other spectacularly violent events were widely reported: the brutal murder of Collins Khosa, a 40-year-old black man from Alexandra, Johannesburg, on April 10; the femicide of 28-year-old and eight-months-pregnant Tshegofatso Pule in Johannesburg on June 8; and the eviction scandal of Bulelani Qolani on 1 July 2020, who was violently evicted by four law enforcement officers, while being naked and washing himself in his shack in Khayelitsha, a large settlement on the outskirts of Cape Town. All three spectacularly violent events, which all created a widely mediatised furore, not only happened in the context of the raging COVID-19 crisis in South Africa, but they were also directly related to South Africa's lockdown regulations. Collins Khosa, for example, was allegedly choked and slammed against a concrete wall inside his own house by soldiers from the South African National Defence Force (SANDF) (Brown, 2020). They were enforcing lockdown rules and had accused Khosa of buying and drinking alcohol in public – which was then considered a minor crime under the lockdown rules, which instituted a ban on the sale of alcohol (but allowed drinking at home) (Taylor, 2020). The alcohol ban had been introduced, and later re-introduced, with the aim of reducing the burden on hospitals and clinics of alcohol-related injuries (Wassermann & Moynihan, 2020). A few hours after his encounter with the soldiers, Khosa died from head injuries. He was also one of, at least, 12 other police or soldier killings during the lockdown, while some 230000 people had been charged or arrested for lockdown-related offences by late May 2020 (Businesstech, 2020). Khosa's murder sparked public debate about the slow, ongoing militarised policing crisis in South Africa, which dates back to the most violent apartheid policing of the apartheid era. Much like George Floyd's murder, Khosa's death enabled a transient media visibility of ongoing, and often forgotten or disputed, security force brutality.

Tshegofatso Pule was found stabbed and hanging from a tree in a suburb of Johannesburg after she had gone missing on 4 June 2020. With one of the highest femicide rates in the world, and more than 20 other women murdered in the weeks of May and June, President Ramaphosa denounced gender-based violence as 'the second pandemic that we have to contend with' (Gerber, 2020). Lockdown conditions had created a more dangerous condition for women, and cases of domestic violence significantly increased following the introduction of lockdown in late March 2020 (Adebayo, 2020; BBC News, 2020). Described as a 'twin pandemic' to COVID-19, or as a 'shadow pandemic' or 'invisible pandemic', gender-based violence sharply increased with the national lockdown implementation, 'with 87,000 gender-based violence complaints in the first month' (Nduna & Tshona, 2021; Warah, 2021; Mlambo-Ngcuka, 2020). In the first three weeks of the lockdown alone, more than 120 000 women had also called the South African National helpline for GBV (Udo, 2020). Femicides, rapes, and domestic violence have in recent years reached extraordinarily high levels in South Africa, but the lockdown and the COVID-19 crisis also intensified these brutal crimes, especially against poor and working-class black women in the townships. When asked by a CNN reporter about whether the state was doing enough to address gender-based violence, long-time activist Ilitha Labantu replied: 'Not at all. I don't think they are serious about it. If they could deal with GBV – gender-based violence – exactly the way they are dealing with COVID-19, we would be far' (CNN, 2020).

Despite the lockdown, municipalities together with law enforcement officials and private security companies, such as the notorious Red Ants in Johannesburg, also continued to demolish homes and evict people (Neille, 2020). In early April 2020, for instance, a group of urban dwellers had built shacks on an unoccupied site in Empolweni, a settlement in Khayelitsha, Cape Town. Many of these occupiers had recently lost their jobs as taxi drivers and food sellers in the informal economy and had been evicted by landlords from their backyard dwellings because they could not afford their rents anymore, all as a result of the lockdown (Eviction Lawyers South Africa, 2020). 'They say it's lockdown, and we must stay inside our homes, but then they take our homes', reads the statement of one Empolweni evictee in a news reportage (Christianson, 2020). A High Court order issued on 17 April 2020 considered the evictions by the City of Cape Town as unlawful (Ayanda, 2020), and 49 households were allowed to remain on the site and confiscated building materials were returned so that the housing structures could be rebuilt (Christianson, 2020). A nation-wide moratorium on evictions had already been declared to halt all evictions and home demolitions during the national disaster. On 1 July 2020, however, a widely shared video emerged from the same community that showed Bulelani Qolani being dragged naked from his shack by the City of Cape Town law enforcement officers, who prevented him from getting back inside to put on clothing while they demolished his structure (Kassen & Fisher, 2020). 'What distinguished this moment of evictions', writes journalist William Shoki on the platform *Africa Is a Country*, 'from all the rest that South Africans are used to is that Qolani was naked – and what are usually unnoticed acts of ordinary cruelty became a recorded episode of spectacular dehumanization' (Shoki, 2020). In July 2022, the Western Cape High Court ruled the eviction of Qolani as unlawful and unconstitutional.

Gender-based violence, security force brutality, and continuous evictions are merely some features of the 'slow dyings' and steady violence, or what Lauren Berlant has termed 'the crisis ordinary', which most impoverished black South Africans experience throughout their lives; this was merely amplified by the COVID-19 lockdowns. According to Lauren Berlant, the 'crisis ordinary' is an everyday condition which involves living 'in extended crisis, with one happening piling on another' (Berlant, 2011: 7). Berlant goes on to write in her book *Cruel Optimism* that 'the genre of crisis is itself a heightening interpretive genre, rhetorically turning an ongoing condition into an intensified situation in which extensive threats to survival are said to dominate the reproduction of life' (Berlant, 2011: 7). In similar ways, the spectacularised media coverage around COVID-19 threats and deaths, as well as the reportage of Khosa's and Pule's murders and Qolani's eviction, also rhetorically turn an ongoing condition of slow violence into an intensified and amplified situation – into an instant media spectacle. As a genre of crisis, these 'cruel stories' and spectacularly violent events are not singularities but momentary portals that elicit debates and actions about enduring hardships and violence. For millions of South Africans in the townships, however, the 'crisis ordinary', following Berlant, means that they must constantly find new tactics, resources, and skills 'for adjusting to newly proliferating pressures to scramble for modes of living on' (Berlant, 2011: 8). Lockdowns made this new scramble particularly tough and troublesome. So, while the South African government was seen to act decisively by introducing a hard lockdown in the early phase of the pandemic, these actions both obscured and intensified the ongoing slow violence and 'crisis ordinary' experienced by millions of South Africans.

Susan Levine and Lenore Manderson (2021) have discussed how South Africa's harsh lockdown measures, and with it the constraints on mobility enforced by a state military apparatus, recall a particular system of institutionalised racism that echoes the controls enforced under apartheid. What the authors term as 'a spatial economy of proxemics' is marked by social distancing, curfews, constraints on movement, and social engagement. Described as 'a shift from an ethics of intimacy to an ethics of proximity', the new COVID-19 government response or ethics of proximity merely 'reinforces inequality already mapped by the epidemics of HIV, tuberculosis, cardio-metabolic disease, and gender-based violence, and serves as an ugly reminder of the role of segregation in … the racist ideas of pollution under apartheid' (Levine & Manderson, 2021: 395). In other words, the continuous crisis conditions of security force brutality, gender-based violence, movement constraints, and displacement, as they were intensified and triggered by South Africa's national lockdown measures, bear testimony to unique, and also uncanny, historical resemblances in South Africa.

July unrests, Basic Income Grants, and the COVID-19 crisis

In July 2021, following the imprisonment of former President Jacob Zuma, KwaZulu-Natal and Gauteng witnessed the dramatic eruption of 'riots' that caused R50 billion of estimated losses due to damage caused by the looting, damage to and destruction of shopping malls and dozens of business premises. The spectacular violence of July 2021, for a while, displaced concerns with COVID-19. It was only when the dust had settled a couple of weeks later that COVID-19 once again began to re-emerge in media and public visibility. In an opinion piece in the *Daily Maverick*, the political scientist Prof. Susan Booysen wrote that by making R38-billion available for social relief, the government had 'fused COVID-19 recovery and compensation action for the R50-billion of estimated losses due to damage and destruction' (Booysen, 2021). In other words, the government's response targeted the damage to business, livelihoods, and jobs, caused by both COVID-19 and the July unrests:

> There was safety in the fusion with COVID-relief. The temporary reintroduction of the Social Relief of Distress Grant was announced. The Unemployment Insurance Fund (UIF)'s COVID-19 temporary relief was extended with a fund of R5.3-billion. The Department of Employment and Labour is drafting a directive to assist the 75 000 workers who lost their jobs due to the riots but who do not qualify for UIF temporary employer/employee relief scheme. The SOE South African Special Risks Insurance Association (SASRIA) will assist insured businesses to recover (through a R4-billion capital injection). There will be additional funds to help the uninsured, especially small businesses.

This 'fusion' of the multiple crises of COVID-19, staggering levels of structural unemployment, long-term economic stagnation and the massive damage caused by the unrests, suggested that government was ready to collapse these crises together rather than responding to them as singular events and separate problems. Moreover, some analysts and activists, who responded to what they labelled as 'food riots', demanded the introduction of a BIG, a variation of proposals that had been put forward since the late 1990s. These converging crises of July 2021 provided BIG advocates and activists with an opportunity to once again mobilise around this welfare intervention at a time when government seemed to be signalling that it was now ready to take these proposals seriously (Majavu, 2021b; New Frame, 2021).

During the continuous lockdowns and waves of infection, millions of impoverished South Africans were, in part, able to sustain themselves through the meagre COVID-19 social relief of distress grant of R350 per month (Majavu, 2021b). But this was insufficient in a context when the country's unemployment rate, including staggering youth unemployment, was at a historical high of around 42%. The fact that the relief grant was first terminated on 30 April 2021 was identified by journalists, political analysts, and activists as one of the triggers for the food riots (Majavu, 2021b). In other words, chronic poverty and massive unemployment revealed themselves to be another major 'crisis within a crisis'. It was only with the spectacular spectre of violent revolution in the streets that government appeared to apply its mind to the long-standing BIG idea, a proposal that seeks to recognise the reality of structural unemployment, chronic poverty, and hunger that is unlikely to go away any time soon. BIG was suggested to be paid to all South Africans irrespective of age or income. As early discussions have demonstrated, it is still unclear whether BIG is part of the repertoire of social democratic, Keynesian, and labor-rights movement arguments, or rather an expression of a more elaborate neoliberal agenda that equally appears to be pro-poor and pro-welfare (Ferguson, 2015). Although some critics still viewed BIG as a mere band-aid, it was clear that the overlapping 'slow crises' that culminated in the July 2021 unrests convinced some within the South African government to take seriously social relief measures that had previously been off the table. As the *Daily Maverick* journalist Anna Majavu noted a couple of months before the 'riots', families would not survive without the special COVID-19 grant of R350 per month, which was about to come to an end. As the title of Majavu's op ed put it: 'No COVID-19 grant, no food on the table' (Majavu, 2021a). Two months later, following the explosion of the 'food riots', the Minister of Social Development and other senior state officials, including President Ramaphosa, were signalling that the introduction of some form of BIG was being seriously considered by government. The multiple and overlapping 'slow crises', underpinned by massive structural unemployment and chronic poverty, had come home to roost; government seemed to be left with little option but to act decisively, as it had at the onset of COVID-19.

Conclusion: 'The Omicron crisis' in the context of global vaccination inequality

In this chapter, we did not seek to provide definitive answers as to why this most recent global crisis of COVID-19 became the target of such intensive, draconian, and wide-ranging governmental responses in South Africa, and elsewhere in the world. We could perhaps speculate that it had something to do with the spectacular global media coverage of the COVID-19 deaths and overwhelmed ICU wards throughout the world, including the advanced industrial countries of the Global North (Perrino, 2020). It could also be seen to be an outcome of the devastating speed with which the virus spread to so many parts of the world following its initial outbreak in China. But rather than entering into such speculative terrain, the chapter has limited itself to highlighting the contingent and conjunctural relationship between slow, enduring structural crises, and the spectacular, episodic and seemingly singular eruptions of 'crisis', along with their 'blind spots' and tendencies towards restoring social and political stasis.

We suggest, following Julie Livingston (2019) and Nancy Fraser (2021), and of course Karl Marx before them, that capitalism generates its own conditions of perpetual crises through its self-devouring and cannibalistic logics, which ultimately corrode its own conditions of possibility, and stability. As Fraser notes,

> Capitalist society, conceived expansively to include all the necessary background conditions for a capitalist economy – nonhuman nature and public power, expropriable populations and social reproduction – all non-accidently subject to cannibalization by capital, [are] all now under the wrecking ball and reeling from it.
>
> (Fraser, 2021: 126)

Amitav Ghosh (2021) goes even further by arguing that not only capitalism but the wider geopolitical struggles over dominance lie at the heart of a planetary crisis which disproportionally affects countries in the global South. He writes:

> In this sense, climate change, mass dislocations, pollution, environmental degradation, political breakdown, and the COVID-19 pandemic are all cognate effects of the ever-increasing acceleration of the last three decades. Not only are these crises interlinked – they are all deeply rooted in history, and they are all ultimately driven by the dynamics of global power.
>
> (Ghosh, 2021: 158)

In the context of South Africa, it would seem that the underlying system of racial capitalism and political power could well be seen as a centuries-old 'crisis machine' that continues to generate both ongoing, chronic 'slow crises', and singular episodes of spectacular crisis. As we have shown in this chapter, COVID-19 served to both surface *and* submerge the multiple, and nested, crises of this self-devouring system.

How intricately multiple epidemics or health crises are interwoven with the persistence and proliferation of the COVID-19 virus, was highlighted in late 2021 once again, when a potentially new crisis surfaced with the discovery of the Omicron variant. Various South African scientists suspected that the new mutation originated among a number of unvaccinated and immunocompromised persons with untreated HIV (Aizenman, 2021; Healy, 2021). It was surmised that the coronavirus could linger and undergo multiple genetic changes in HIV patients' bodies over a series of months, without their impaired immune systems being able to overcome the virus. Infectious disease specialist Prof. Jonathan Li, who was also one of the first to detect coronavirus mutations among HIV-immunocompromised patients, spoke of a dangerous 'syndemic' – that is 'the confluence of two epidemics with the potential to worsen outcomes for both' (Healy, 2021). South Africa's patients with untreated HIV could, according to Bioinformatics researcher Professor Tulio de Oliveira at Stellenbosch University, 'become a factory of variants for the whole world' (Healy, 2021). For some observers and commentators, a variety of countries worldwide reacted to the detection of the new variant with a travel ban for Southern Africa only seemed to reaffirm the 'age-old' fear and stigmatisation of Africa as a place of pathology and disease.

Some of the responses to the travel ban from a number of South African scientists, activists, and politicians, including the President of South Africa, indicted Western countries for creating the conditions for this crisis by hoarding vaccines and failing to support African countries in tackling the pandemic. They also claimed that as long as a stark global vaccination inequality persisted, and as long as African countries remained stigmatised as places of multiple crises, or 'crisis within crisis', – marked by poverty and malnutrition, unreliable healthcare, failed states, and weak state programs – it would also remain a potentially dangerous place for the continuous proliferation of new variants among immunocompromised populations.

In other words, these responses to the travel ban attributed the Omicron crisis to the unjust machinations of 'vaccine apartheid' as well as a long history of unequal relations between Europe and Africa. As Matthew Gandy (2021) discussed in his article entitled 'Zoonotic City', the likely scenario is that COVID-19 becomes 'an endemic disease of poorer communities, of the immuno-compromised and of older demographics'. According to Gandy, this is due to the 'lack of international cooperation' in tandem with 'manifestations of "vaccine nationalism"' that prevent countries in the global South from accessing adequate and sufficient medicines (Gandy, 2021: 11). Harsha Walia (2021) puts it even more succinctly, and provocatively, by saying that 'flattening the curve' would require 'flattening all inequality'. In terms of the political rhetoric of President Ramaphosa, travel ban responses to the Omicron variant in Europe and North America conjured up the spectre of histories of colonial paternalism on the African continent. For ordinary working-class and poor people living in townships and informal settlements, however, this new variant was simply another aspect of their everyday experiences of multiple, slow crises.

By early 2022, while countries in Europe, North America, and many other parts of the world were deeply concerned that the transmissibility of the new Omicron variant could overwhelm their health systems, some South African scientists and government health officials were also hinting that the new variant, with its relatively mild symptoms and low hospitalisation and death rates, could signal the shift of COVID-19 from a 'pandemic' to an 'endemic' (Madhi, Abdullah & Myers, 2022). The government's response to the discovery of the Omicron variant in South Africa in November 2021 did not result in an immediate change in the country's Adjusted Alert Level 1, which had been in place since 1 October 2021. Meanwhile, the country's media responded to this development by shifting its focus to other national stories and crises that surfaced in early January 2022 – the burning down of key buildings in the parliamentary precinct on 2 January, the release of the Zondo Commission Report on State Capture two days later, the ongoing factional battles within the ruling ANC, and numerous other 'crises within crisis'. It remains to be seen what governmental responses will emerge in South Africa, and the rest of the world, in the face of relentless waves of slow and spectacular crises and in a world still reeling from COVID-19.

Acknowledgements

We are grateful for the insightful comments and suggestions on earlier drafts of this chapter from Peter Redfield, Cymene Howe, Kamala Visweswaran, Rebecca Henderson, and Thomas Koelble. We are also grateful for the helpful comments from the editors and reviewers of this chapter.

Notes

1 Masco had argued that the nuclear crisis is fast, short, and immediate, whereas the climate crisis unfolds slowly and unpredictably but with 'accumulative and accelerating effects'. Joseph Masco, 'The Six Extinctions: Visualizing Planetary Ecological Crisis Today'. See https://www.youtube.com/watch?v=hgGRHY7kbgw.
2 It is questionable, however, whether the characterisation of the social and economic consequences of lockdowns as 'side effects' has not been devastating in itself. Writing about contaminated waterways through pharmaceutical waste, Joseph Masco explores the meaning of side effects, and concludes that

> the alchemy of the "side effect" concept splits effects of a molecule into a desired (treatment) and undesired (side effect). Thus, the language of the side effect installs a value system as well as a hierarchy within a molecule's range of biological consequences.

Joseph Masco, 'Side Effect' (December 3, 2013), *Somatosphere*, See http://somatosphere.net/2013/side-effect.html/.

References

(2020). HIV and AIDS in South Africa. *Avert*. Retrieved from https://www.avert.org/professionals/hiv-around-world/sub-saharan-africa/south-africa.

(2020). South African president: We're battling two pandemics. *CNN*. Retrieved from https://edition.cnn.com/videos/world/2020/07/13/south-africa-ramaphosa-gender-based-violence-coronavirus-mckenzie-pkg-intl-ldn-vpx.cnn.

(2020, 12 September). Long read: SA lockdown failed on multiple fronts. *New Frame*. Retrieved from https://www.newframe.com/long-read-sa-lockdown-failed-on-multiple-fronts/.

(2020, 17 June). Global fund survey: Majority of HIV, TB and malaria programs face disruptions as a result of COVID-19. *The Global Fund*. Retrieved from https://www.theglobalfund.org/en/covid-19/news/2020-06-17-global-fund-survey-majority-of-hiv-tb-and-malaria-programs-face-disruptions-as-a-result-of-covid-19/.

(2020, 17 June). Tshegofatso Pule killing: South African man on murder charge. *BBC News*. Retrieved from https://www.bbc.com/news/world-africa-53076289.

(2020, 22 May). 230,000 cases opened against people for breaking South Africa's lockdown rules. *Businesstech*. Retrieved from https://businesstech.co.za/news/lifestyle/400831/230000-cases-opened-against-people-for-breaking-south-africas-lockdown-rules/.

(2021, 30 July). The politics of a basic income. *New Frame*. Retrieved from: https://www.newframe.com/the-politics-of-a-basic-income/.

Adebayo, B. (2020, 19 June). South Africa has the continent's highest Covid-19 cases. Now it has another pandemic on its hands. *CNN*. Retrieved from https://www.cnn.com/2020/06/19/africa/south-africa-gender-violence-pandemic-intl/index.html.

Ahmann, C. (2018). 'It's exhausting to create an event out of nothing:' Slow violence and the manipulation of time. *Cultural Anthropology*, 33(1), 147.

Aizenman, N. (2021, 1 December). The mystery of where omicron came from – and why it matters. *NPR*. Retrieved from https://www.npr.org/sections/goatsandsoda/2021/12/01/1055803031/the-mystery-of-where-omicron-came-from-and-why-it-matters?

Anderson, W. (2021). The model crisis, or how to have critical promiscuity in the time of Covid-19. *Social Studies of Science*, 51(2), 167–188.

Beaubien, J. (2020, 9 June). Modelers suggest pandemic lockdowns saved millions from dying of COVID-19. *NPR News*, Retrieved from https://www.npr.org/sections/goatsandsoda/2020/06/09/872441984/modelers-suggest-pandemic-lockdowns-saved-millions-from-dying-of-covid-19.

Berlant, L. (2011). *Cruel Optimism*. Durham, NC: Duke University Press.

Bhan, G., Caldeira, T., Gillespie, K., & Simone, A. (2020, 3 August). The pandemic, southern urbanisms and collective life. *Society & Space*. Retrieved from https://www.societyandspace.org/articles/the-pandemic-southern-urbanisms-and-collective-life.

Booysen, S. (2021, 30 July). South Africa's July riots and the long shadow of Jacob Zuma fall over party and state. *Daily Maverick*. Retrieved from https://www.dailymaverick.co.za/opinionista/2021-07-30-south-africas-july-riots-and-the-long-shadow-of-jacob-zuma-fall-over-party-and-state/.

Brown, R. L. (2020, 8 June). An ocean apart, similar stories: US protests hit home in South Africa. Retrieved from https://www.csmonitor.com/World/Africa/2020/0608/An-ocean-apart-similar-stories-US-protests-hit-home-in-South-Africa.

Caduff, C., & Bonilla, Y. (2020, 2 July). Covid, Twitter, and critique: An interview with Carlo Caduff. *American Anthropologist*. Retrieved from http://www.american-anthropologist.org/2020/07/02/covid-twitter-and-critique-an-interview-with-carlo-caduff/.

Caduff, C. (2020). What went wrong: Corona and the world after the full stop. Retrieved fromhttps://www.academia.edu/42829792/What_Went_Wrong_Corona_and_the_World_after_the_Full_Stop [Accessed July 2020].

Caduff, C. (2014). Pandemic prophecy, or how to have faith in reason. *Current Anthropology*, 55(3), 296–315.

Christianson, B. (2020, 23 April). Lockdown means 'eviction' for many back-yard dwellers. *New Frame*. Retrieved from https://www.newframe.com/lockdown-means-eviction-for-many-backyard-dwellers/.

Collier, S. J., & Lakoff, A. (2015). Vital systems security: Reflexive biopolitics and the government of emergency. *Theory, Culture & Society*, 32(2), 19–51.

Davis, R. (2020, 15 June). Social Solidarity may be the only way through for SA in times of Covid-19. Retrieved from https://www.dailymaverick.co.za/article/2020-06-15-social-solidarity-may-be-the-only-way-through-for-sa-in-covid-19-times/.

Dorward, J. et al. (2021, 14 February). The impact of the COVID-19 lockdown on HIV care in 65 South African primary care clinics: An interrupted time series analysis. *The Lancet*, 8(3), E158–E165, Retrieved from https://www.thelancet.com/journals/lanhiv/article/PIIS2352-3018(20)30359-3/fulltext.

Erikson, S. (2019). Global health futures? Reckoning with a pandemic bond. *Medicine Anthropology Theory, An Open-Access Journal in the Anthropology of Health, Illness, and Medicine*, 6(3), 77–108.

Eviction Lawyers South Africa (2020, 14 April). Khayelitsha residents 'evicted twice' during lockdown. Retrieved fromhttps://evictionlawyerssouthafrica.co.za/uncategorized/khayelitsha-residents-evicted-twice-during-lockdown/.

Ferguson, J. (2015). *Give a Man a Fish*. Reflections on the New Politics of Distribution. Duke University Press.

Ferguson, J. (2009). The uses of neoliberalism. *Antipode*, 41(S1), 175 ff.

Fraser, N. (2021). Climates of capital: For a trans-environmental eco-socialism. *New Left Review*, 127, (January).

Gandy, M. (2021). The zoonotic city: Urban political ecology and the pandemic imaginary. *International Journal of Urban and Regional Research*. 10.1111/1468–2427.13080.

Gerber, J. (2020, 24 July). New GBV bill proposes obtaining protection orders online. *News24*. Retrieved from https://www.news24.com/news24/SouthAfrica/News/new-gbv-bill-proposes-obtaining-protection-orders-online-20200724.

Ghosh, A. (2021). *Nutmeg's Curse. Parables For a Planet in Crisis*. Chicago, IL: The University of Chicago Press.

Giddy, J. (2020, 9 June). Talking about pandemics – what is 'unprecedented'? *Daily Maverick*. Retrieved from https://www.dailymaverick.co.za/article/2020-06-09-talking-about-pandemics-what-is-unprecedented/.

Haffajee, F. (2020, 15 July). The day the bottom fell out of South Africa – a triple pandemic has hit us. *Daily Maverick*. Retrieved from https://www.dailymaverick.co.za/article/2020-07-15-the-day-the-bottom-fell-out-of-south-africa-a-triple-pandemic-has-hit-us/#gsc.tab=0.

Hasan, M. & Roy, A. (2020, 21 April). Mehdi Hasan and Arundhati Roy on India, Narendra Modi, and the Coronavirus. *The Intercept*. Retrieved from https://www.youtube.com/watch?v=xBOg7AlrY4U.

Healy, M. (2021, 3 June). As COVID-19 collides with HIV/AIDS, the pandemic may be taking an ominous turn. Retrieved from https://www.latimes.com/science/

story/2021-06-03/why-reaching-herd-immunity-in-the-u-s-wont-be-enough-to-protect-us-from-covid-19.

Kassen, J. & Fisher, S. (2020, 2 July). Bulelani Qholani wants dignity back after being dragged naked from home. Retrieved from https://ewn.co.za/2020/07/02/bulelani-qholani-wants-dignity-back-after-being-dragged-naked-from-home.

Lakoff, A. (2010). Two regimes of global health. *Humanity: An International Journal of Human Rights, Humanitarianism, and Development*, 1(1), 59–79.

Lakoff, A. (2008). The generic biothreat, or, how we became unprepared. *Cultural Anthropology*, 23(3), 399–428.

Levine, S. & Manderson, L. (2021). Proxemics, COVID-19, and the ethics of Care in South Africa. *Cultural Anthropology*, 36(3), 391–399. https://doi.org/10.14506/ca36.3.06.

Livingston, J. (2019). *Self-devouring Growth: A Planetary Parable as Told from Southern Africa*. Durham, NC: Duke University Press.

Madhi, S.A., Abdullah F., & Myers, J. (2022, 7 January). South Africa has changed tack on tackling COVID: Why it makes sense. *Daily Maverick*. Retrieved from https://www.dailymaverick.co.za/article/2022-01-07-south-africa-has-changed-tack-on-tackling-covid-why-it-makes-sense/.

Majavu, A. (2021a, 13 July). Food riots show the need for a basic income. *New Frame*. Retrieved from https://www.newframe.com/food-riots-show-the-need-for-a-basic-income-grant/.

Majavu, A. (2021b, 3 May). No Covid-19 grant, no food on the table. *New Frame*. Retrieved from https://www.newframe.com/no-covid-19-grant-no-food-on-the-table/.

Mandavilli, A. (2020, 3 August). 'The Biggest Monster' Is Spreading. And It's Not the Coronavirus. *New York Times*. Retrieved from https://www.nytimes.com/2020/08/03/health/coronavirus-tuberculosis-aids-malaria.html.

Masco, J. (2019). Crisis in Crisis. In: Hetherington, K. (Eds.). *Infrastructure, Environment, and Life in the Anthropocene*. Durham, NC: Duke University Press.

Masco, J. (2016), The Crisis in Crisis. *Current Anthropology*, 58 (S15), S65–S76.

Mlambo-Ngcuka, P. (2020, 6 April). Violence against women and girls: The shadow pandemic. Retrieved from https://www.unwomen.org/en/news/stories/2020/4/statement-ed-phumzile-violence-against-women-during-pandemic.

Mostowlansky, T., & Caduff, C. (2020, May). On Pandemic Prophecy, Unsustainable Lockdowns and the Magic of Numbers: A Conversation with Carlo Caduff. *Allegra Lab*. Retrieved from https://allegralaboratory.net/on-pandemic-prophecy-unsustainable-lockdowns-and-the-magic-of-numbers-a-conversation-with-carlo-caduff/.

Msomi, N. et al. (2020, 1 December). Africa: Tackle HIV and COVID-19 together. Retrieved from https://www.nature.com/articles/d41586-021-03546-8.

Ndamane, A. (2020, 18 April). Evicted Empolweni residents set to rebuild after high court victory. Retrieved from https://www.iol.co.za/news/south-africa/western-cape/evicted-empolweni-residents-set-to-rebuild-after-high-court-victory-46868520.

Nduna, M. & Tshona, S.O. (2021). Domesticated poly-violence against women during the 2020 Covid-19 lockdown in South Africa. *Psychology Studies*, 66, 347–353. https://link.springer.com/article/10.1007/s12646-021-00616-9.

Neille, D. (2020, 22 April). Gauteng demolitions: Red Ants in all-out war on the poor. *Daily Maverick*. Retrieved from https://www.dailymaverick.co.za/article/2020-04-22-gauteng-demolitions-red-ants-in-all-out-war-on-the-poor/.

Neville, K. J., & Martin, S. J. (2022). Slow justice: A framework for tracing diffusion and legacies of resistance. *Social Movement Studies*, DOI: 10.1080/14742837.2022. 2031955.

Nixon, R. (2011). *Slow Violence and the Environmentalism of the Poor.* Cambridge, MA: Harvard University Press.

Perrino, S. M. (2022). Narrating pandemics across time and space. *Anthropology and Humanism*, 0(0), Wiley Online Library. https://doi.org/10.1111/anhu.12377.

Ralph, M., & Singhal, M. (2019). Racial capitalism. *Theory Social*, 48, 851–881. https://doi.org/10.1007/s11186-019-09367-z.

Robins, S. (2014). Slow activism in fast times: Reflections on the mass media after apartheid. *Journal for Southern African Studies*, 40(1), 91–110.

Robinson, C. (2005). *Black Marxism: The Making of the Black Radical Tradition*. Chapel Hill: University of North Carolina Press.

Rogan, M., & Skinner, C. (2020, 15 July). The Covid-19 crisis and the South African informal economy 'Locked out' of livelihoods and employment. Retrieved https://cramsurvey.org/about/.

Roitman, R. (2013). *Anti-Crisis*. Durham, NC: Duke University Press.

Samimian-Darash, L. (2013). Governing Future Potential Biothreats: Toward an Anthropology of Uncertainty. *Current Anthropology*, 54(1), 1–22.

Schimke, K. (2020, 14 May). Glenda Gray: The woman heading up South Africa's sub-team of Covid-19 pandemic research advisors. *South African Medical Research Council (SAMRC)*. Retrieved from https://www.samrc.ac.za/news/glenda-gray-woman-heading-south-africa%E2%80%99s-sub-team-covid-19-pandemic-research-advisors.

Shepherd, N. (2019). Making sense of 'day zero': Slow catastrophes, anthropocene futures, and the story of cape town's water crisis. *Water*, 11(9), 1744; https://doi.org/10.3390/w11091744.

Shoki, W. (2020) The existing order of things. *Africa Is a Country*. Retrieved from https://africasacountry.com/2020/07/the-existing-order-of-things.

Taylor, D. (2020, 29 May). Report clearing soldiers in South African Man's death sparks anger. Retrieved from https://www.voanews.com/a/africa_report-clearing-soldiers-south-african-mans-death-sparks-anger/6190133.html.

Tswanya, Y. (2019). *African News Agency*. Retrieved from https://www.iol.co.za/capetimes/news/sa-has-fifth-highest-burden-of-tb-globally-20074421.

Udo, F. (2020). COVID-19 Lockdown: South Africa battles the deadly epidemic of gender-based violence. *Institute for African Women in Law*. Retrieved from https://www.africanwomeninlaw.com/post/covid-19-lockdown-south-africa-battles-the-deadly-epidemic-of-gender-based-violence.

Vigh, H. (2008). Crisis and chronicity: Anthropological perspectives on continuous conflict and decline. *Ethnos*, 73(1), 5–24. doi: 10.1080/00141840801 927509.

Walia, H. (2021). *Border and Rule. Global Migration, Capitalism, and the Rise of Racist Nationalism*. Halifax, NS: Fernwood Publishing.

Warah, R. (2021, 1 July). The invisible pandemic: COVID-19s toll on African women and girls. Retrieved from https://www.one.org/africa/blog/invisible-pandemic-gender-based-violence/.

Wassermann, H. & Moynihan, R. (2020, 22 July). South Africa's lockdown is so strict, alcohol and tobacco sales are banned and some are resorting to smoking tea. Retrieved from https://www.businessinsider.com/in-worlds-strictest-lockdown-south-africa-banned-alcohol-sales-again-2020-7.

Webster, D. (2022, 10 March). Tuberculosis: South Africa's forgotten killer. Retrieved from https://www.newframe.com/tuberculosis-south-africas-forgotten-killer/ [Accessed March 2022].

Wolf, M. (2012). Zoonoses: Towards an urban epidemiology. In: Matthew Gandy (Eds.), *Urban Constellations*. Berlin: Jovis.

World Health Organisation. (2019). Global tuberculosis control. Retrieved from www.who.int/tb/publications/global_report/en/.

6 Mobilising the public sector to combat COVID-19, and the pandemic's effect on public sector governance

Vinothan Naidoo

Introduction

COVID-19 swept through the world like a perfect storm in the early months of 2020. It generated unprecedented policy and administrative strain for countries like South Africa, which had to defend itself against a global public health crisis alongside an economic slump, a public finance crisis, and a society shouldering a high burden of communicable diseases. The coronavirus presented an extraordinary test for South Africa's government institutions to mount a coordinated response to avert the risk of precipitous deaths, accelerating economic decline, and significant disruption to public service delivery. It also threatened to scupper the ambitious plans of President Cyril Ramaphosa to rebuild the ethical integrity of South Africa's public sector, following a significant deterioration in governance quality under Jacob Zuma.

The most astonishing feature of COVID-19 was the dramatic way that it forced the hand of world leaders to 'lock-down' their societies. The global call to 'flatten the curve' became a universal rallying cry to prevent severe disruption to the provision of medical care and to avert the risk of public health facilities being overrun with emergency room admissions. South Africa instituted one of the most rapid and strict lockdowns in the world (Gustafsson, 2020). This was driven by the lethal combination of an under-resourced public health sector and the risk of severe illness faced by scores of South Africans with compromised immuno-health caused by the country's high prevalence of diseases such as tuberculosis and HIV/AIDS. Yet, lockdown also had to contend with the acute scarcity for millions of South Africans of the most basic social and economic amenities to mount an effective defence against the virus whilst confined to stay-at-home orders.[1]

Introducing a rapid country-wide lockdown of restrictions and prohibitions to mitigate the public health and non-health effects of the coronavirus reverberated across all government departments. It was the single biggest test for the public sector to internally coordinate its actions and break out of the silos for which it has long been criticised. COVID-19 forced public sector organisations to reckon with the narrow jurisdictional and operational routines through which they have historically operated and to act with agility

DOI: 10.4324/9781003294931-6

and pragmatism to marshal a collective response in a race to stem the spread of infection. Analysing how and why South Africa framed and executed its public sector response to COVID-19 matters, because it revealed how the choice of a centralised disaster-managed response, on the one hand, facilitated the need for speed and overcame the paucity of information. On the other hand, it also generated concerns about policy and institutional incoherence and overreach. In addition, the pandemic accentuated deficiencies that have long afflicted South Africa's public sector, namely capacity, ethical integrity, and financial sustainability, which is likely to hinder meaningful efforts in the short-term to shift the public sector towards increased use of technological platforms.

Activating South Africa's public-sector machinery to combat COVID-19: A centralised disaster-managed approach

COVID-19 provoked unprecedented governmental responses around the world. The use of 'lockdowns', 'shutdowns', 'stay-at-home orders', and an array of compulsory prohibitions on public and private activities were employed throughout the world, from high and middle-income countries to the least-developed countries. There was a visible degree of reactive policy mimicry in the use of lockdowns, compared to informed policy learning, as governments were under pressure to take urgent action with very little information at hand. Despite the widespread use of lockdowns, trying to mitigate their consequences revealed striking differences between lower and higher-income countries. The most obvious difference relates to comparative public health expenditure, which according to some accounts showed that low and middle-income countries were spending considerably less on public health as a percentage of GDP compared to their higher-income counterparts, pre-COVID (Voituriez and Chancel, 2021). This suggests that middle and lower-income countries had considerably more to lose without enforcing lockdowns, yet they were not necessarily going to benefit from these measures either by shoring up already weak public health systems. The best they could hope for was avoiding system collapse.

The turn to lockdowns also highlighted the prominence of centrally driven or 'centre of government' (CoG) arrangements to coordinate the government machinery to respond to a pandemic (Kunicova, 2020). The overarching lesson from how various countries employed CoG mechanisms to fight COVID-19 is that trans-national learning that feeds into 'good practice' is a necessary but insufficient marker of success – the structure and character of CoG mechanisms must also demonstrate 'good fit' with individual country contexts. Good practice features might include hands-on executive leadership, clearly defined roles, responsibilities, and interface between policy command and operational structures, as well as public awareness campaigns. Good fit factors would include the size and constitutional structure of a country, e.g., its multi-layered governance architecture, public sector capacity, inequality/levels of development, as well as public trust in government (Kunicova, 2020).

This chapter contends that South Africa's CoG approach struggled to marry good practice with domestic good fit considerations. On the one hand, hands-on executive leadership was clearly demonstrated by President Ramaphosa, cabinet ministers, and provincial premiers, resulting in highly visible and sustained level of public awareness. On the other hand, the choice to deploy a centralised disaster-managed approach to configure the institutional response to COVID-19 resurrected a historical tendency in South Africa to construct overly complex and hierarchical coordination arrangements to drive joined-up responses to major policy problems (Naidoo, 2013). Although this was enabled by the country's centralised inter-governmental architecture, which exhibits a high degree of functional overlap between national, provincial, and municipal governments, it also limited the flexibility and discretion for sub-national authorities to adapt their COVID-19 responses to changing local conditions (Rosenkranz et al., 2021).

The coronavirus crisis reached South Africa's shores in March 2020. It led to the rapid imposition of far-reaching measures beginning with a national disaster declaration and culminated in the start of a nationwide stay-at-home order, or 'lock-down'. The imposition of a lock-down was unprecedented in South Africa's democratic history and had immediate consequences for the country's public sector, ranging from the mobilisation of the police services and military to enforce lock-down measures, to the disruption of public service provision as a result of adjusted workplace and delivery arrangements for government services. In the latter case, the Department of Public Service and Administration (DPSA) issued a plethora of circulars, guidelines, and measures throughout 2020 to mitigate the impact of COVID-19 on public servants. This ranged from revised health and safety protocols in the workplace to provisions governing the shift to remote working and adjustments to other human resource practices.

President Cyril Ramaphosa's State of the Nation Address (The Presidency, 2020a) on 13 February 2020 reprised his administration's efforts to instil confidence in South Africa's public sector institutions, which had been wracked by corruption, financial mismanagement and 'state capture'. He also outlined an ambitious agenda for building a 'capable state'. This phrase had first been used in the National Development Plan (2012) to describe wide-ranging reforms to improve the professionalism, competency, and integrity of the public sector. President Ramaphosa highlighted specific interventions that had been introduced as part of the capable state agenda, notably the creation of new coordinating structures in the Presidency to expedite private investment and public sector delivery. He could not have foreseen how dramatically the Presidency would have to scramble to respond to a nationwide emergency that was only weeks away, drawing on structures that were not designed to lead a whole-of-government response to fight a rapidly spreading global health pandemic.

Centrally coordinating the public sector's COVID-19 response adopted a dual approach. In the first instance, it worked through existing cabinet and governmental coordinating structures which had long been in existence to facilitate inter-ministerial and inter-governmental coordination. This included cabinet 'clusters' or inter-ministerial committees[2] in shared sectors along with their administrative counterparts. These joined-up structures had been used to varying effects since the early 2000s to promote horizontal coordination amongst cabinet departments. It also relied on existing inter-governmental structures such as the President's Coordinating Council, which was used to facilitate vertical coordination between national, provincial, and local governments.

In the second instance, COVID-19 also saw the creation of new ad hoc structures to inform and convene a whole-of-government response to the particularities of the pandemic. Chief among these was the 'National Coronavirus Command Council' (NCCC), which acted as a kind of 'wartime' inner cabinet structure to enable virus-related matters to be discussed and recommendations sent to the full cabinet (Hunter, 2020). A Ministerial Advisory Committee on the coronavirus, falling under the purview of the Ministry of Health, was also established to supply the NCCC with technical advice from health experts. The blending of pre-existing and new ad hoc central coordinating bodies signalled the importance of a robust central government response to the crisis, yet it also resulted in unwieldy,[3] top-heavy and rigid coordination arrangements in which ad hoc structures were essentially grafted onto existing structures which cascaded out from the centre of government. This obscured the locus and lines of executive authority and transparency (Rosenkranz et al., 2021).

Chief among these criticisms were concerns about overly centralised decision-making and the legality of new coordinating structures, which appeared to hold considerable sway in determining how the government should respond, and what the public should accept. Questions were raised about the constitutionality of the NCCC and its relationship to cabinet, with the President admitting that the body was not established by any Act of Parliament but constituted a committee of cabinet (Ngalwana, 2020; Mkhwanazi, 2020; Rosenkranz et al., 2021). The constitutionality of the NCCC as well as aspects of the Disaster Management Act (2002) regulations – to be discussed later in this chapter - was also challenged in the courts.[4] Others noted that despite presidential replies to questions by members of parliament confirming that the NCCC was merely a committee of cabinet with no independent authoritative powers, public messaging sometimes implied otherwise. This 'blur[red] the lines of executive governance', and fuelled concerns about the pandemic being used to upend existing working arrangements in cabinet, curb deliberation, and frustrate transparency and parliamentary oversight (Merten, 2020). Moreover, the decision to eventually incorporate all cabinet departments into the NCCC in order to resolve confusion effectively rendered this ad hoc structure redundant.

Concerns about the government's centrally coordinated approach generated wider public criticism about a lack of public deliberation and engagement, and a strict control over information dissemination (Staunton, Swanepoel and Labuschaigne, 2020: 3, 10). Muller (2021) cast this in normative terms, observing that the haste with which the government implemented an aggressive lockdown strategy was continuously justified on 'scientific' grounds, or what he referred to as 'performative scientism'. Muller's appraisal of this strategy emphasised the confidence and moral rectitude of politicians in a strategy that appeared to mimic international trends. This was justified by the fear of a human catastrophe, which was sharply juxtaposed against the country's policy prevarication around HIV and AIDS over a decade earlier. Muller's critique focused on the damaging short and longer-term consequences of how 'performance scientism' can limit transparency and debate in high-level decision-making structures to sustain a preferred narrative and confine the space for wider policy deliberation on alternative, more balanced, and less drastic interventions.

Singh (2020: 441) drew similar conclusions about the cloistered and narrowed disciplinary composition of South Africa's Ministerial Advisory Committee on COVID-19. This risked not only eroding public trust, but also marked a sharp disjuncture between the societal-wide impact of its decisions, and the absence of a more diverse set of non-health sciences voices in its decision-making, potentially '...rob[bing] SA policymakers of valuable insights that could prove invaluable in the country's fight against the pandemic'. This sentiment was echoed in an editorial by Hofman and Madhi (2020: 698), drawing on a statement by the Academy of Science of South Africa's (ASSAf) standing committee on Health, who argued that 'experts' advising government on combating the pandemic 'should not be confined to clinicians and epidemiologists'.

The decision to employ the Disaster Management Act (DMA) (2002) as the legislative instrument through which to enforce the lockdown had major repercussions for the complexity of the government's coordinated response. When President Ramaphosa announced measures that the government would be taking in response to the first confirmed cases of coronavirus in South Africa, he prefaced his remarks by acknowledging what had already become a global health emergency. He invoked the DMA, which allows for the declaration of a national state of disaster (The Presidency, 2020b). The scale of the nationwide restrictions and prohibitions he would announce would certainly constitute a 'disaster' in any general sense of the term, but South Africa's disaster management legislation and the specialised network of structures it created across national, provincial, district and local government had never foreseen a killer infectious virus scenario of the scale and intensity of COVID-19. South Africa's disaster management legislation is overseen by the National Department of Cooperative Governance and Traditional Affairs

(CoGTA). Disaster Management is also a shared national and provincial legislative competency. The national department houses a National Disaster Management Centre, and there are disaster management offices at the provincial level, as well as in district and metropolitan municipalities.

Although the DMA provided the legal mechanism to institute severe restrictions and prohibitions that accompanied a lockdown, there were doubts about whether the Act's framing of a disaster allowed public sector organisations to respond appropriately. Padayachee et al. (2020: 16) stated that

> [t]here is a failure to consider a health pandemic as a national disaster in itself that can impact on all sectors and all aspects of life … the Act tends to focus on administrative structures and institutional arrangements and the 'what to do' with limited focus on how to implement….

This implied that the Act was at best a blunt instrument, a rough blueprint for the public sector to follow. Moreover, although the government's disaster management architecture clearly has a role to play in mitigating the effects of a health pandemic, and mirrored the role that civil protection agencies played in responding to COVID-19 in other countries (OECD, 2020a), this role should – in keeping with the thrust of the DMA – ideally be to support an epidemiologically-led (health) risk mitigation strategy by mobilising emergency response measures, rather than being used to pre-emptively impose restrictions on freedom of movement, trade, social and educational activities.

The sustainability of the DMA-led lockdown strategy was clearly sparking concerns amongst the public health fraternity. Madhi et al. (2020) argued that the effectiveness of an extended lockdown had limited effects on the transmission of the virus; in other words, it had a shelf-life, a point by which diminishing returns would begin to creep in and generate significant economic and other health care shocks. They advocated for a non-lockdown strategy consisting of more robust public health interventions to track/test, trace, and contain infection as well as protect those in the population at greatest risk of severe disease. A more aggressive public health strategy would then be used to inform what the authors described as a 'risk-based economic strategy'.

There were also wider constitutional concerns about using the DMA as a vehicle to combat COVID-19. This noted the exceedingly broad[5] regulatory powers granted to the Minister of CoGTA under the DMA, which – as highlighted by Ngalwana (2020), are starkly evident in S 27(2)(n) which empowers the minister to take 'steps that may be necessary to prevent an escalation of the disaster, or to alleviate, contain and minimise the effects of the disaster'. This should be juxtaposed against the narrower interpretation of a 'disaster' based on how the DMA has traditionally been used, and the decision not to use more sector-specific legislation such as the International Health Regulations Act (IHRA)[6] (1974). For Ngalwana, the constitutionality of South Africa's COVID-19 interventions comes down to a rationality test between the wide scope and magnitude of a DMA-framed intervention and the more targeted policy aim of flattening the infection curve.

The clarity and scope of CoGTA's role in mobilising the DMA to fight a pandemic were also questioned in relation to other cabinet and inter-governmental actors. In a briefing to Parliament, the Deputy Minister of CoGTA stressed that the department was empowered only to formally declare a state of disaster, mobilise its institutional resources to coordinate a government response to the disaster and issue directives within the ambit of its own jurisdictional area, e.g., inter-governmental and municipal planning, support, and traditional leadership. The department's disaster management powers did not explained the Deputy Minister, 'usurp' or supersede the powers of other cabinet departments to issue directives within the scope of their own jurisdictional areas (Parliamentary Monitoring Group, 2020a). This seems to have placed CoGTA in the invidious position of being the face and custodian of an unprecedented national disaster response, but without the legal right and sometimes informational knowledge to enforce or explain the length and breadth of measures taken by a host of other departments. This compares with a conventional[7] 'disaster' scenario which would typically be more localised and span fewer government institutions. One of the most unusual features of the public sector response to COVID-19 was how it elevated the national visibility of CoGTA, which is a department that usually operates behind the scenes in a supporting and facilitating role.

The ambiguity surrounding CoGTA's role was evident in the wording of the disaster declaration itself, which empowered the department to issue directives that 'augment[ed]' existing measures undertaken by other organs of state to assist and protect the public to mitigate the consequences of the disaster (DCGTA, 2020). This implied that the department was not empowered to directly coordinate the actions of other organs in the public sector, something which Van Niekerk (2014: 865) traced to the institutional placement of disaster management powers in a line department rather than at the political apex of government (i.e., office of the head of state/Presidency). This is something that he believed 'constrained' the implementation of disaster management actions.[8]

Conversely, the legal powers that the DMA conferred on CoGTA to institute regulations and directives to assist and protect the public and property could, in the context of a public health pandemic, evince broad interpretation and generate direct and far-reaching consequences for the actions of its departmental counterparts, rather than merely augmenting their efforts. This would ordinarily have been a difficult line for CoGTA to tread, yet the department was able to close ranks with its cabinet counterparts in contesting a lawsuit brought by private citizens which challenged disaster management regulations.[9]

Efforts to mark a clear separation between the role of CoGTA's network of constitutive disaster management structures and the role of the Presidency, cabinet, and the NCCC, did not appear to filter down to the sub-national level. In other words, the same degree of institutional separation was not evident in the overlapping roles between provincial and municipal disaster management structures and command councils convened by provincial and municipal executive authorities (Parliamentary Monitoring Group, 2020b). South Africa's hierarchical inter-governmental model allowed the national government to act swiftly to impose a tiered national lockdown system under a state of disaster, which empowered it to issue provincial-specific prohibitions facilitated by wide functional overlap between national, provincial, and local governments.

This did not stop provincial premiers from adopting a more public footing to defend their constituents and their provincial health infrastructure against the shifting effects of COVID-19.[10] However, this occasionally courted conflict with DMA regulations overseen by the national CoGTA. Examples include the Western Cape provincial government's opposition to a continued blanket ban on alcohol sales (Businesstech, 2020a), and the Western Cape's opposition to a ban on accessing beaches and other outdoor recreational areas (Dayimani, 2021). In the KwaZulu-Natal province, the Premier was described as engaging in rumours and speculation about a need to shift to a harder lockdown, with a spokesperson for CoGTA indicating that no such plans were in the works (Businesstech, 2020b). Such points of tension later escalated, with the Premier of the Western Cape arguing that it was time to end the national state of disaster and afford provinces the flexibility to manage COVID-19 in line with provincial-specific public health and economic conditions (Western Cape Office of the Premier, 2021).

The pandemic's effect on South Africa's public sector

The adoption of a centrally orchestrated disaster-managed response framed how the public sector responded to the pandemic. The net effect is that a more targeted public health-led infection control strategy to contain and mitigate the effects of the virus was substituted in the interest of speed, and in the context of informational scarcity, for a more top-heavy, whole-of-government response. The consequences of the centralised disaster-managed response also compromised the government's ability to project and maintain the policy and institutional coherence. The pandemic also heightened systemic challenges that South Africa's public sector has been struggling with for years, namely financial sustainability, its capacity to deliver, and its ethical integrity. Each of these issues will now be discussed in-turn.

The public sector's financial sustainability

COVID-19 came at a particularly inauspicious time for South Africa's public sector, which had already been subject to increased scrutiny by the Department of Finance over its escalating cost to the fiscus. The remuneration of public servants, or the 'wage bill', had reached unsustainable levels according to the state. By the time COVID-19 hit, a process had already begun to try to curb the public-sector wage bill, stemming from longstanding criticisms about wastage and inefficiency. This had put the state on a collision course with public sector unions with respect to wage negotiations. The additional fiscal demands, which the pandemic suddenly imposed, including the reallocation and appropriation of substantial emergency funding, upended the process of negotiating a more financially viable wage agreement with public servants. Instead, the government failed to implement the final year of a three-year wage agreement negotiated in 2018, citing affordability concerns, which ultimately triggered court action by public sector unions (Magubane, 2021).

The economic slowdown caused by the pandemic put the South African fiscus under severe strain in order to mitigate the effects on households by mobilising emergency expenditure programmes. South Africa's public finances were already under pressure from expenditure pressures driven by wages, State-owned Enterprise bailouts, and rising debt servicing costs (Bhorat et al., 2020: 19). This is also evident in the commentary which seemed to echo the proverbial chickens coming home to roost metaphor. De Villiers, Cerbone and Van Zijl (2020) praised the government for its quick and decisive action to lock down the country to stem the rapid spread of infection. However, they also acknowledged that years of ill-disciplined fiscal management, including State-owned Enterprise (SoE) bailouts, monies lost to corruption, and a runaway public-sector wage bill had effectively backed the government into a political corner. It was unable to manage the economic consequences of lockdown's widening gap between shrinking revenues and growing welfare payments, and unable to cost-cut itself out of the woods without a credible long-term economic recovery plan. In this sense, COVID-19 catapulted to the fore long-simmering concerns about public sector financial management.

The employment conditions of public servants can elicit polarising views in South Africa, where the public-sector wage bill often draws sharp rebukes from the public, who point to the disjuncture between the state's remuneration of public servants and the poor quality of public services they receive. This usually evokes an equally robust defence by public sector unions, which cite inordinate demands, insufficient resources to meet those demands, and political interference and graft, as adversely affecting the working conditions of public servants. In an opinion piece, Moffat (2021) argued that giving public servants an above-inflation increase was unsustainable and potentially immoral in the midst of a 'COVID-19 pandemic-induced economic crisis'. Citing the economic devastation that COVID-19 had inflicted on the jobs market, he added that public servants should 'be more grateful to still have their jobs'. Offering a wider and more comparative perspective, Hasnain (2020) argued that governments should be cautious about asking public servants to accept cuts in order to fund emergency COVID mitigation and relief efforts. This was partly due to the relative cushioning that public sector salaries provided for vulnerable groups such as women and lower-skilled workers, and because a large proportion of the public sector workforce carries out essential services (health, education, policing, welfare), which took on a heightened level of importance during the pandemic.

The coronavirus has had a disruptive and debilitating effect on South Africa's army of front-facing public sector workers, including public health practitioners, teachers, correctional service, and police officials. The heightened risk of exposure faced by these workers has strained working conditions which were already stretched by capacity shortages and unrelenting demands. It also drew a sharp contrast with their management-level counterparts who could more easily shift to alternative modes of working (i.e., remote working) in order to mitigate workplace risk (Kiewet, 2020a). The disproportionate impact of COVID-19 on South Africa's public sector workforce has also heightened concerns about the under-resourcing of front-line 'care-work', including community health workers, home-based care providers, and early childhood development practitioners, along with nurses and social workers. The Public Servants Association (PSA, 2020), which represents a large proportion of South Africa's public service workforce, acknowledged this as a lesson laid bare by the pandemic, especially a reluctance to formalise the many workers performing primary care jobs by absorbing them into full-time state employment. This is despite significant resources being allocated to the employment of home-based care and early childhood development workers as part of an Expanded Public Works Programme, since 2004.

Containing public sector wage increases in a context of stagnant growth in employee numbers, deepening debt, and non-commensurate productivity, reached critical levels under COVID-19 (OECD, 2020b; Intellidex, 2020). But efforts to reduce unsustainable compensation spending are bound to be unpopular with public sector unions, who represent the bulk of the very front-line workers that South Africans have relied on to keep the state functioning. This was also combined with the private sector-laced language of using COVID-19 to re-imagine how the public sector operates. Management consultants have leveraged the pandemic to advocate for major reforms in how the public sector operates. However, some of these ideas already enjoy wide purchase, despite achieving limited local traction, e.g., improving governance quality and pursuing greater operational efficiencies, relaxing regulatory obstacles in an increasingly tight fiscal environment, and fostering public trust (PWC, 2020; Accenture, 2020). This harkened back to the 'New Public Management (NPM)' doctrine of the 1980s and 1990s, except that it is stripped of NPM's innovative managerial techniques and focused squarely on cost containment and shedding unnecessary functions. South African policymakers did not fully embrace this market-based public sector paradigm in the mid-1990s, or at least did so quite cautiously (Cameron, 2009). Therefore, it is hard to see how even the impact of COVID-19 will change perceptions about minimising the role and scope of what the public sector should do when there seem to be competing agendas between the need for a fiscally restrained state and a more professional and capacitated state.

While these are not inherently binary positions, they were bound to diverge in the heightened politicised atmosphere of post–COVID-19 labour negotiations. This was evident in Finance Minister Tito Mboweni's 2021 Budget speech, which exhibited a difficult balancing act between fiscal restraint, which was clearly the dominant theme, and negotiating a 'fair' multi-year compensation agreement with public sector unions (Mboweni, 2021). The Public Servants Association (2021), which represents nearly a quarter of a million public sector workers, argued prior to the tabling of the budget that the primary challenge facing the public sector was enhancing the capacity – expressed in the parlance of 'professionalisation' – of front-line workers (e.g., health workers, educators, prison wardens, border management, etc.), and redressing the costs of financial mismanagement, and corruption on service delivery. The message from unions seemed clear: even after COVID-19, wage containment is neither a panacea for a sustainable public sector nor is it even desirable in the face of capacity deficits on the frontline, and the damage inflicted by financial mismanagement.

The public sector's capacity to deliver

The public sector's capacity to deliver has long been its Achilles heel, the weakest point in its institutional machinery. COVID-19 has exacerbated this weakness, notwithstanding calls for public servants to hasten the adoption of remote working and digital delivery platforms. This is partially due to the significant disparities in access to services in South Africa, which means that a large swathe of the population depends on direct interaction with public servants to obtain services. We know anecdotally that front-line service delivery was slowed considerably by limits on the number of people congregating in private and public facilities, which resulted in longer queues and processing times for services such as IDs, passports, vehicle licensing, social grants, etc. This also placed front-line public servants at greater risk of exposure to infection. It also amplified the disparity between the urban poor and higher-income groups, with the former experiencing greater difficulties complying with public health protocols such as social distancing and self-isolation, and hand hygiene, in the context of crowded and poorly resourced settlements whose inhabitants overwhelmingly rely on public transport (Staunton, Swanepoel, and Labuschaigne, 2020: 3). COVID-19 may have also exploited already low levels of public trust in government institutions, which frustrated the government's efforts to tackle the pandemic by limiting the extent and willingness of the public to comply with government directives (Devermont, Mukulu, 2020). A recognition of declining public trust in government may have also contributed partially to the adoption of a paternalistic and economically risky hard lockdown strategy, along with concerns about an under-capacitated public health system (Hirsch, 2020).

The pre-pandemic challenges faced by the public sector were heightened by the risks that public servants experienced on the COVID-19 frontline, and the political minefield of pandemic regulations that public institutions have had to negotiate to enforce compliance and render services. This was most acute in the public health sector, the leading edge of the government's response. Yet, despite staffing constraints in its workforce, South Africa had already tried to expand the reach of its public health machinery by mobilising an auxiliary army of semi-formal community health workers (CHW) in partnership with NGOs to combat the effects of HIV/AIDS (Schneider, Hlophe, and Van Rensburg, 2008). South Africa's history of epidemic management produced a cohort of community health workers who were instrumental in early-phase infection prevention and management through ground-level screening, testing, and treatment. This aided the state's efforts to communicate and conduct localised screening for COVID-19. The expansion of testing to map the scope of local transmission occurred in conjunction with community health workers being deployed for home visitations, resulting in an estimated 28,000 CHWs screening 900,000 people during April 2020 (Wadvalla, 2020; Bhorat et al., 2020: 3). The COVID-19 crisis also prompted innovative strategies to ensure that HIV positive patients continued to receive their ART medication, whilst minimising their risk of infection and placing an added burden on already stretched clinical services. This included extending the period of ART prescriptions, adjusting the supply chain of medication to enable the dispensing of medication over fewer patient visits, and home delivery of medication. (Uevrard, 2020; Davies, 2020).

Despite efforts by the public health sector to innovate and adapt its wider infection management services to mitigate the risks of COVID-19, Staunton, Swanepoel and Labuschaigne's (2020: 2) likening of South Africa's response to coronavirus as being between a proverbial rock and a hard place was an apt description of an acute dilemma facing the government: how to moderate the wave of sickness that was likely to be unleashed on an under-performing public health sector, without courting severe economic disruption. The demands on the country's public health sector did not give the government room to ameliorate this dilemma, with the authors noting that most of South Africa's population relies on an under-resourced and poorly administered public health sector. They cited a report by the Office of Health Standards Compliance (2018) that covered the 2016–2017 period, which showed that 62% of 851 public sector health establishments were not compliant with norms and standards for quality healthcare.

Apart from the public health sector, the effects of a prolonged – if risk-adjusted – strategy of stay-at-home orders were probably most acutely felt at the local/municipal level of government. It is here that COVID-19 seemed to worsen the strains of delivering public services across areas with significant inequalities and infrastructure backlogs, affecting everything from disruption and delays to planning, budgeting, public participation and basic service provision, as well as a reduction in revenue income (DPME, 2020b). According to a Department of Planning, Monitoring and Evaluation (DPME) (2020a: 27) survey which examined the effects of the coronavirus on South African municipalities, 78% of sampled municipalities said they were not well prepared to mitigate periods of reduced revenue, and nearly the same proportion indicated that having to redirect funds would have a moderate to high impact on service delivery. The DPME (2020a: 31) added that the pandemic has 'exposed many failures of municipalities in the provision of basic services to communities especially in informal settlements and rural areas'.

The Public Service Commission (2020) initiated a rapid survey in 2020 to investigate how COVID-19 was affecting the service delivery processes of a cross-section of government departments. This ranged from high-volume public-facing sectors such as health, education, home, and correctional affairs, to departments providing crucial social and economic support to members of the public and businesses. The constraints of deploying ICT technologies to circumvent physical interaction with the public were clearly evident in the experience of some departments, and, seemed to cut both ways: on the one hand, digital platforms and the credibility of the information contained therein did not always prove to be effective in verifying applicants' eligibility to access benefits or facilitate smooth interfacing between departments to meet extraordinary demands. On the other hand, there were also limits on the use and take-up of digital platforms by members of the public, and cases where technology could not overcome the challenge of extending services to far-flung areas.

The public sector's ethical integrity

The ethical integrity of South Africa's public sector has been battered by years of fraud, corruption, and conflicts of interest. Despite nascent efforts by President Cyril Ramaphosa to take a harder line on prosecuting government officials for engaging in corruption, the significant ramping up of state spending to combat the Coronavirus also fell prey to already weak internal controls in the public sector. There have been many instances of alleged interference or collusion by high-ranking government officials in the negotiation of pandemic spending contracts, including the procurement of materials such as personal protective equipment. The most high-profile of these involved the national Minister of Health, Dr Zweli Mkhize, who for many South Africans was the most visible face of the government's response to the pandemic through his regular appearances on television. Dr Mkhize resigned as Health Minister following allegations that he was involved in the awarding of a multi-million rand contract by the Department of Health to a private communications company staffed by former aides. Questions about the contract have not been limited to the minister's role, and have also encompassed the role that senior public servants in the department may have played in the irregular awarding of the contract (Kahn, 2021). The minister's alleged undue influence in pandemic spending was one of several high-profile cases of alleged corruption, which had earlier included President Ramaphosa's own spokesperson as well as the provincial health minister in Gauteng (Tandwa, 2020).

Reports of alleged corruption involving politicians are no longer breaking news in South Africa, where the public has become cynically accustomed to such revelations. The public sector's endemic problem of weak integrity controls and financial mismanagement in the procurement of goods and services was severely tested by COVID-19, with a report by the Auditor-General (AG) highlighting many instances of irregularities in the procurement of personal protective equipment (PPE). This resulted in the AG (2020: 11) 'recommend[ing] that these contracts be investigated, as such circumstances can be a red flag for fraud or abuse of the supply chain management process'. The urgency of pandemic relief spending also worsened existing bottlenecks in the public sector's administration of entitlement programmes, such as the incorrect disbursement of unemployment relief funds to larger numbers of people, and validation errors in the disbursement of social relief grants. In the former case, several senior officials in the Unemployment Insurance Fund were suspended pending a forensic investigation into the payment of COVID relief funds (eNCA, 2020). In the latter case, there were reportedly thousands of ineligible beneficiaries who received a special COVID social relief of distress grant, including persons employed in government or receiving income from other sources. This was attributed to poor data quality and a heightened risk of fraud and corruption (Public Service Commission 2020: 15, 24).

Conclusion

South Africa's centrally driven disaster-managed approach to the pandemic enabled the government to marshal its existing institutional machinery to swiftly and aggressively keep the transmission of the coronavirus in check. Hands-on executive leadership and regular briefings by the President and Cabinet were visible throughout the pandemic response, as well as at the provincial level. This approach enabled the government to buy time to allow the country's overstretched public health system to sustain the impact of a virus that threatened to wreak havoc amongst South Africa's immuno-compromised population. But this approach also came with a host of costs – confusing and cumbersome institutional arrangements for coordinating the response, which obscured the locus and lines of authority, impeded agile decision-making, and limited transparency. Compounding these factors were already low levels of public trust in the government sector, fuelled by persistent ethical breaches and financial mismanagement, and uneven public sector capacity leading to strained labour relations.

As the pandemic matured in South Africa, including a fourth wave of infections in December 2021, the country remained at the lowest risk-adjusted level amid increasing calls to end the national state of disaster. Clearly, COVID-19 management fatigue had set in along with a desire to resuscitate dampened economic activity. President Ramaphosa had already announced that the government had started a process of amending public health regulations to allow the country to lift the national state of disaster and shelve the DMA (The Presidency, 2021). On 5 April 2022, the president announced the termination of the national state of disaster and explained that the focus would shift to finalising new regulations to the National Health Act to manage COVID-19 going forward. Yet the shelving of the DMA and shifting pandemic planning to the DoH has elicited accusations that the new regulations are largely transferring broad restrictive measures introduced in the early days of the pandemic under the DMA, and contain unrealistic measures which fail to account for what has been learned to date about what worked, what did not, and at what cost (Mandelson et al., 2022).

In an address to the South African Association of Public Administration and Management, former Minister of the DPSA Geraldine Fraser-Moleketi (2020) opined that the public sector should not '…revert to "business as usual" after the [COVID] crisis', and that the public sector advocates ought to seize the opportunity to "reinvent" the public service. It would be trite to simply pass this off as a proverbial *never waste a crisis* comment because the unprecedented defensive strategies adopted by countries can be said to have forced every sector to re-visit their operating models. The ironic feature of the former minister's comment is that South Africa's public sector has for years struggled even to attain an acceptable level of business-as-usual in the eyes of its citizens. Therefore, it can be agreed that reverting to business-as-usual is simply not acceptable for the public sector, not because the COVID-19 crisis has created a catalyst for revolutionary change, but because of what the crisis has revealed about the failure of the public sector to adhere to traditional values. In this regard, Fraser-Moleketi's words should not be misinterpreted as reformist but rather as introspective. She speaks, in particular, about COVID-19 reinforcing a more activist role for the public sector, undergirded by the extraordinary efforts of front-line public servants. This ought to be the business-as-usual which has to date eluded many parts of South Africa's public sector.

COVID-19 significantly disrupted and stretched the day-to-day output and internal operations of public sectors across the globe. This was accentuated in South Africa, where pre-pandemic front-line public sector delivery had already been experiencing severe strain. COVID-19 produced something of a reckoning for global public sectors, and no less so for South Africa, thrusting into the spotlight a post-modern conception of managing public service delivery via digitised formats compared to more traditional bricks and mortar platforms. Yet the public-facing officials who have traditionally manned these offices, ironically given the new discourse, have not had the luxury or the protections afforded to their work-at-home counterparts in a pandemic scenario. And this has not been confined to just public health workers but includes a myriad of street-level officials ranging from immigration officers to sanitation workers, teachers to police, labour inspectors to social workers, and officials engaged in the delivery of entitlement programmes – even under staggered socially-distanced office conditions. Moreover, this is also the segment of South Africa's public sector workforce that will be hit hardest by a moratorium on agreed-to wage increases resulting from the pandemic's impact on government revenues. The net effect of COVID-19 is therefore likely to hinder any meaningful effort to re-cast South Africa's public sector in a post-modern mould of automation. Fixing the problems that have for years hampered the traditional delivery of front-line services and re-building trust with citizens must take precedence.

To this end, the release of a draft implementation framework for professionalising the public service in December 2020, may be instructive. The document addressed a set of longstanding issues aimed at improving the capacity, skills, and ethical integrity of South Africa's public sector through instituting reforms in recruitment, performance, and career management (NSG, 2020). What was striking about the timing of the document's release was how COVID-19-neutral it all appeared; that is to say, these issues remained 'issues' with or without the existence of a pandemic. While COVID-19 did not generate these problems, it clearly intensified the stresses and strains experienced by a public sector which is on a journey towards professionalisation. The pandemic has undoubtedly pushed some government departments to adopt 'business unusual' methods for rendering services, but it has more often than not highlighted the difficulties of breaching the digital divide to improve the pace and scale of service delivery because of the very constraints that the professionalisation document highlights.[11]

Notes

1 The absence of poor quality social and economic infrastructure and household assets for many South Africans is illustrated in the findings of an Afrobarometer survey (see Isbell, 2020).

2 Including the NATJOINTS and PROVJOINTs cluster of police, defence and state security agencies.

3 Rosenkranz et al. (2021: 69) similarly found that the institutional arrangements to manage COVID-19, amongst other things, produced a 'clutter of institutions with…fuzzy boundaries', and resulted in a duplication of reporting.

4 In *Esau and Others v Minister of Co-operative Governance and Traditional Affairs and others*, in the Western Cape High Court.

5 These powers were challenged in *Esau and Others v Minister of Co-operative Governance and Traditional Affairs and others*. The applicants argued that the Minister of CoGTA did not engage in an adequate public consultation/participation process to obtain inputs by affected persons and sectors whose activities and operations would be adversely affected by these regulations.

6 It is doubtful that the IHRA can be viewed as an alternative response framework compared to how the DMA was used to direct COVID-19 infection mitigation and suppression efforts. The former is largely limited to disease containment and mitigation at ports of entry, and the collection and sharing of epidemiological data with the WHO.

7 The unconventional nature of CoGTA's role was acknowledged by its Deputy Minister in a portfolio committee briefing: 'The Deputy Minister's sense was that the Ministry and Department were better prepared to deal with natural

disasters such as fires and droughts, but they did not have the same level of experience in epidemiological disasters and were having to learn very fast how to deal with the reality' (Parliamentary Monitoring Group, 2020a).

8 Rosenkranz et al. (2021: 63, 69) similarly argue that locating disaster management powers within CoGTA diluted its 'convening power', and suggested that the National Disaster Management Centre could be relocated to the office of the President.

9 *Esau and Others v Minister of Co-operative Governance and Traditional Affairs and others.*

10 See Kiewit, L. (2020b). Fighting COVID-19: The rise of the premiers.

11 In a blogpost, William Gumede (2020) argued that COVID-19 underscored the imperative of fixing the professionalisation and wider 'governance' deficiencies in a post-pandemic scenario, and that South Africa's ability to mitigate its damaging after-effects will be inextricably tied to this task.

References

(2020a, 11 August). New push to relax South Africa's alcohol ban at provincial level. *Businesstech.* Retrieved from https://businesstech.co.za/news/business/424208/new-push-to-relax-south-africas-alcohol-ban-at-provincial-level/ [Accessed 17 May, 2021].

(2020b, 27 October). Government dismisses talk of harder lockdown for South Africa. 27 October. *Businesstech.* Retrieved from https://businesstech.co.za/news/government/443952/government-dismisses-talk-of-harder-lockdown-for-south-africa/ [Accessed 17 May, 2021].

Accenture (2020). *Public Service for a new era: a practical action guide for outmaneuvering uncertainty.* Retrieved from https://www.accenture.com/_acnmedia/PDF-127/Accenture-Public-Service-New-Era.pdf [Accessed 3 February, 2021].

Auditor General (2020). *Auditor-general reports significant faults in procurement and contract management processes of COVID-19 relief package.* Media release, 9 December. Retrieved from https://www.agsa.co.za/Portals/0/Reports/Special%20Reports/COVID-19%20Special%20report/2020%202nd%20COVID-19%20Media%20Release%20FINALISEDFN.pdf [Accessed 5 February, 2021].

Bhorat, H. et al. (2020). *The economics of COVID-19 in South Africa: early impressions.* DPRU Working Paper 202004, Development Policy Research Unit, University of Cape Town.

Cameron, R. (2009). New Public Management reforms in the South African Public Service: 1999–2009. *Journal of Public Administration, 44*(4.1), 910–942.

Dayimani, M. (2021, 31 January). Cape Town breach protest: ANC wants arrests, while Winde calls ban 'nonsensical'. *News24.* Retrieved from https://www.news24.com/news24/southafrica/news/cape-town-beach-protest-anc-wants-arrests-while-winde-calls-ban-nonsensical-20210131 [Accessed 20 May, 2021].

Department of Cooperative Governance and Traditional Affairs. (2020). *Disaster Management Act, 2002, Declaration of a National State of Disaster.* Government Gazette, 15 March 2020, No.43096.

Department of Planning, Monitoring and Evaluation. (2020a). *Presentation on the measures implemented by the South African Government to combat the Coronavirus disease (COVID– 19) during the Pre-disaster and Disaster phases.* 19 August. Pretoria: DPME.

Department of Planning, Monitoring and Evaluation. (2020b). *2nd report of the DPME on measures implemented by the South African Government to combat the Coronavirus disease (COVID – 19) during the disaster phase.* Pretoria: DPME.

De Villiers, C., Cerbone, D., Van Zijl, W. (2020). The South African Government's Response to COVID-19. *Journal of Public Budgeting, Accounting & Financial Management*, *32*(5), 797–811.

Devermont, J., Mukulu, T. (2020, 12 May). South Africa's bold response to the COVID-19 Pandemic. *Center for Strategic and International Studies.* Retrieved from https://www.csis.org/analysis/south-africas-bold-response-COVID-19-pandemic [Accessed 18 January, 2021].

(2020, 2 September). Nxese says entire UIF management is suspended. *eNCA.* Retrieved from https://www.enca.com/news/labour-minister-says-entire-uif-management-suspended [Accessed 6 July, 2021].

Fraser-Moleketi, G. (2020). *Address by Geraldine J Fraser-Moleketi on Public Service and COVID-19: the future implications. South African Association of Public Administration and Management,* 29 May 2020. Retrieved from http://saapam.co.za/address-by-geraldine-j-fraser-moleketi-on-public-service-and-COVID-19-the-future-implications/ [Accessed 2 February, 2020].

Gumede, W. (2020, 15 June). South Africa needs a new governance model post–COVID–19. Retrieved from https://www.wits.ac.za/COVID19/COVID19-news/latest/south-africa-needs-a-new-governance-model-post-COVID-19.html [Accessed 20 February, 2021].

Gustafsson, M. 2020. How does South Africa's COVID-19 response compare globally? A preliminary analysis using the new OxCGRT dataset. Stellenbosch Economic Working Papers: WP07/2020. Bureau for Economic Research, University of Stellenbosch.

Hasnain, Z. (2020, 6 April). What about public sector wage bill cuts to finance coronavirus response? *World Bank Blogs.* Retrieved from https://blogs.worldbank.org/governance/should-public-sector-wages-be-cut-finance-coronavirus-response [Accessed 3 February, 2020].

Hirsch, A. (2020, 28 April). South Africa – can its achievement in containing COVID-19 lead to sustained success in dealing with the crisis? *OECD Development Matters.* Retrieved from https://oecd-development-matters.org/2020/04/28/south-africa-can-its-achievement-in-containing-COVID-19-lead-to-sustained-success-in-dealing-with-the-crisis/ [Accessed 18 January, 2021].

Hofman, K., Madhi, S. (2020). The unanticipated costs of COVID-19 to South Africa's quadruple disease burden. *South African Medical Journal*, *110*(8), 698–699.

Hunter, Q. (2020, 13 May). EXPLAINER: What exactly is the National Coronavirus Command Council? *New24.com.* Retrieved from https://www.news24.com/news24/SouthAfrica/News/explainer-what-exactly-is-the-national-coronavirus-command-council-20200513. [Accessed 22 April, 2021].

Intellidex. (2020). *The Public Sector Wage Bill – an evidence-based assessment and how to address the challenge.* Retrieved from https://www.intellidex.co.za/wp-content/uploads/2020/11/Intellidex-Public-Sector-Wage-Bill-Nov-2020.pdf [Accessed 11 December, 2020].

Isbell, T. (2020). COVID-19 lockdown in South Africa highlights unequal access to services. Afrobarometer Dispatch, No. 358. Afrobarometer.

Kahn, T. (2021, 8 June). Zweli Mkhize offers to go on special leave. *Business Day*. Retrieved from https://www.businesslive.co.za/bd/national/health/2021-06-08-zweli-mkhize-offers-to-go-on-special-leave/ [Accessed 4 July, 2021].

Kiewet, L. (2020a, 16 July). Civil service edges closer to COVID cliff. *Mail & Guardian*. Available from https://mg.co.za/coronavirus-essentials/2020-07-16-civil-service-edges-closer-to-COVID-cliff/ [Accessed 2 February, 2021].

Kiewet, L. (2020b, 16 April). Fighting COVID-19: The rise of the premiers. *Mail & Guardian*. Available from https://mg.co.za/article/2020-04-16-fighting-COVID-19-the-rise-of-the-premiers/ [Accessed 4 July, 2021].

Kunicova, J. (2020). *Driving the COVID-19 response from the center: institutional mechanisms to ensure whole-of-government coordination*. Working paper, World Bank Governance Global Practice. Washington, DC: World Bank.

Madhi, S. A. et al. (2020, 9 April). South Africa needs to end the lockdown: here's a blueprint for its replacement. *The Conversation*. Retrieved from https://theconversation.com/south-africa-needs-to-end-the-lockdown-heres-a-blueprint-for-its-replacement-136080 [Accessed 18 January, 2021].

Magubane, K. (2021, 25 August). Union lawyers tear into govt's argument that 2018 wage agreement is 'invalid'. *News24*. Retrieved from https://www.news24.com/fin24/Economy/union-lawyers-tear-into-govts-argument-that-2018-wage-agreement-is-invalid-20210825 [Accessed 19 October, 2022].

Mandelson, M. et al. (2022, 22 March). The incoherent and illogical new government COVID-19 regulations are the real state of disaster. *Daily Maverick*. Retrieved from https://www.dailymaverick.co.za/article/2022-03-22-the-incoherent-and-illogical-new-government-COVID-19-regulations-are-the-real-state-of-disaster/ [Accessed 2 October, 2022].

Mboweni, T. 2021. Minister Tito Mboweni: 2021 Budget Speech. Retrieved from https://www.gov.za/speeches/minister-tito-mboweni-2021-budget-speech-24-feb-2021-0000#:~:text=This%202021%20budget%20framework%20puts,avoid%20a%20sovereign%20debt%20crisis. [Accessed 19 October, 2022].

Mkhwanazi, S. (2020, 10 June). National Coronavirus Command Council not established by any law – Ramaphosa. *IOL*. Retrieved from https://www.iol.co.za/news/politics/national-coronavirus-command-council-not-established-by-any-law-ramaphosa-49214144 [Accessed 13 January, 2020].

Merten, M. (2020, 10 June). Who is in charge – the NCCC or the Cabinet? Ramaphosa unveils the blurring of democratic practice at the highest level. *Daily Maverick*. Retrieved from https://www.dailymaverick.co.za/article/2020-06-10-who-is-in-charge-the-nccc-or-the-cabinet-ramaphosa-unveils-the-blurring-of-democratic-practice-at-the-highest-level/ [Accessed 23 April, 2021].

Moffat, C. (2020, 17 August). Extraordinary times require extraordinary measures on public sector pay. *Business Day*. Retrieved from https://www.businesslive.co.za/bd/opinion/2020-08-17-extraordinary-times-require-extraordinary-measures-on-public-sector-pay/ [Accessed 2 February, 2021].

Muller, S. M. (2021). The dangers of performative scientism as the alternative to anti-scientific policymaking: A critical, preliminary assessment of South Africa's COVID-19 response and its consequences. *World Development*, *140*, 105290.

Naidoo, V. (2013). The challenges of policy coordination at a programme level: why joining-up is hard to do. *Development Southern Africa*, *30*(3), 386–400.

National School of Government. (2020). *A National Implementation Framework towards the Professionalisation of the Public Service.* Draft, 8 December. Government Gazette, No. 44031.

Ngalwana, V. (2020, 2 May). Do COVID-19 regulations pass the constitutionality test in SA? *IOL.* Retrieved from https://www.iol.co.za/sundayindependent/analysis/do-COVID-19-regulations-pass-the-constitutionality-test-in-sa-47474336 [Accessed 18 January, 2021].

OECD. (2020a) *Building resilience to the COVID-19 pandemic: the role of centres of government.*

OECD. (2020b). *OECD Economic Surveys, South Africa,* July 2020, Overview. Retrieved from http://www.treasury.gov.za/comm_media/press/2020/20200731%20OECD%20Economic%20Survey%20SA%202020.pdf [Accessed 2 February, 2021].

Office of Health Standards Compliance. (2018). *Annual Inspection Report 2016–2017.* Pretoria.

PWC. (2020). *Where next for government in South Africa? An opportunity for change. COVID-19 Government and Public Sector.* Retrieved from https://www.pwc.co.za/en/assets/pdf/Where%20Next%20for%20Government%20in%20South%20Africa.pdf [Accessed 2 February, 2021].

Padayachee, A. et al. (2020). *Position Paper: Priority setting for interventions in pre- and post-pandemic management: the case of COVID-19.* South African Technology Network. Retrieved from https://www.newssite.co.za/dhen/satn-COVID-19-position-paper.pdf [Accessed 2 January, 2021].

Parliamentary Monitoring Group. (2020a). *Ministry and Deputy on Disaster Management Regulations and their Amendments.* 21 April. Retrieved from https://pmg.org.za/committee-meeting/30103/ [Accessed 4 February, 2021].

Parliamentary Monitoring Group. (2020b). *Question NW1299 to the Minister of Cooperative Governance and Traditional Affairs.* Retrieved from https://pmg.org.za/committee-question/14461/ [Accessed 18 January, 2021].

The Presidency. (2021). *Statement by President Cyril Ramaphosa on progress in the national effort to contain the COVID-19 pandemic.* 28 November. Retrieved from http://www.thepresidency.gov.za/speeches/statement-president-cyril-ramaphosa-progress-national-effort-contain-COVID-19-pandemic-7 [Accessed 7 December, 2021].

The Presidency. (2020a). *State of the Nation Address.* 13 February. Retrieved from https://www.gov.za/speeches/president-cyril-ramaphosa-2020-state-nation-address-13-feb-2020-0000 [Accessed 4 February, 2021].

The Presidency. (2020b). *Statement by Presidency Cyril Ramaphosa on measures to combat COVID-19 epidemic.* 15 March. Retrieved from http://www.thepresidency.gov.za/press-statements/statement-president-cyril-ramaphosa-measures-combat-COVID-19-epidemic. [Accessed 4 February, 2021].

Public Servants Association of South Africa. (2021). *Budget Vote: PSA input on Budget Vote to be delivered by Minister of Finance Tito Mboweni. Media release.* 22 February. Retrieved from https://www.psa.co.za/media-statements [Accessed 25 February, 2021].

Public Servants Association of South Africa. (2020). *Coronavirus and Implications for the Public Service.* 14 April. Retrieved from https://www.psa.co.za/docs/default-source/psa-documents/psa-opinion/coronavirus-and-implications-for-the-public-service.pdf?sfvrsn=d13ce776_1 [Accessed 16 February, 2021].

Public Service Commission. (2020). *Report on Lessons Learnt and State Capacity to facilitate Ethical, Efficient, Economic and Effective Service Delivery during the Post the COVID-19 pandemic.* Pretoria: PSC.

Rosenkranz, B., Anelich, L., Harrison, P., Mubangizi, C. B., Ndevu, Z., Rabie, B., Rumbold, K. (2021). Leadership, governance, and institutional arrangements. *South Africa COVID-19 Country Report, First edition*. DPME (Department of Planning, Monitoring and Evaluation), GTAC (Government Technical Advisory Centre) & NRF (National Research Foundation), Pretoria: June.

Schneider, H., Hlophe, H., Van Rensburg, D. (2008). Community health workers and the response to HIV/AIDS in South Africa: Tensions and Prospects. *Health Policy and Planning*, *23*, 179–187.

Singh, J. A. (2020). How South Africa's Ministerial Advisory Committee on COVID-19 can be optimised. *South African Medical Journal*, *110*(6), 439–442.

Staunton, C., Swanepoel, C., Labuschaigne, M. (2020). Between a rock and a hard place: COVID-19 and South Africa's response. *Journal of Law and the Biosciences*, *7*(1), 1–12.

Steytler, N. (2020). *Federalism and the COVID-19 crisis: a perspective on South Africa. Forum of Federations*. Retrieved from http://www.forumfed.org/wp-content/uploads/2020/05/SouthAfrica_COVID.pdf [Accessed 27 January, 2021].

Tandwa, L. (2020, 22 October). ANC Gauteng recommends Masuku, Diko head to provincial DC over Covid-19 corruption allegations. *News24*. Retrieved from https://www.news24.com/news24/southafrica/news/anc-gauteng-recommends-masuku-diko-head-to-provincial-dc-over-covid-19-corruption-allegations-20201022 [Accessed 19 October, 2022].

Uevrard, J., Davies, M-A. (2020, 20 July). COVID-19 promotes innovative HIV service delivery in Cape Town. *The Conversation*. Retrieved from https://theconversation.com/COVID-19-promotes-innovative-hiv-service-delivery-in-cape-town-142583 [Accessed 8 December, 2021].

Van Niekerk, D. (2014). A critical analysis of the South African Disaster Management Act and Policy Framework. *Disasters*, *38*(4), 858–877.

Voituriez, T., Chancel, L. (2021). Developing countries in times of COVID: comparing inequality impacts and policy responses. Issue Brief 2021/01. World Inequality Lab, United Nations Development Programme.

Wadvalla, B. A. (2020). COVID-19: decisive action is the hallmark of South Africa's early success against coronavirus. *BMJ* 2020;369:M1623. Retrieved from https://www.bmj.com/content/369/bmj.m1623 [Accessed 20 April, 2021].

Western Cape Office of the Premier. (2021). *Premier Alan Winde calls to end National State of Disaster and save jobs. South African Government*. Retrieved from https://www.gov.za/speeches/premier-alan-winde-calls-end%C2%A0national-state-disaster-and-save-jobs-8-sep-2021-0000 [Accessed 10 September, 2021].

7   COVID-19 vaccines

Triumphs and tragedies

Keymanthri Moodley

Introduction

Colliding pandemics of viral outbreaks, mistrust and social injustice created a perfect storm since December 2019 when the emergence of a new coronavirus, SARS-Cov-2, became evident. The public health crisis that followed was set against a backdrop of lapses in global health governance, contentious health guidance and unprecedented societal lockdowns. The social isolation, death, sadness, anxiety and uncertainty that followed were devastating in many respects.

Much to our detriment, public health literacy, a long-neglected component of the health environment, was suboptimal, enhancing vulnerability to misinformation that was spread irresponsibly via social media – now widely referred to as the infodemic. This in turn contributed to the erosion of trust in medicine, science and governments. Public health establishments globally were understaffed and poorly equipped and infection control measures were exposed even in private health establishments as they became overwhelmed. Political expediency often trumped science and ethics in decision-making. Marginalised communities became more isolated. Ethnic and gender-based violence was unmasked in various settings.

Against this tragic backdrop to the pandemic, medical scientists, epidemiologists, bioinformaticians, clinicians, health researchers and front-line responders soldiered on in hospitals, laboratories and on research sites. Pre-pandemic health inequity was seamlessly drawn into the COVID-19 pandemic. This global health phenomenon played itself out in the form of COVID testing capacity of low- and middle-income countries (LMICs), availability of hospital beds, critical care beds, medical personnel, oxygen supplies and eventually, COVID-19 vaccines. From a public health perspective, the tide of this pandemic turned significantly after the development and administration of carefully tested vaccines together with natural immunity in those who were infected during earlier waves of infection. Compared to the first and second waves of infection in South Africa and globally, the third, fourth and subsequent waves of infection were less severe, with substantially less death, illness, hospitalisation and intensive care requirements in countries

DOI: 10.4324/9781003294931-7

with moderate to high vaccination rates. Hybrid immunity played a significant role in decoupling infection from death and hospitalisation (Madhi et al. 2022; Moghadas et al., 2021; Lin et al., 2022). This medical triumph was lauded in scientific and non-scientific circles alike despite the global inequity in access and supply of vaccines.

Although the health systems of high-income countries (HICs) were overwhelmed too, the impact of the pandemic on health systems in LMICs was simply catastrophic. Globally, strict triage criteria were established for access to intensive care units (ICUs) and eventually, extremely limited vaccine supplies had to be fairly distributed in the face of unprecedented simultaneous global demand. The asymmetric distribution of vaccines was blatant throughout the pandemic.

Global vaccine inequity

Although an efficacious COVID-19 vaccine was widely recognised as a global game changer required by the global community urgently and synchronously, the distribution of vaccines during the pandemic was far from fair or just (Moodley, 2021).

Lapses in global governance have led to asymmetrical vaccine distribution with high-income countries (HICs) accessing disproportionate quantities of limited vaccine supplies. Vaccine nationalism, stockpiling of limited vaccine supplies by HICs and profit-driven strategies of global pharmaceutical manufacturers (Hassan) have brought into sharp focus global health inequities and the plight of low-and-middle-income countries (LMICs) in Africa.

Vaccine manufacturing capacity in Africa is limited to one country – Senegal – where only one vaccine – the Yellow Fever vaccine – has historically been produced (Makenga, 2019). Consequently, the fair distribution of extremely limited supplies of an efficacious COVID-19 vaccine, once approved for marketing, is likely to pose both public health and procurement challenges. Sadly, not all were first in line to receive it.

COVID-19 vaccine supplies in South Africa

On 1 February 2021, South Africa was fortunate to procure its first delivery of the AstraZeneca (AZ) vaccine from the largest vaccine manufacturer in the world, the Serum Institute of India. However, a million doses of the vaccine arrived at a cost levied by AstraZeneca of $5.25 per dose, more than double the $2.16 per dose paid by European Union countries to AZ. The explanation for the price difference was that SA had not contributed financially to research and development of vaccines (Kahn, 2021). Yet SA had hosted a clinical trial of the AZ vaccine and was still unable to secure a fair pricing agreement (Porteous, 2021), violating the fundamental principles of post-trial access and benefit sharing in research (Moodley, 2021).

These are firmly entrenched research ethics principles, justified by collaborative partnership, which is a quintessential research ethics requirement and one of the key principles that contribute to the ethical conduct of research in developing countries (Emanuel, 2004). Collaborative partnership requires a fair distribution of both tangible and intangible rewards of research among the partners (Emanuel, 2004). Resentment, mistrust and a sense of exploitation are inevitable if those who bear the burdens of research, that is, research participants, do not benefit.

Due to a small trial of the AZ vaccine in South Africa, concerns were raised that the vaccine could not sufficiently protect against the 501Y.V2 variant. The trial enrolled mostly young adults, so generalisability to older people was limited. Consequently, the research results could only be extrapolated to the prevention of mild and moderate disease and not to the prevention of severe diseases (Madhi, 2021). The SA government then decided to resell the AZ vaccines to the African Union, given that they would be ineffective against certain virus variants (Mkhize, 2021). The diversion of AZ vaccine supplies to other African countries raised deep ethical concerns and could have contributed to vaccine hesitancy in some recipient African countries, (Venter, 2021) such as Uganda and Malawi. The destruction of nearly 20,000 expired AZ vaccine doses due to poor uptake exacerbated vaccine hesitancy in countries such as Malawi (Muhumuza, 2021; News 24).

Several clinical trials had been hosted in SA, so the Johnson and Johnson (J&J) COVID-19 vaccine was rolled out in the form of a phase 3B 'implementation trial' to healthcare workers in February 2021, given that they were the group at the highest risk. As an open-label trial, all participants were offered an active vaccine (Moodley et al., 2021 SAMJ).

In the months that followed, large quantities of Pfizer vaccines were purchased and donated to South Africa. Cold chain requirements were maintained and Pfizer vaccines were offered to high-risk adults by May 2021 followed by adolescents 12 years and older. As the vaccine supply increased, rollout of vaccines was extended to other groups and eventually became available to everyone 12 years and older by October 2021. Currently, two vaccine doses are available three weeks apart and a booster dose may be obtained three months after the second dose.

Suboptimal vaccine uptake

Despite adequate vaccine supplies since 2021, together with education campaigns and improved access via additional vaccine sites and pop-up sites across the country, South Africa remained way below the target of 300,000 doses per day by December 2021. During January 2022, vaccine uptake remained at under 70,000 doses a day while in March 2022, this increased to around 90,000 doses per day. Under these circumstances of poor uptake, the potential for vaccine wastage is significant. During 2021, media publications already alluded to undisclosed wastage (Tshikalange, 2021, The Citizen, 2021). This ought to have been a red flag for government to introduce mandates since vaccine wastage in a context where so many countries have suboptimal supplies, is unethical. Recent reports from the SA Department of Health indicate that the country has 30 million vaccine doses for 2022. While the Johnson and Johnson vaccines will probably expire in 2023, approximately 400,000 Pfizer vaccines are at risk of wastage due to expiry dates of March 2022 if vaccine uptake does not improve in SA. Further vaccines, almost seven million doses of Pfizer vaccines, expired in June-July 2022 (Crisp, 2022). Even more alarming is the possibility that vaccines for children aged 5 to 11 years, once approved in SA, will be unaffordable. This is because children require a smaller dosage compared to adults, which is available in different vials and that requires different syringes and needles to draw up (Malan, 2022). The pandemic has already used up the health budget to the extent that many qualified young doctors are unemployed as funding for salaries is not available.

Strategies to increase vaccine uptake

The ideal scenario is for vaccine uptake to occur on a voluntary basis to ensure that everyone is protected. To date, the altruistic approach has not worked and vaccine uptake remains suboptimal. Ongoing public engagement efforts appear to be insufficient to increase uptake of vaccines substantially. Project Last Mile supported the National Department of Health in South Africa to raise awareness around COVID-19 vaccines using mass media channels from September 2021 to January 2022. This extended to using digital media such as TikTok to engage a younger audience. Over this period vaccine uptake increased from 10% of fully vaccinated South Africans to 27% but remained suboptimal (USAID, 2021). Other options include nudges to encourage behaviour modification, offering incentives and vaccine mandates. Incentives are being provided in some contexts to encourage vaccination. Monetary incentives (Allen, 2021), food vouchers, retail discounts and lower life or medical insurance premiums (Buthelezi, 2021), are examples.

However, in other settings less attractive measures are being implemented. These include unpleasant alternatives like weekly COVID-19 testing for the unvaccinated and wearing of N95 masks to nudge people in the right direction. Several studies have demonstrated that incentives increase vaccine uptake by two to five percentage points (Campos-Mercade et al., 2021; Kluver, 2021). This will not boost immunity at a population level to a satisfactory extent. There are further challenges with incentivising health behaviour. It has the potential to raise suspicion and fuel mistrust (Cooper, 2021). Furthermore, adults ought to be sufficiently motivated to protect and improve their own health without being offered incentives, yet this does not always occur in practice. Furthermore, a dangerous precedent could be set to achieve other health-related outcomes for other diseases. Nudges and incentives are not sufficiently powerful to drive vaccine uptake at the scale required to bring the pandemic under control like vaccine mandates that can increase vaccine uptake by around 18 percentage points (Community Preventive Services Task Force). In SA, the private health insurer, Discovery Limited has successfully increased vaccine uptake amongst employees from 22% in September 2021 to 94% in November 2021 (Businesstech, 2021). Globally, studies are now emerging to demonstrate the efficacy of vaccine mandates (Mills, 2021). Despite this, there is considerable vaccine hesitancy (Cooper, 2021).

Arguments against vaccines

Vaccine hesitancy in South Africa

Surveys in SA to explore willingness to accept COVID-19 vaccines have yielded interesting results. Vaccine acceptance levels ranged from 52% to 82% in different surveys. The most common explanations for unwillingness to vaccinate were concerns about side effects (25%) as well as about the overall effectiveness of the vaccine (18%). Only 7% of the study sample was influenced by conspiracy theories (Cooper, 2021).

Some predisposing medical conditions may exacerbate side effects after taking COVID-19 vaccines. However, there are very few conditions that can be classified as medical exemptions and these include a severe allergic reaction to the first dose of a COVID-19 vaccine, allergy to specific components of a vaccine and a few other medical indications such as a prior diagnosis of an autoimmune inflammatory condition affecting the neurological, haematological or cardiovascular systems such as Guillain Barre syndrome and immune thrombocytopaenic purpura (ITP). Some medical conditions may be associated with a bleeding risk (haemophilia or Von Willebrand's disease) – especially intramuscular bleeding post-vaccination (UCT Draft Vaccine Policy, 2021).

Religious objections

Most major world religions promote vaccination making authentic religious objections rare. Religious teachings generally support vaccination as an 'act of love' and a moral obligation towards fellow human beings (Watkins, 2021). Some groups have raised arguments based on a misperception that COVID-19 vaccines contain aborted foetal cells. Decades ago, these cells were used to create 'immortal' cell lines for vaccines and other drug research including research for several processed food additives. Many commonly used drugs were developed based on this type of research such as Aspirin, Brufen, Tylenol, Benadryl, Azithromycin and Zoloft (Zimmerman, 2021). If people were to claim a religious objection based on aborted foetal cell-associated research, they would then have to refuse to take a wide range of medication that they have already been using for decades. Consequently, such arguments fail the test of consistency and authenticity (Wynia et al., 2021).

Mandatory vaccine policies are justifiable on the basis of a public health ethics framework based on the principles of limited autonomy, social justice and the common good.

Justification for vaccine mandates

Access, safety and efficacy

In order to implement vaccine mandates in high-risk environments, a pre-requisite is a free, accessible supply of safe and effective COVID-19 vaccines. Despite global vaccine inequity, this condition was met in SA by July 2021 (Moodley, 2021, 2022). There were over 3,000 vaccination centres widely distributed throughout the country as well as supplemental pop-up vaccine sites, yet access via primary healthcare providers and hospital outpatient departments could be improved.

Breakthrough infections due to the Omicron variant created concern about vaccine efficacy in partially and fully vaccinated people, especially those with comorbidities. However, two doses of the vaccines currently available in South Africa (Pfizer and Johnson and Johnson) have proven efficacy in reducing severe illness and death. Booster doses increase protection. Some argue that rapid development of COVID-19 vaccines means that safety and efficacy standards were compromised. However, mRNA technology has been in development for the past 20–30 years. Furthermore, billions of COVID-19 vaccine doses have been administered globally in the real world and have mostly been safe and are protecting against severe disease and death in most cases with serious side effects being experienced only by a minority with underlying risk factors (Polack et al., 2020; Anand, 2021; Takuva et al., 2021; Barda et al., 2021). For most people, these side effects are temporary and reversible. Natural COVID-19 infections may be mild, moderate or severe. For those with underlying conditions, obesity and other risk factors, irrespective of age, the impact on health could be severe and persist long after the acute infection.

In addition to 'Long COVID' other complications, that are more debilitating have been described. A recent study analysed data from 11 million people who had natural COVID-19 infections. The study found that those who had contracted COVID-19 were at increased risk of cardiovascular disease – cerebrovascular disorders (strokes), dysrhythmias, ischaemic and non-ischaemic heart disease, pericarditis, myocarditis, heart failure and thromboembolic disease. These risks were detected among people who were not hospitalised during the acute phase of the infection and increased if they were hospitalised or admitted to intensive care. This study provides evidence that 'the risk and one-year burden of cardiovascular disease in survivors of acute COVID-19 are substantial' and that this risk increases with the severity of the initial COVID-19 infection (Xie et al., 2022).

Another study has shown concerning evidence of brain damage after natural COVID-19 infections. In this study published in *Nature* on 7 March 2022, brain scan data on 785 patients aged 51–81 years were analysed. The scans were examined before and after patients contracted COVID-19 (Douaud et al., 2022). Although evidence was found of reduced grey matter in the brain and reduced brain size, the impact on cognitive function is uncertain. This will become clearer in follow-up studies in those who have had natural infections.

Those who spread misinformation about COVID-19 vaccines often cite rare side effects experienced by a minority of people. What they fail to do is compare the prevalence of those side effects with the short-, medium- and long-term effects of natural infection. Overall, comparing the complications of natural COVID-19 infection, with vaccine side effects, the risk-benefit assessment favours vaccines as a safer option.

A public health ethics approach

Once the safety and efficacy of COVID-19 vaccines were established, a public health ethics approach became the most appropriate framework to guide decision-making and policy development. This approach is based on the principles of solidarity, effectiveness, efficiency, proportionality and transparency (Schroder-Back et al., 2014). It is intended to save lives during a public health emergency, to use limited resources efficiently, to create social cohesion in the public interest and to contribute to building public trust.

Furthermore, the approach is supported by a human rights framework. The Siracusa principles on the Limitation and Derogation Provisions in the International Covenant on Civil and Political Rights were adopted by the United Nations, Economic and Social Council in 1985 have reference (United Nations, 1985). These principles are now firmly enshrined in international human rights law and standards and are reflected in Section 36 of the South African Constitution (SA Constitution, 1996) dealing with the limitation of rights. According to these principles, any restriction on human rights must be based on law. The National Health Act No. 61 of 2003[9] (NHAct, 2003) via regulations relating to notifiable medical conditions and the Disaster Management Act apply. Furthermore, restrictions on individual rights imposed via vaccination must be based on a legitimate objective and must be strictly necessary for the achievement of the policy objective. In the case of COVID-19, the objectives of reducing the risk of transmission of infection, reducing severe disease, minimising death and preserving health systems and health personnel are unambiguously in the public interest. Various reports now suggest that the reported death toll due to COVID-19 is almost three times higher across the globe. South Africa currently reports approximately 113 000 deaths due to COVID-19 while the Medical Research Council (SAMRC) has 326 671 excess deaths documented, of which 85–95% are ascribed to COVID-19 (Farber, 2022). Restriction of individual rights under these circumstances is therefore legitimate.

The South African Bill of Rights (Section 36) specifies that any limitation of rights must be 'reasonable and justifiable in an open and democratic society based on human dignity, equality and freedom' and that the restriction must be proportional to the purpose of the limitation. Most importantly, such restrictions must be based on scientific evidence and should not be arbitrary, discriminatory or unreasonable.

A public health ethics approach supports the limitation of individual rights for the greater good and promotion of solidarity. Several pieces of legislation in SA similarly support vaccine mandates under pandemic conditions (de Vos, 2021; Cheadle, 2021; Moodley, 2021). Despite this, the South African government has failed to implement mandates. Consequently, vaccine mandates are being promoted and implemented mainly in private organisations (Gore, 2021). In operationalising vaccination, according to the Siracusa principles and the limitation clause of the Constitution, the least restrictive and intrusive means must be used. Options that are less restrictive than mandates include nudges and incentives. However, there is evidence as discussed earlier, that these approaches are minimally effective.

The right to a safe working environment

In corporate settings and other occupational environments, guidelines for implementing vaccine mandates are based on the rights of employees and employers to a safe working environment (Department of Labour). Implementation of vaccine policies must be underscored by procedural justice. A process of risk assessment must be initiated in the workplace. This must be followed by employee engagement and consideration of exemptions and alternatives.

To date, there have been several legal challenges to vaccine mandates in various work environments. However, the Commission for Conciliation, Mediation and Arbitration (CCMA), has so far supported vaccine mandates and ruled in favour of employers (Medical Brief, 2022). There are still cases under review at the time of writing.

Other considerations to support vaccine mandates

The immunosuppressed remain vulnerable

For four decades the African continent has had to fight a ravaging Human Immunodeficiency Virus (HIV). Over the past two years, HIV and COVID-19 become synergistic pandemics in South Africa. Almost 8 million of our population of 60 million is HIV-infected (Freer, 2021). During the past two years, clinics and hospitals were less accessible to non-COVID patients and hence access to antiretroviral treatment has been suboptimal. Unsurprisingly, many HIV-infected people have low CD4 counts and are at risk of contracting other infections, including COVID-19. Research has shown that HIV infection resulted in doubling of mortality from COVID-19. Consequently, this group of patients remains at high risk for COVID-19 and must be prioritised for vaccines and boosters (Davies, 2020). Some HIV-infected patients are not able to clear the virus as quickly as others. This allows the virus to mutate for months potentially creating new variants.

Children remain a vulnerable population in Africa

Globally, more children were hospitalised during the 4th wave of infections due to the high transmissibility of the Omicron variant (Wang et al., 2022). This was exacerbated in sub-Saharan African countries, where children with underlying health conditions experienced higher morbidity and mortality related to infection with the Omicron variant compared to high-income countries (Nachega et al., 2022). Vaccine rollout started in adults in South Africa in February 2021, while children 12 years and older were offered vaccines recently and uptake has not been sufficient. With schools reopening in SA, this is a high-risk group to trigger further outbreaks. In the Western Cape alone, only 19, 27% of those 12–17 years are vaccinated with at least one dose (Western Cape DOH, 2022). Given that SA has a culture of multi-generational households, the youth risk infecting older family members who are also likely to have a higher prevalence of comorbidities. Most importantly, compared to the previous three waves, more younger people died of COVID-19 during the recent fourth wave (Crisp, 2022).

Although there is interest in vaccinating younger children (5–11 years), this has not commenced in South Africa at the time of writing. Multiple factors merit consideration here. The Pfizer vaccine is currently the only approved vaccine for use in this age group. Our medicines regulatory body (SAHPRA) still needs to approve the use of the Pfizer vaccine in this age group. Current reports suggest that the reduced dosage selected for this group is not inducing a sufficient immune response (Dorabawila, 2022). Establishing a balance between safety and efficacy is imperative. Even if the vaccine is approved for this age group, funding for the vaccine for these children is questionable. Since this age group will require a dose of vaccine that differs from adults, new different vials of Pfizer vaccine, different syringes and needles will need to be purchased requiring a new financial investment (Malan, 2022).

Moving beyond vaccines, children are at risk of developing a range of mental health problems related to the pandemic. The social isolation during lockdowns, school closures, online education and restricted interaction with other children are likely to impact negatively on mental health. More concerning, the widespread emergence of COVID-19 orphans due to the loss of parents and caregivers is likely to become more and more important (Hillis et al., 2022).

Health systems remain under pressure

Despite the Omicron variant being more severe based on its genetic makeup, the severity of the disease that resulted clinically was significantly reduced due to prior natural infections and vaccines. Consequently, healthcare institutions coped with the fourth wave of admissions. However, the national burden of all-cause disease in SA must not be forgotten. South Africa has a high burden of diseases that substantially increase the risk of developing severe COVID-19 infection, including tuberculosis, HIV and non-communicable diseases (Mayosi et al., 2012). During the four waves of COVID-19 infection, hospitals prioritised patients acutely ill with the infection and diverted treatment away from other non-COVID conditions like cancer and chronic diseases (hypertension, diabetes, HIV) and de-escalated elective procedures and surgery. As a result, many patients with chronic conditions were neglected, chronic treatment was interrupted and illnesses spiralled out of control. In the first two waves of infection, this was unavoidable to a large extent. However, as vaccines became available in early 2021, the de-escalation of care for non-COVID-19 patients became less and less justifiable. The harsh reality and consequence of unvaccinated patients occupying hospital beds and ICUs unnecessarily became more apparent (Mendelsohn et al., 2021).

The fifth wave of infection occurred in May 2022. South Africa currently has fewer therapeutic options for acute COVID-19 infection. In some HICs, monoclonal antibodies are routinely used in hospitals to treat COVID-19 symptoms. This is not the case in South Africa. Even though expensive antiviral drugs like Paxlovid may become available in some settings to treat COVID-19 in the first 3 days of symptom onset, this will not be an option in SA due to potentially high costs and lack of early testing and diagnosis. Another huge burden on healthcare systems in the aftermath of the first four waves of infection are post-viral syndromes. Also referred to as 'long COVID', patients are debilitated by symptoms that linger for several months after natural infection. This is already straining clinical services globally including in SA (Mendelsen et al., 2020).

Even more concerning are the long-term cardiovascular complications of natural COVID-19. Consequently, many hospitals and medical practices could become busier than in pre-pandemic times (Xie, 2022). Other studies have shown that natural COVID-19 infection causes significant brain damage (Douaud, 2022).

Compassion fatigue amongst healthcare professionals

Healthcare professionals (HCPs) around the world are physically and emotionally exhausted. SA is no exception. Unsurprisingly, they are becoming less sympathetic towards those who deliberately decline vaccines, especially in the absence of medical contraindication to justify an exemption (Ngqakamba, 2021; Moodley, 2021 SAMJ). During the first three waves of infection, many HCPs witnessed severe illness or death at catastrophic levels. This continued during the fourth wave, predominantly amongst the unvaccinated or partially vaccinated. (Moodley, 2021).

Thousands of non-COVID-19 patients have been deprived of timeous care or access to ICU because critical care units have been overrun by non-compliant COVID-19 patients despite an abundant vaccine supply in SA. During the first wave of infections access to ICU beds and ventilators was limited. Criteria were developed to help critical care doctors to decide who could get access to beds when demand surged. These criteria did not include vaccine status. In future waves, if many patients are competing for the last bed in an ICU, will vaccination status as a surrogate for prognosis become an important deciding factor? Since the basis for triage criteria is the prognosis, it can be argued that a fully vaccinated person may have a better chance of recovery from severe COVID-19 compared to an unvaccinated person, all other factors being equal (Ebrahim, 2021). These decisions are both ethically complex and logistically challenging. It would be necessary to carefully document reasons for declining vaccines in medical records. Counselling efforts by health professionals, where medical contra-indications do not exist, must be included. In the absence of such information, using vaccination status as a triage criterion may not be easily defensible.

During recent surges of infection, the unvaccinated or partially vaccinated have filled hospital beds and ICUs. The death rate in the United States is about 13-fold higher in unvaccinated patients compared to those who have had 2 doses (Johnson et al., 2021). In South Africa, 90% of deaths in patients hospitalised for COVID-19 were either unvaccinated or partially vaccinated (Ebrahim, 2021). Although it is unlikely that fully vaccinated and boosted patients will develop severe COVID-19 disease in future waves, the partially vaccinated will be at risk. What remains concerning is the number of patients with non-COVID-19 illnesses requiring hospitalisation or critical care and who may be unfairly denied access to ICU and high-care facilities that are full of unvaccinated patients with COVID-19. Such a scenario may prompt the revision of ICU triage guidelines.

Duties and obligations of healthcare professionals

Based on a foundational principle of medical ethics, *primum non nocere* or *first do no harm*, healthcare professionals are duty-bound to protect patients and prevent harm. This includes ensuring that they do not infect patients with a wide range of communicable diseases. Patient safety is a primary ethical obligation. Likewise, reducing risk to colleagues in the healthcare environment is imperative and reducing risk to family members at home would be the right thing to do.

The South African Constitution in Section 23 indicates that 'Everyone has a right to fair labour practices'. The use of the word 'Everyone' means that employers and employees are included. Consequently, employers would need to institute policies to ensure a safe working environment for all. Although the preferable approach would include encouragement and counselling of all medical and care staff regarding the benefits of vaccination, there would be legal and human rights considerations that must be taken into account in the context of public interest, the Disaster Management Act and the National

Health Act. Competing entitlements in the Bill of Rights can be resolved through the appropriate application of Section 36 of the South African Constitution in which limitation of rights in the interest of the public good may occur.

Are vaccine mandates necessary on university campuses?

Vaccine mandates on university campuses have generated considerable debate in South Africa. These areas are high risk because they involve congregate activities in indoor lecture venues and in residences. Ventilation may not always be ideal depending on the type of air-conditioning systems at different institutions as well as the ability to open windows. Academic and administrative staff and postgraduate students who are older, with or without comorbidities, could be at risk in multigenerational contexts. Those with immunosuppression from a wide range of causes including HIV are also at risk.

Most academic programs require in-person interaction and interruptions must be avoided at all costs. Outbreaks at academic institutions will potentially involve large numbers of students and staff making these settings high risk for 'superspreader' events. Irrespective of whether new variants cause less severe disease, those who are symptomatic will need to isolate for a minimum of a week. Where many students are involved from different disciplines, the potential for disruption of teaching and/or examinations is substantial.

Some of the country's leading universities such as the University of the Witwatersrand and the University of the Western Cape implemented vaccine mandates since 1 March 2022 (Makhafola, 2021) while others are in the process of policy development and stakeholder engagement. Hybrid teaching works well for the privileged with devices and data. Transitioning from online teaching to in-person education is imperative in South Africa given the digital divide between privileged and historically disadvantaged students. Vaccine mandates on university campuses are in the best interests of students and staff alike.

Vaccine mandates for international travel

Since the onset of the pandemic and after the availability of safe and efficacious vaccines, international travel has been impossible without proof of COVID-19 vaccination, even post-Omicron. Long before the current pandemic, Yellow Fever vaccination was mandatory for entry into some countries. Annex 7 of the International Health Regulations (2005) provides an 'overarching legal framework that defines countries' rights and obligations in handling public health events and emergencies that have the potential to cross borders (WHO, 2005). Intended to protect the rights of travellers and airline staff, these regulations are legally binding in 196 countries. Article 31 of the IHR allows governments to require 'proof of vaccination or other prophylaxis, legitimising vaccine mandates in the context of international travel.' Consequently, vaccine mandates for airline travel are likely to be required for several months until COVID-19 is no longer regarded as a public health threat.

Sustainability of COVID-19 vaccine supplies in South Africa

One of the most powerful lessons that we have learnt from this pandemic is the need for self-sufficiency. Asymmetrical vaccine distribution globally occurred because major manufacturing vaccine plants are predominantly located in high-income countries. Even though the Serum Institute of India is the largest vaccine manufacturer in the world, the local demand in India during the Delta wave meant that supplies for the rest of the world had to be limited. Their vaccine manufacturing capacity was further impacted by a fire at the plant. This impacted the WHO pooled procurement initiative – COVAX or the COVID-19 Global Vaccine Access Facility which was intended to support global vaccine access. Sadly, this mechanism to improve access to vaccines for LMICs was not sufficient to meet the global need time-ously. Wealthy countries secured bilateral deals with vaccine manufacturers during vaccine development, invested in development and proceeded with vaccine rollout in their own countries significantly derailing vaccine delivery to COVAX.

Sharing of intellectual property (IP) and technology transfer was a blatant omission in the solidarity needed during this pandemic. Given the threat to public health globally, temporary waivers on some intellectual property rights on COVID-19 vaccines ought to have been implemented to allow local manufacturers to produce vaccines. The application for waivers by South Africa and India was repeatedly opposed by HICs until fairly recently when partial waivers were granted. The IP restrictions on the

> manufacture and production of COVID-19 vaccines have been partially waived for the next five years, after an agreement was reached on 17 June by participating countries attending the 12th Ministerial Conference of the World Trade Organisation (WTO) in Geneva, Switzerland.
>
> (Medical Brief, 2022)

The waivers do not apply to therapeutics and diagnostics.

Only one mRNA COVID-19 vaccine manufacturer, Moderna, decided not to enforce a patent on its vaccine in 2020. Although this meant that LMICs could develop their own versions of the vaccine using less expensive resources, many countries could not do this without knowledge and tech-nological transfer. On 8 March 2022, Moderna extended its promise indef-initely to 92 LMICs who are recipients of vaccines via the WHO COVAX program. South Africa is not one of these countries. Even in the 92 countries where patents were not filed, licensing fees could be required (Park, 2022 Time). In July 2021, WHO established an mRNA vaccine technology hub as part of its Initiative for Vaccine Research. Afrigen, a South African bio-tech company, learnt the technology but it took 8 months to develop its own mRNA version of the COVID-19 vaccine. This occurred in February 2022 supported by funding of around $ 100 million over the next five years from Europe. This occurred without access to animal testing data, assays, quality control tests and process parameters from Moderna. Because the SA vaccine has been developed from scratch it will still need to undergo testing for safety and efficacy in clinical trials planned to start in November 2022. If all goes well, the Afrigen mRNA vaccines will only be available for commercial use in 2024 (Park, 2022). Perhaps too late for this pandemic but possibly in time for the next pandemic.

Global solidarity and social justice

Many tourists from the global north who were fully vaccinated and, in some cases, additionally protected with booster doses, were privileged to travel to various countries in Africa, between the third and fourth waves of infection and even during the fourth surge. This occurred even though healthcare and front-line workers had not yet been vaccinated in some African countries. Despite widespread notifications of COVID-19 pro-tocols in SA, many privileged tourists blatantly disregarded mandatory masking policies in African countries. And when the Omicron variant was announced in November 2021, some fled back to their HICs, in some cases taking the variant with them thereby crippling their own health sys-tems and economies. Omicron has provided the evidence for why vaccine nationalism does not work making this approach ethically indefensible (Moodley, 2022).

Research is another domain where vulnerability to exploitation persists. Throughout the pandemic, South African scientists have contributed genomic sequencing data. Despite this valuable contribution, reciprocal advantage in access to vaccines or antiviral therapies did not follow. Paradoxically, travel restrictions were slapped onto several southern African countries (Luke, 2021) fuelling mistrust in international scientific collaboration.

Conclusion

The COVID-19 pandemic has unmasked deep-seated inequities in health, particularly in the distribution of vaccines. In the first three waves of infec-tion, our health systems were overwhelmed necessitating alcohol restrictions to minimise trauma admissions and to save beds for those with acute COVID infections. The combined effect of natural immunity and vaccines, warm weather and a younger population resulted in a less severe fourth or 'Omicron' wave in South Africa. Unlike healthcare systems in the global north, our hos-pitals were busy but not completely overwhelmed during the recent outbreak. Despite this good outcome, a cautiously optimistic approach is warranted.

South Africans carry a high burden of chronic disease that increases the risk of developing severe COVID-19 infection. This risk exists even if the next variant, predicted to appear in late April or May 2022 (Meterlerkamp, 2022), is equally or less transmissible than Omicron. Long COVID, neurological damage and cardiovascular complications of COVID-19 (Xie et al., 2022) remain chronic health challenges.

Apart from health impacts, socio-economic impacts could potentially be catastrophic as clinical severity is unpredictable at the time a new variant is announced. Globally the unvaccinated account for the majority of people with severe infections and are the majority of patients requiring ventilation and critical care. Consequently, they are and have been blocking beds for patients with serious non-COVID conditions. Vaccines, including boosters, remain the mainstay of prevention and mandates will improve vaccine uptake, protect health and health systems and promote economic revival. A combination of non-pharmacologic measures and high vaccine coverage will prepare us better for future waves. Self-interest and 'pandemic individualism' are incompatible with a successful outcome to this public health crisis (Dwyer, 2022).

Undoubtedly, our safest option now is to ensure that as many South Africans as possible are vaccinated and receive boosters. Vaccine mandates for high-risk congregate settings will help us to achieve this end. The choices we make now will shape the world for decades to come.

References

Anand P, Stahel VP. (2021). Review the safety of COVID-19 mRNA vaccines: a review [published correction appears in Patient Saf Surg. 2021 May 18;15(1):22]. *Patient Saf Surg.* 2021;15(1):20. Published 2021 May 1. doi: 10.1186/s13037-021-00291-9 https://www.ncbi.nlm.nih.gov/pmc/articles/PMC8087878/

Barda N, Dagan N, Ben-Shlomo Y, Kepten E, Waxman J, Ohana R, et al. (2021). Safety of the BNT162b2 mRNA COVID-19 Vaccine in a Nationwide Setting. *NEJM.* 2021 doi: 10.1056/nejmoa2110475

Businesstech. (2021). Why Discovery introduced mandatory vaccines in South Africa and why some workers said no. 2021 Dec 1. https://businesstech.co.za/news/business/543028/why-discovery-introduced-mandatory-vaccines-in-south-africa-and-why-some-workers-said-no/

Buthelezi L. (2021). Discovery Life will charge unvaccinated people more for new policies. 29 July 2021. https://www.news24.com/fin24/companies/discovery-life-will-charge-unvaccinated-people-more-for-new-policies-heres-why-20210729

Campos-Mercade P, Meier AN, Schneider FH, Meier S, Pope D, Wengström E. (2021). Monetary incentives increase COVID-19 vaccinations. *Science.* 2021 Nov 12;374(6569):879–882. doi: 10.1126/science.abm0475. Epub 2021 Oct 7. PMID: 34618594.

Cheadle H. (2021). Mandatory vaccine policies will survive a constitutional challenge. *The Daily Maverick.* 2021 November 10. https://www.dailymaverick.co.za/article/2021-11-10-mandatory-vaccine-policies-will-survive-a-constitutional-challenge-legal-expert-halton-cheadle/

Community Preventive Services Task Force. (2016). Increasing appropriate vaccination: vaccination requirements for childcare, school and college attendance. https://www.thecommunityguide.org/sites/default/files/assets/Vaccination-Requirements-for-Attendance_1.pdf

Constitution of the Republic of South Africa. No 108 of 1996. https://www.gov.za/sites/default/files/images/a108-96.pdf

Cooper S, van Rooyen H, Wiysonge CS. (2021). COVID-19 vaccine hesitancy in South Africa: how can we maximize uptake of COVID-19 vaccines? *Expert Rev Vaccines*. 2021 Aug;20(8):921–933. doi: 10.1080/14760584.2021.1949291. Epub 2021 Jul 12. PMID: 34252336.

Crisp N. (2022). Acting Deputy Director General. Department of Health. Cape Talk Radio interview with John Maytham. 2022 February 8. https://lifepodcasts.fm/podcasts/144-afternoon-drive-with-john-maytham/episode/598632-the-sinopharm-roll-out

Davies MA. (2020). HIV and risk of COVID-19 death: a population cohort study from the Western Cape Province, South Africa. *medRxiv* [Preprint]. 2020 Jul 3:2020.07.02.20145185. doi: 10.1101/2020.07.02.20145185. PMID: 32637972; PMCID: PMC7340198. https://pubmed.ncbi.nlm.nih.gov/32637972/

Department of Employment and Labour. (2021). Employment and Labour Minister issues new direction with regard to vaccination in the workplace. https://www.labour.gov.za/employment-and-labour-minister-issues-new-direction-with-regard-to-vaccination-in-the-workplace

Department of Health. (2021). Strategies to address COVID-19 vaccine hesitancy and promote acceptance in South Africa. https://sacoronavirus.co.za/2021/04/12/strategies-to-address-covid-19-vaccine-hesitancy-and-promote-acceptance-in-south-africa/

de Vos P. (2021a). The Government could and should compel vaccinations in South Africa for the greater good. *The Daily Maverick*. 2021 February 7. https://www.dailymaverick.co.za/opinionista/2021-02-07-the-government-could-and-should-compel-vaccinations-in-south-africa-for-the-greater-good/

de Vos P. (2021b). The law and the greater good: why I support a COVID-19 vaccine requirement at UCT. *The Daily Maverick*. 2021 September 15. https://www.dailymaverick.co.za/article/2021-09-15-the-law-and-the-greater-good-why-i-support-a-covid-19-vaccine-requirement-at-uct-part-two/

Dorabawila V, Hoefer D, Bauer UE, Bassett MT, Lutterloh E, Rosenberg ES. Effectiveness of the BNT162b2 vaccine among children 5–11 and 12–17 years in New York after the Emergence of the Omicron Variant. *medRxiv* 2022.02.25.22271454; doi: 10.1101/2022.02.25.22271454

Douaud G, Lee S, Alfaro-Almagro F. et al. (2022). SARS-CoV-2 is associated with changes in brain structure in UK Biobank. *Nature*. doi: 10.1038/s41586-022-04569-5

Dwyer J. (2022). Pandemic Individualism. *Impact Ethics*. 2022 February 3 https://impactethics.ca/2022/02/03/pandemic-individualism/

Ebrahim Z. More than 90% of hospital deaths in the 4th wave are unvaccinated. IOL. 2021, Dec, 17. https://www.news24.com/health24/medical/infectious-diseases/coronavirus/covid-19-more-than-90-of-hospital-deaths-in-4th-wave-are-in-unvaccinated-partially-vaccinated-people-20211217

Emanuel EJ, Wendler D, Killen J, Grady C. (2004). What Makes Clinical Research in Developing Countries Ethical? The Benchmarks of Ethical Research, *The Journal of Infectious Diseases*. 189(5):930–937, doi: 10.1086/381709Top of Form

Farber T. (2022). Nearly 300 000 dead from COVID-19 in South Africa. *Sunday Times.* https://www.timeslive.co.za/sunday-times/news/2022-02-13-nearly-300000-dead-from-covid-19-in-sa--and-the-threat-is-not-over/

Freer J, Mudaly V. (2022). HIV and COVID-19 in South Africa. *BMJ* 2022; 376:e069807 doi: 10.1136/bmj-2021–069807 https://www.bmj.com/content/376/bmj-2021-069807

Gore A. (2021). Why we are mandating vaccines for Discovery's SA based employees. *Business Day*, 2021 September 6. https://www.businesslive.co.za/bd/opinion/2021-09-05-adrian-gore-why-we-are-mandating-vaccines-for-discoverys-sa-based-employees/Bottom of Form

Hassan F. (2020). The Great COVID-19 vaccine heist. *The Daily Maverick*. https://www.dailymaverick.co.za/article/2020-12-06-the-great-covid-19-vaccine-heist/

Hillis SD, Unwin HJT, Chen Y, Cluver L, Sherr L, Goldman PS, et al. (2021). Global minimum estimates of children affected by COVID-19-associated orphanhood and deaths of caregivers: a modelling study. *The Lancet.* 398(10298): 391–402. doi: 10.1016/S0140-6736(21)01253-8

Johnson AG, Amin AB, Ali AR, Hoots B, Cadwell BL, Arora S, et al. (2021). COVID-19 Incidence and Death Rates Among Unvaccinated and Fully Vaccinated Adults with and Without Booster Doses During Periods of Delta and Omicron Variant Emergence — 25 U.S. Jurisdictions, April 4–December 25, 2021. MMWR Morb Mortal Wkly Rep 2022; 71: 132–138. doi: 10.15585/mmwr.mm7104e2external icon

Kahn T. (2021). COVID-19 shots from Serum Institute of India. *Business Day.* 21 January 2021, https://www.businesslive.co.za/bd/national/health/2021-01-21-exclusive-sa-paying-huge-premium-for-covid-19-shots-from-serum-institute-of-india/

Klüver H, Hartmann F, Humphreys M, et al. (2021). Incentives can spur COVID-19 vaccination uptake. *Proceedings of the National Academy of Sciences.* 118(36): e2109543118; doi: 10.1073/pnas.2109543118; https://www.pnas.org/content/118/36/e2109543118 (accessed 10 September 2021)

Lin DY, Gu Y, Wheeler B, Young H, Holloway S, Sunny SK, Moore Z, Zeng D. Effectiveness of COVID-19 Vaccines over a 9-Month Period in North Carolina. *N Engl J Med.* (2022). Mar 10;386(10):933–941. doi: 10.1056/NEJMoa2117128. Epub 2022 Jan 12. PMID: 35020982; PMCID: PMC8781317.

Luke D. (2021). Tourists won't be back in South Africa anytime soon – and fears of travel bans hurt tourism industry in the long run. *Business Insider.* https://www.businessinsider.co.za/south-africa-travel-bans-hurt-tourism-industry-in-the-long-run-2021-12

Madhi S. (2021). Results from Novavax vaccine trials in the UK and South Africa differ: why and does it matter? https://theconversation.com/results-from-novavax-vaccine-trials-in-the-ukand-south-africa-differ-why-and-does-it-matter-154293

Makhafola G. (2021). UFS joins Wits and UWC in implementing vaccine mandates for staff students on campus. *News24.* 2021. https://www.news24.com/news24/southafrica/news/ufs-joins-wits-and-uwc-in-implementing-vaccine-mandate-for-staff-students-on-campus-20211127

Malan M. (2022). Wait, donate, demolish: Why millions of SA's vaccines will never be used. Bhekisisa. 2022 February 25. https://bhekisisa.org/health-news-south-africa/2022-02-25-wait-donate-demolish-why-millions-of-sas-vaccines-will-never-be-used/

Mayosi BM, Lawn JE, van Niekerk A, Bradshaw D, Abdool Karim SS, Coovadia HM (2012). Lancet South Africa team. Health in South Africa: changes and challenges since 2009. *Lancet*. 2012 Dec 8;380(9858):2029–43. doi: 10.1016/S0140–6736(12)61814-5. Epub 2012 Nov 30. PMID: 23201214 https://pubmed.ncbi.nlm.nih.gov/23201214/.

Medical Brief. (2022). CCMA again rules in favour of employers over mandatory vaccinations. 2022 February 2. https://www.medicalbrief.co.za/ccma-again-rules-in-favour-of-employers-over-mandatory-vaccinations/

Medical Brief. (2022). Solidarity's urgent application to stop vaccine mandate dismissed by labour court. 2022 February 9. https://www.medicalbrief.co.za/solidaritys-urgent-application-to-stop-vaccine-mandate-dismissed-by-labour-court/

Mendelsohn AS, de SA A, Morden E, Botha B, Boulle A, Paleker M, et al. (2021). COVID-19 wave 4 in Western Cape Province, South Africa: Fewer hospitalisations, but new challenges for a depleted workforce. *SAMJ*, [S.l.], dec. 2021. ISSN 2078–5135. Available at: http://www.samj.org.za/index.php/samj/article/view/13484.

Mendelsen, M, Nel J, Blumberg J, Madhi S, Dryden M, Stevens W, et al. (2020). Long-COVID: An evolving problem with an extensive impact. *SAMJ*, [S.l.], 111(1): 10–12, Nov. 2020. ISSN 2078–5135. http://www.samj.org.za/index.php/samj/article/view/13141. doi: 10.7196/SAMJ.2020.v111i11.15433.

Meterlerkamp T. (2022). South Africa's fourth wave is waning but don't celebrate just yet say experts. *The Daily Maverick*. 2022 Jan 18. https://www.dailymaverick.co.za/article/2022-01-18-south-africas-fourth-wave-is-waning-but-dont-celebrate-just-yet-say-experts/

Mills MC, Ruttenauer T. (2021). The effect of mandatory COVID-19 certificates on vaccine uptake: synthetic-control modelling of six countries. *The Lancet Public Health*. 7(1): E15–E22. doi: 10.1016/S2468-2667(21)00273-5

Mkhize Z. (2021). Media Statement: The Minister of Health, Dr Zweli Mkhize, is pleased to announce that the sale of the Astra Zeneca vaccines that we had acquired has been concluded. Twitter, 21 March 2021. https://twitter.com/DrZweliMkhize/status/1373647784625238023

Moodley K. (2020). Tough Choices about who gets access: the ethical principles guiding South Africa. The Conversation, April 2020 https://theconversation.com/tough-choices-about-who-gets-icu-access-the-ethical-principles-guiding-south-africa-135227

Moodley K. (2021). Why COVID-19 Vaccines should be mandatory in South Africa. The Conversation. August 10. https://theconversation.com/why-covid-19-vaccines-should-be-mandatory-in-south-africa-165682

Moodley K. (2022). The ethics behind mandatory COVID-19 vaccination post-Omicron: the South African context. *South African Journal of Science*. 118(5/6). doi: 10.17159/sajs.2022/13239

Moodley K. (2021). Vaccine mandates in South Africa: where are they most needed? *The Conversation*. 2021 December 7. https://theconversation.com/vaccine-mandates-in-south-africa-where-are-they-most-needed-173253

Moodley K. (2021). COVID-19: 'A pandemic of the unvaccinated'? – compassion fatigue among healthcare professionals in South Africa. *SAMJ*, [S.l.]. 111(11): 1040–1041, Oct. 2021. ISSN 2078–5135. Available at: http://www.samj.org.za/index.php/samj/article/view/13398

Moodley K, Rossouw T. (2021). What could fair allocation of an efficacious COVID-19 vaccine look like in South Africa? *Lancet Global Health.* 9(February). doi: 10.1016/S2214-109X(20)30474-5

Moodley K. (2022). Vaccine inequity is unethical. *Nature Human Behaviour.* 6:168–169. doi: 10.1038/s41562-022-01295-w.

Moghadas SM, Vilches TN, Zhang K, Wells CR, Shoukat A, Singer BH, Meyers LA, Neuzil KM, Langley JM, Fitzpatrick MC, Galvani AP. (2021). The Impact of Vaccination on Coronavirus Disease 2019 (COVID-19) Outbreaks in the United States. *Clin Infect Dis.* Dec 16; 73(12): 2257–2264. doi: 10.1093/cid/ciab079. PMID: 33515252; PMCID: PMC7929033.

Muhumuza R. (2021). In Africa, vaccine hesitancy adds to slow rollout of doses. https://apnews.com/article/world-news-public-health-health-kampala-coronavirus-vaccine-7ca6c2cfb013174cf3faa35904fc7c26

Nachega JB, Sam-Agudu NA, Machekano RN, et al. (2022). Assessment of clinical outcomes among children and adolescents hospitalized with COVID-19 in 6 Sub-Saharan African countries. *JAMA Pediatr.* Published online January 19, 2022. doi: 10.1001/jamapediatrics.2021.6436 https://jamanetwork.com/journals/jamapediatrics/fullarticle/2788373

Ngqakamba S. (2021). 'Compassion fatigue': Mpumalanga doctor refuses to see unvaccinated patients. *News24,* 2021 September 7. https://www.news24.com/news24/southafrica/news/compassion-fatigue-mpumalanga-doctor-refuses-to-see-unvaccinated-patients-20210907

News24. (2021). 'Malawi to destroy 16 000 expired COVID-19 vaccines', (14 April 2021). https://www.news24.com/news24/africa/news/malawi-to-destroy-16-000-expired-covid-19-vaccines20210414.

Polack FP, Thomas SJ, Kitchin N, Absalon J, Gurtman A, Lockhart S, et al. (2020). Safety and Efficacy of the BNT162b2 mRNA COVID-19 Vaccine. *N Engl J Med.* 2020 Dec 31; 383(27): 2603–2615. doi: 10.1056/NEJMoa2034577. Epub 2020 Dec 10. PMID: 33301246; PMCID: PMC7745181. https://pubmed.ncbi.nlm.nih.gov/33301246/

Porteous R. (2021). AstraZeneca's COVID vaccine no-profit pledge rings hollow. *Mail and Guardian.* 2021. https://mg.co.za/health/2021-01-21-astrazenecas-covid-vaccine-no-profit-pledge-ringshollow/

Rappeport A. (2021). The Biden administration wants states and cities to pay people $100 to get vaccinated. 29 July 2021 https://www.nytimes.com/2021/07/29/us/politics/100-dollars-covid-vaccine-biden.html

Republic of South Africa. National Health Act 61 of 2003. https://www.gov.za/documents/national-health-act

Republic of South Africa. Disaster Management Act, 2002. Declaration of a National State of Disaster. Government Gazette No. 43096:313. 15 March 2020. https://www.gov.za/sites/default/files/gcis_document/202004/43217gon457s.pdf

Schröder-Bäck P, Duncan P, Sherlaw W, et al. (2014). Teaching seven principles for public health ethics: towards a curriculum for a short course on ethics in public health programmes. *BMC Med Ethics.* 15: 73. doi: 10.1186/1472-6939-15-73

Stellenbosch University. (2021). Have your say about intended vaccine rule. 2021 December 8. https://www.sun.ac.za/english/Lists/news/DispForm.aspx?ID=8810

Takuva S, Takalani A, Seocharan I, Yende-Zuma N, Reddy T, Engelbrecht I, et al. (2021). Safety of the single-dose Ad26.CoV2.S vaccine among healthcare workers in the phase 3b Sisonke study in South Africa. *medRxiv* 2021.12.20.21267967; doi: 10.1101/2021.12.20.21267967

Tshikalange S. (2021). Low wastage of covid-19 vaccines in Gauteng at 0.12%. *Timeslive*. 2021 July https://www.timeslive.co.za/news/south-africa/2021-07-07-low-wastage-of-covid-19-vaccines-in-gauteng-at-012/

TheCitizen.(2021).COVIDvaccineswasted-Gauteng2021November16https://www.citizen.co.za/news/covid-19/2909983/3636-covid-vaccines-wasted-gauteng/

United Nations, Economic and Social Council, Siracusa Principles on the Limitations and Derogation of Provisions in the International Covenant on Civil and Political rights. UN Doc. E/CN.4/1985/4(1985) https://www.refworld.org/pdfid/4672bc122.pdf

University of Cape Town. (2022). Call for comment on draft UCT vaccine mandate policy. 2022 December 21. https://www.news.uct.ac.za/article/-2021-12-20-call-for-comment-on-draft-uct-vaccine-mandate-policy

USAID. (2021). Using private sector approaches to amplify COVID-19 vaccine communications. https://www.usaid.gov/southern-africa-regional/news/applying-private-sector-approaches-amplify-covid-19-vaccine-communications-27

Venter WDF, Madhi SA, Nel J, Mendelson M, van den Heever A, Moshabela M. (2021). South Africa should be using all the COVID-19 vaccines available to it – urgently. *South Africa Medical Journal*. : 1–3. http://www.samj.org.za/index.php/samj/article/view/13238

Watkins D. (2021). Pope Francis urges people to get vaccinated against COVID-19. *Vatican News*. https://www.vaticannews.va https://www.vaticannews.va/en/pope/news/2021-08/pope-francis-appeal-covid-19-vaccines-act-of-love.html

Wang L, Berger NA, Kaelber DC, Davis PB, Volkow ND, Xu R. (2022). COVID infection severity in children under 5 years old before and after Omicron emergence in the US. doi: 10.1101/2022.01.12.22269179

Western Cape Department of Health. COVID-19 Dashboard https://coronavirus.westerncape.gov.za/vaccine-dashboard

World Health Organisation. International health Regulations. https://www.who.int/health-topics/international-health-regulations#tab=tab_1

Wynia MK, Harter TD, Eberl JT. (2021). Why a universal COVID-19 vaccine mandate is ethical today. 2021. *Health Affairs Blog*. https://www.healthaffairs.org/do/10.1377/hblog20211029.682797/full/

Xie Y, Xu E, Bowe B. et al. (2022). Long-term cardiovascular outcomes of COVID-19. *Nature Medicine*. doi: 10.1038/s41591-022-01689-3

Zimmerman RK. (2021). Helping patients with ethical concerns about COVID-19 vaccines in light of fetal cell lines used in some COVID-19 vaccines. *Vaccine*. 39(31): 4242–4244. doi: 10.1016/j.vaccine.2021.06.027 https://www.ncbi.nlm.nih.gov/pmc/articles/PMC8205255/

8 Police legitimacy and the SAPS's policing of the COVID-19 pandemic

Guy Lamb

Introduction

In 2020 and 2021, the SAPS featured prominently in the South African government's response to the COVID-19 pandemic. That is, the SAPS were the principal government agency responsible for the execution of many of the COVID-19 mitigation regulations relating to public spaces (especially during the periods of 'hard' lockdown). The police were also required to quell protest action, criminality, and collective violence that was associated with the pandemic and government's efforts to contain it. The government's decisive response to pandemic in March 2020 did initially receive considerable praise (Stiegler & Bouchard, 2020). However, there was extensive criticism of how the police in South Africa pursued their mandate, with available research indicating that the SAPS had been overly reliant on the use of force in their efforts to maintain order and compel South Africans to comply with the COVID-19 regulations throughout 2020 and 2021 (Lamb, 2022; Langa & Leopeng, 2020).

The South African situation was not unique as studies of police work during the height of the COVID-19 pandemic in many other countries have indicated that the police were expected to implement unpopular measures that restricted population movement and social interaction. These circumstances, ultimately led to police behaviours that impacted police-community relations both negatively and positively, especially police legitimacy (Maskály, Ivković, & Neyroud, 2021). As noted by Laufs and Waseem (2020:4), 'effective police responses to public crises can put people out of harm's way and ensure public safety and well-being, [but] ineffective police response can undermine public trust and confidence in the police'.

In Australia, assertive police practices in relation to COVID-19 controls have been linked to a weakening of police legitimacy (Mazerolle & Ransley, 2021). In Nigeria, it has been suggested that lockdown measures created new opportunities for police corruption (Onuoha, Ezirim, & Onuh, 2021). In Pakistan, insufficient police leadership resulted in rank-and-file police using informal methods of policing and more regularly resorting to the excessive use of force in an attempt to compel populations to adhere to COVID-19

DOI: 10.4324/9781003294931-8

control regulations (Waseem, 2021). Conversely, in New Zealand, it has been suggested that an empathetic (Jones, 2020) and consistent policing approach combined with widespread community buy-in (Deckert et al., 2021) towards the implementation of COVID-19 controls adopted by the New Zealand Police, reinforced police legitimacy.

This chapter will analyse the relationship between the actions of the SAPS during the height of the COVID-19 pandemic and police legitimacy in 2020 and 2021. It will build on my earlier work on police legitimacy in South Africa (Lamb, 2021a), which demonstrated that between 1994 and 2020 SAPS personnel engaged in behaviours that often eroded public trust in the police. Apparently, South African communities, especially in socioeconomically disadvantaged areas, regularly experienced indifference, low levels of professionalism, and incompetence from the police. In addition, it was shown that trust in the police, and subsequently police legitimacy, had been further undermined by pervasive corruption within the SAPS, and militarised approaches to police work which had resulted in numerous incidents of excessive use of force (Lamb, 2021a:102–103). As with my previous work on police legitimacy, select aspects of the 'trust-diminishing' police behaviours framework constructed by Goldsmith (2005) will be used to analyse the SAPS's approach to policing during the COVID-19 pandemic.

The police and legitimacy

In democracies, a central element of police work is that of *policing by consent*, which in basic terms is an arrangement where citizens collectively assign some of the responsibilities for law enforcement and the maintenance of social order to the police, and thereafter not only recognise the authority of the police to take such action in the interests of public safety, but also recognise the common obligation to obey the police (Jones et al., 1996; Reiner, 2010). Moreover, such an understanding infers that populations recognise that the police have the power to use force within the confines of the law. Such consent is derived and sustained by public trust in the police where the police and their actions are regarded as being legitimate by the people that they are mandated to serve (Tyler, 2004). However, such legitimacy is typically dependent on the nature of the police's institutional culture (Terrill, Paoline, & Gau, 2016), and on whether the police are regarded by communities as being fair and just, combined with the nature of social order at the local level (Bradford, Jackson, & Hough, 2013; Macdonald & Stokes, 2006).

Studies on police legitimacy have demonstrated that police legitimacy can have a positive influence on police effectiveness (Tankebe, 2013; Tyler, 2004). That is, it can lead to closer social relations between the police and communities, especially in situations where police and community members actively collaborate to address problems that contribute to criminal offending (Kääriäinen & Sirén, 2011; Morgan & Newburn, 1997), and where there is transparency and accountability in terms of police actions (Kochel & Skogan, 2021). In addition, police legitimacy can result in an improved commitment to the rule of law by populations and an increased inclination of ordinary people to cooperate with the police and report crime (Hough et al., 2010). Nonetheless, as noted by Herbert (2006), police legitimacy is often a site of contestation between the public and the police, as in some contexts, the enforcement of the law (and perceptions thereof) by the police may alienate certain populations groups.

Goldsmith (2005) has identified ten 'trust-diminishing' behaviours that have been exhibited by the police in various environments which have to potential to weaken police legitimacy. These behaviours are as follows: Neglect, indifference, incompetence, petty corruption, extortion, discrimination, inconsistency, intimidation, excessive force, and brutality. Subsequent studies of police legitimacy have reaffirmed the negative impact that these 'trust-diminishing' police behaviours have had on police legitimacy, especially coercive police practices (Bayley, 1995; Tyler, Jackson, & Mentovich, 2015; Zoorob, 2020), police militarisation (Jones, 2020; Mummolo, 2018) and corruption (Jackson et al., 2014; Reisig & Lloyd, 2009). With a view to assessing the impact of the SAPS's policing of COVID-19 control and containment measures in 2020 and 2021 on police legitimacy in South Africa, this chapter will use Goldsmith's framework to describe and discuss the actions and behaviour of members of the SAPS with a particular focus on the excessive use of force by police personnel and corruption amongst the police.

The SAPS and its police work

The SAPS was established through the South African Police Service Act (No. 68 of 1995) with the mandate to guarantee the safety and security and uphold the fundamental Constitutional rights of everyone in South Africa, as well as closely cooperate with crime-affected communities (Republic of South Africa, 1995). Currently, there are close to 145,000 sworn SAPS officials, which represents a police-population ratio of 1:413 (South African Police Service, 2022), with the police consistently receiving one of the largest allocations of total government spending compared to most other departments annually (National Treasury, 2021).

The SAPS has retained considerable hierarchical and militarised legacies from the colonial and apartheid periods in South Africa with police work being commanded in a top-down manner from the SAPS Headquarters in Pretoria through a system of provincial and cluster structures to the station level. Military-style personnel ranking, terminology, operational strategies, and practices have been used by the police (Altbeker, 2009). There were superficial attempts to demilitarise the police in the late-1990s, but such labours were short-lived as elevated violent crime levels and declining public confidence in the police resulted in the SAPS adopting the National Crime Combatting Strategy (NCCS) in 2000 and framing police work in a context of a 'war on crime' (Steinberg, 2014). The SAPS have pursued community policing approaches through community policing forums in more than 1 100 police station areas, but in reality, these efforts have largely been undertaken in support of the SAPS's overall martial policing orientation (Benit-Gbaffou, Fourchard, & Wafer, 2012; Pelser, 2000), and the SAPS, in numerous statements to the media has regularly bemoaned the inadequate cooperation from residents in high-crime areas.

These developments resulted in the repurposing of apartheid-era styles of belligerent policing in an attempt by the police leadership to stabilise crime levels and leverage greater public support for the police, especially from the early 2000s (Lamb, 2018). A key strategy was the use of high-density operations, which typically takes the form of saturating targeted areas with police (and sometimes includes soldiers), followed by roadblocks, robust interactions with residents, and mass arrests of those regarded as having broken the law (Steinberg, 2014). In such operations and well as with respect to police responses to protests and labour strikes, police personnel were frequently implicated in the excessive use of force, particularly between 2008 and 2018, which undermined police legitimacy (Lamb, 2022).

South Africa's stark income inequalities are mirrored in its policing practices and resource allocation as wealthier areas with relatively lower levels of crime have received a disproportionately greater share of police capital (Redpath & Nagla-Luddy, 2015). This in turn has further entrenched existing disparities in relation to poverty, inequality, and criminality (Samara, 2003). The quality of service provided by the SAPS has also been unequal across policing areas, with there being lower levels of police performance combined with more forceful policing actions in poorer areas (Hornberger, 2013). Added to this, key categories of violent crimes, such as murder, attempted murder, and robbery (with aggravated circumstances) have increased by more than 20% between 2010/11 and 2020/21 (South African Police Service, 2021a). Such a situation has, according to IPSOS data, negatively affected public sentiment in terms of whether South Africans feel that the police have adequately responded to crime, with there being a decline in positive perceptions from 43% in 2010 to 33% in 2019 (IPSOS, 2021).

There is consensus among policing scholars focusing on South Africa that corruption within the South African Police Service (SAPS) has been endemic and systemic since its inception in the mid-1990s, with anti-corruption strategies generally being regarded as ineffective (Faull, 2007; Kutnjak Ivković & Sauerman, 2015; Newham, 2002; Newham & Faull, 2011). Such corruption has been diverse in nature and has affected all levels of police work, such as the payment bribes by beat cops to 'look the other way'; the intentional loss of dockets by clerks and detectives in exchange for cash or gifts; police personnel illegally benefiting from SAPS procurement processes; and police collusion with organised criminal groups. The upper echelons of the SAPS leadership have also been embroiled in a series of corruption scandals, with four SAPS National Commissioners and at least three provincial commissioners having been removed from public office due to alleged corruption and improper behaviour since 2008. In 2018, Robert McBride, the head of the South African police watchdog, the Independent Police Investigative Directorate (IPID), stated in a verbal report to South Africa's Parliamentary Portfolio Committee on Police that the SAPS were being governed by a 'matrix of corruption', which had become the 'biggest threat to national security', as it had drastically eroded the ability of the police 'to contain serious and violent crime' (McBride, 2018). One basis of public opinion data, the 2019 Global Corruption Barometer reported that the SAPS was the most corrupt government institution in South Africa (AfroBarometer & Transparency International, 2019).

Combatting COVID-19: Stick with what you know

The rapid global spread of the COVID-19 pandemic in 2020 combined with the relatively short time that the South African police were given to prepare an implementation plan to compel the general population to comply with the lockdown regulations, meaning that the leaders and strategists responsible for policing ultimately resorted to using the SAPS's tried-and-tested area-based crime combatting strategy. More specifically, the SAPS's high-density policing approach became government's primary lockdown compliance strategy.

At the onset of the 'hard' lockdown period, the decision to apply existing crime-fighting strategies to enforce lockdown regulations appeared to be relatively rational on the part of government as there was considerable similarity between the crime-combatting approach that had been pursued by the government since the late-1990s and the public health approach to mitigating the spread of pandemics, as advocated by specialist epidemiologists and the South African Department of Health. That is, both the crime and pandemic control approaches entail surveillance and data analysis of a specific problem which is then used to identify problem hotspots or spatial clusters of infection/crime and thereafter targeted, area-specific containment and prevention measures are undertaken (Lessler et al., 2017; Sherman et al., 2014). Furthermore, the high-density template was familiar to police commanders and most operational personnel, which meant the security forces could be deployed in large numbers from the start of the 'hard' lockdown.

Combining the war on crime with a war on a virus

The SAPS has frequently used a war metaphor to describe its policing response to violent crime in general, but also in relation to how it intends to reduce levels of gender-based violence. Moreover, since the mid-1990s, government has also made considerable references to warfighting with respect to how it intends to deal with a range of societal and governance challenges, such as poverty, corruption, as well as drug and alcohol abuse. Such militaristic language has often been used as form of propaganda to convey to the public that government is taking these matters seriously and planning to devote resources towards resolving or 'defeating' the problem. However, a militaristic framing of a government's ideological approach to social control, and policing in particular, often emphasises 'the use of force and threat of violence as the most appropriate and efficacious means to solve problems' (Kraska, 2007:503).

The way the South African government designed and announced the national lockdown in March 2020 was a strong indication that its response to the pandemic would have a fundamental warlike framing. That is, the martial-sounding National Corona Virus Command Council was established in terms of the National Disaster Management Act (2002), with the policing of the lockdown regulations being mandated by the National Joint Operational and Intelligence Structure (NATJOINTS), which had previously adopted militaristic strategies to national crises (Lamb, 2022). Furthermore, during an address to SANDF soldiers in Johannesburg prior to their deployment to enforce the COVID-19 regulations, President Ramaphosa donned a SANDF uniform and declared, with reference to COVID-19: '[W]e will…wage a war against an invisible enemy'. Ramaphosa also made use of the war metaphor whilst addressing members of the G20 in late March 2020, in which the South African President stated: 'We have a disease spreading throughout the world. We must fight this common enemy. At war, it pays no benefit to fight among one another' (Meyer, 2020). Ramaphosa made frequent references to the war metaphor throughout the lockdown period, emphasising that a warlike response was essential for 'saving lives'.

There were clear signs at the onset of the lockdown period that government's warlike framing of its response to COVID-19 was not mere propaganda, in that the use of force, and the threat thereof, was envisaged to be the central mechanism through which the regulations would be enforced. For instance, investigative journalists reported that during the process of devising the lockdown regulations that some senior security force officials had advocated that security force officials be indemnified for their various actions during the lockdown period, even though such provisions would be unconstitutional (Daily Maverick, 2020). In addition, following 55 arrests for alleged violations within the first 24 hours of lockdown, the Minister of Police, Bheki Cele, who referred to the police as 'ground forces', warned in a press briefing:

> [W]hat is happening here is not the war against any citizen … It's a war against this enemy called Coronavirus. But whoever is breaking the law, whoever is not working with South Africa … is joining the enemy against the people of South Africa…If you don't walk with us then we will pull you to walk with us.

Furthermore, later in the press briefing (in response to a question from a journalist relating to the SAPS' alleged use of excessive force), Cele quipped: 'Oh, you believe they are using more force? Wait, wait until you see more force' (eNCA, 2020b). Concerns about government's militarised responses to containing the pandemic were raised publicly by various commentators and opposition political parties but government officials generally dismissed these concerns as overreactions. (Times Live, 2020).

In the days preceding the commencement of the 'hard' lockdown, it became evident that senior officials responsible for policing and justice were of the view that a key objective of the National Disaster regulations, other than 'saving lives', was the combatting of crime. For instance, on 20 March 2020, a joint media statement by the Minister of Police (Bheki Cele) and the Minister of Justice and Correctional Services (Ronald Lamola) categorically indicated that the 'enforcement' of these measures would be aligned to one of the SAPS' primary objectives, namely 'stamping the authority of the state' (Cele & Lamola, 2020). This objective dates back to the launch of Operation *Fiela*-Reclaim in 2015, which was borne out of concern by government that it lacked sufficient legitimacy and influence in many poor, high-crime areas. Within the space of a few weeks, the 'saving lives' imperative was de-emphasised and much of the discourse about the policing of lockdown increasingly highlighted the supposed crime reduction and compliance effects of these measures.

The NATJOINTS' implementation of the lockdown regulations was clearly primed for the crime-combatting approach to take precedence over infection mitigation. For instance, the SAPS, in a presentation to the Parliamentary Portfolio on Police on 29 April 2020, defined the State of National Disaster as a 'security measure' (South African Police Service, 2020b). In the same presentation, the police indicated that they would use some of their standard crime-fighting tools to enforce the lockdown regulations. That is, roadblocks at strategic points; and 'high visibility patrols' in spaces where the police envisaged that the probability of non-compliance were high, such as alcohol outlets (especially taverns and shebeens) and taxi ranks. Furthermore, the SAPS reported that their chief concern during the lockdown period had been 'instability related to job and food insecurity' and criminal offending, such as looting and theft (South African Police Service, 2020b). The implicit implication of this was that the police were viewing large sections of the South African population as being potentially criminal and that these individuals should be targets of aggressive forms of policing.

The dominance of the crime-combatting objective in the context of containing COVID-19 appeared to have been reinforced by the absence of clear and appropriate guidelines on how the police should implement the lockdown measures in line with South Africa's constitution; as well as inadequate and inconsistent communication from operational leaders to frontline police personnel about how to police pandemic controls. A series of interviews with police undertaken by the *Mail & Guardian* newspaper suggested that some police had resorted to familiar forms of belligerent policing during the lockdown period due to ambiguous messaging, frustration, and punitive views about policing. According to a public order police official:

There's confusion. They want us to keep the people off the street, by issuing fines. But then later, we are told to release them on a warning. And people then just go back out on the streets again. Police are frustrated, and then they become hard-handed.

Another SAPS official stated:

Police are going to do one of two things. They are either going to do nothing because they are confused. Or they are going to *moer* [assault] people. If I had my way, I say *moer* them. Police should be heavy with them.

(Kiewit, 2020)

The primacy of the crime-combatting purpose of lockdown for the police leadership was clearly demonstrated in the Minister of Police's address to SAPS members in Pretoria on 10 July 2020, when Minister Cele acknowledged the difficult circumstances under which the police had been working. No mention was made of 'saving lives', with the speech emphasising roadblocks, high-density operations, and arrests. Of critical importance, the Minister stated:

[C]rime remains your number one enemy. The emergence of COVID-19 means [that] you have to now guard against a second enemy – an invisible one. While the country is on Lockdown, we know that criminals are NOT going [to] 'STAY AT HOME' and they certainly will NOT be sympathetic towards us at this time. So, I call on all of you to continue to decisively deal with both the armed and unarmed enemy.

(Cele, 2020a)

Related to this, from late-April 2020 the Minister of Police began to actively celebrate a reduction in most categories of recorded violent crime, which was being attributed as a key success of the implementation of lockdown regulations. In July 2020, Minister Cele released the quarterly crime statistics and professed that this data demonstrated 'a never-seen-before rosy picture of a peaceful South Africa experiencing a crime holiday' (Waterworth & Chemaly, 2020). Indeed, the SAPS crime data for the period of 1 April to 30 June 2020 showed a significant reduction in most categories of violent crime throughout South Africa between 1 April and 30 June 2020 compared to the same period in previous years but increased again between 1 July and 30 September 2020. However, at the time of writing, it was unclear if these variances in reported criminal offending were directly related to the work of the security forces; or were due to other factors. This could have included: Reduced crime reporting as a result of South Africans being discouraged from visiting police stations; or individuals staying at home due to personal commitments towards preventing COVID-19 transmission rather than out of fear of being accosted and arrested by the police.

People don't listen

A core belief underpinning militaristic governance philosophes is that the general population should be disciplined, rule-abiding, and respectful of authority, and that non-compliant and disrespectful individuals and groups are deserving of punishment (Eastwood, 2018; Eckhardt, 1969; Skjelsbaek, 1979). The Minister of Police and other senior political leaders made frequent references to communities ignoring and defying the lockdown regulations, with Cele frequently stating: 'They do not listen'. In this regard, in an address to members of the security forces in Secunda (Mpumalanga) in early April 2020, Cele indicated that the police and military 'need to be not very kind (sic) to people that don't listen because they are a danger to themselves, and they are a danger to all of us' (eNCA, 2020a). He further stated:

> I hear them [people] crying those cops and soldiers are brutal. Not listening to us is brutality...if you do not want to protect yourself and the rest of us, we must start by protecting you...so we need to push a little bit.
>
> (eNCA, 2020a)

Militaristic beliefs about how South Africa should be governed have also been prevalent in South African society for decades. That is, there has been significant popular support for punitive measures against alleged lawbreakers. This, in turn, has contributed to an enabling environment where the excessive use of force by the police and other security agencies is tolerated by large segments of the South African population (Altbeker, 2007; Hornberger, 2013). Under lockdown, this situation was clearly illustrated in the findings of a survey conducted during April 2020 by Victory Research. The findings, which were based on responses from a representative national sample of 600 South Africans, specified that more than 50% of respondents supported the use of excessive force by the security forces, with 30% agreeing that it was appropriate to 'humiliate' those who did not comply with the lockdown regulations, with 16% indicating that the use of sjamboks in this regard was acceptable (Khumalo, 2020).

Teaching them a lesson

Between March and May 2020, there were numerous allegations of abuse, as well as distribution of video footage on social media of police personnel forcing people in various parts of South Africa to perform demeaning physical exercises such as push-ups, squats, and bunny hops. These exercises were allegedly used as a means of punishment for those persons allegedly not adhering to lockdown regulations, and for those who supposedly disregarded instructions from, and/or were disrespectful towards security force members (Bhengu, 2020; Stone, 2020).

Photographs and videos were circulated via social media platforms of police personnel using rubber rounds, plastic pipes, sjamboks, and in some cases, live ammunition against those suspected of violating the regulations (Reddy, 2020; Singh, 2020). The HSRC survey conducted during the period of 'hard' lockdown (8–24 April 2020) with more than 19,000 respondents found that 25% of the sample had interacted with law enforcement officials, of which more than half indicated that they had 'been treated badly and in a very rough/rude manner' (Human Sciences Research Council, 2020). The worst of the reported cases of excessive use of force by security force personnel generally took place in areas where levels of crime were high, and where the SAPS had previously pursued crackdown forms of policing. In total, between late March and early August 2020, the SAPS arrested and charged 298 252 people for lockdown-related violations, of which 181 579 were released on a warning to appear before a magistrates court, with close to 90% of these arrests taking place between late March and mid-May 2020 (SABC, 2020). Most of the cases related to 'residential-related offences', which in essence entailed persons apprehended by the SAPS that were outside of their places of residence allegedly in contravention of the lockdown regulations (South African Police Service, 2020b).

Civil society organisations and the Parliamentary Portfolio Committee on Police raised concerns about the reports of brutality meted out by the security forces. The United Nations (UN) Human Rights Office publicly expressed unease about the 'disproportionate use of force' by security force members, particularly in poorer areas (Karrim, 2020). The Independent Police Investigative Directorate (IPID) reported that it had investigated 194 cases of alleged excessive use of force by police officials between 26 March and 5 May 2020. This included: ten deaths due to police action; 79 cases of police discharging firearms; and 280 cases of assault. Furthermore, there had been a 32% increase in total cases investigated compared to the same period in 2019 (Independent Police Investigative Directorate, 2020).

In its report to parliament in May 2020, IPID highlighted some of the cases of alleged police brutality, three of which are summarised here. First, on 27 March 2020, a resident of Ravensmead (in Cape Town) was assaulted by SAPS personnel who apprehended the man allegedly purchasing alcohol in violation of lockdown regulations. The man died of a heart attack at his home shortly thereafter. On 1 April 2020, a man that had been arrested for purportedly not following lockdown regulations died in a police cell in Lenasia (in Johannesburg) as a result of sustaining serious injuries. Similarly, on 2 May 2020 in Folweni (in KwaZulu-Natal), two men walking home after drinking alcohol were assaulted by SAPS and SANDF personnel. One of the men subsequently died in the hospital from his injuries (Independent Police Investigative Directorate, 2020).

There were numerous media reports relating to other incidents of police use of excessive force in relation to enforcing lockdown regulations. In Yeoville (in Johannesburg), police fired rubber rounds in an attempt to get people seeking to gain entry into a supermarket to adhere to social distancing regulations (Burke, 2020). In Parkwood (in Cape Town), a community member accused police of stamping his head (Duval, 2020). In Fiksberg (Free State), a journalist was assaulted by police officials after he took a photograph of them (Evans, 2020). In KwaNobuhle (Eastern Cape), an elderly man was walking home with groceries when he was allegedly assaulted and shot at with rubber rounds by police. According to the victim: 'One of the cops standing behind me hit me with a rifle on my head and I fell down'. He shouted, 'We saw you [filming] us and don't talk when we talk' (Mbovane, 2020).

Between 1 and 31 May 2020, the National Coronavirus Command Council permitted ordinary people to leave their homes between 6 am and 9 am for the purposes of exercising. Beaches and parks however remained closed to the public. There were many reports of police acting in a hostile and overly strict manner with regard to the enforcement of the outdoor exercise regulations. A series of incidents in May 2020 in the coastal town of Muizenberg (Cape Town) demonstrated the nature of such overly punitive police behaviour. For example, a family was arrested because a father had entered the beach area to retrieve his 21-month-old daughter who had run onto the sand (Pijoos, 2020).

Large gatherings were not permitted by the National Disaster regulations for much of 2020. Nonetheless, there were various violent and non-violent protests (some of which related to access to food), as well as organised land invasions and community unrest. According to data collected by the Institute for Security Studies, there were 511 protest actions between 27 March and 31 July 2020 due to lockdown restrictions, frustrations relating to crime levels and labour issues (Mlamla, 2020). The police regularly emphasised that gatherings were illegal, and communicated that: 'The *forces* on the ground will not hesitate to take decisive action should people embark on unlawful conduct [unrest and protest action]' (South African Police Service, 2020a). As such, the police frequently responded to protests and collective law-breaking in an assertive and aggressive manner; and between 27 March and 21 August 2020, the SAPS reported that they had arrested 466 people for 'convening' an illegal gathering and another 299 persons for the destruction of property in the context of gatherings (Cele, 2020b).

COVID-19 corruption and the police

In many wealthy, middle and lower-income countries, there were reports of the weakening of anti-corruption measures, abuse of power by government offices, and extensive public and private sector corruption in relation to the procurement of COVID-19 containment resources, such as personal protective equipment (PPE) and materials (Steingrüber et al., 2020). Corruption did not only present a drain on the fiscus, available global studies on vaccination uptake have demonstrated that significant public corruption during the pandemic was correlated with higher COVID-19 risk (Yamen, 2021), related fatality rates (Farzanegan, 2021), and lower vaccination rates (Farzanegan & Hofmann, 2021).

South Africa, which had a recent history of grand-scale corruption and 'state capture' was acutely affected by COVID-related corruption (Mlambo & Masuku, 2020), especially in the health sector and within the SAPS (Corruption Watch, 2021; Heywood, 2021a). In September 2020, the National Treasury's COVID-19 Dashboard revealed that the SAPS had spent R1.56 billion on PPE, hand sanitisers, and disinfecting chemicals. *The Daily Maverick* reported that at least a third of this amount was paid to service providers under suspicious circumstances (Heywood, 2021b). To date, some cases relating to PPE corruption and certain SAPS officials have been before the courts, but these cases were still ongoing at the time of writing.

There were also various incidences of petty corruption amongst some police officials pertaining to violations of COVID-19 regulations and curfews. That is, some police personnel were implicated in the smuggling and illegal sale of alcoholic beverages during the periods of bans on the selling of alcohol (Nyembezi, 2020), as well as the solicitation of bribes in relation to alleged lockdown infringements and during police raids (Eyewitness News, 2021; Knoetze, 2020). There were also allegations of police personnel being responsible for the theft of food parcels that had been earmarked for poverty-stricken communities (Williams, 2020). The findings from research report produced by Corruption Watch indicated that SAPS personnel were regarded as the most corrupt type of government official during lockdown (Corruption Watch, 2020). Between 26 March and 22 April 2020, the Minister of Police reported that 89 SAPS personnel had been arrested for corruption-related offences (Rall, 2020), with the National Police Commissioner indicating on 4 November 2020 that a total of 257 police had been arrested for alleged corrupt activities in 2020 (BusinessTech, 2020).

The July 2021 'riots'

In July 2021, large parts of the KwaZulu-Natal province and some areas in Gauteng province in South Africa were affected by exceedingly high levels of public violence, unrest, and looting. The unrest also triggered a series of vigilante attacks, particularly in Phoenix, a suburb of the City of eThekwini. Three hundred and sixty people died during the episodes of violence. In addition, 161 shopping malls; 161 liquor outlets/distributors; 1,119 retail stores and various court buildings were vandalised and/or damaged. The Banking Industry Association reported that 310 bank branches and 1,227 automatic teller machines were vandalised or destroyed, with cash to the value of R119.4 million being stolen (South African Police Service, 2021b). The SAPS were overwhelmed, and the South African National Defence Force was deployed. It took a week for the authorities to stabilise the violence-affected areas.

These incidents of violence and criminality have been attributed to the COVID-19 lockdown regulations (and the economic and social implications thereof) combined with the consequences of largescale corruption by some commentators and reporters as these measures resulted in a substantial economic downturn, as well as a significant increase in unemployment and poverty (Meyer, 2021; Steinhauser & Aaisha Dadi Patel, 2021). However, no refutable evidence has been presented to date that directly linked the implementation of the COVID-19 regulations to this unrest. Rather, the growing body of evidence, including the findings of the Expert Panel established to investigate the unrest and assess the adequacy of the government's response showed that the violence had been ignited by factional battles within the African National Congress. This evidence however also showed that COVID-19 mitigation measures intensified existing risk factors for collective violence with this violence being largely attributable to the actions of violence entrepreneurs, inadequate intelligence, and weak policing on the part of SAPS (Africa, Sokupa, & Gumbi, 2021; Lamb, 2021b).

Conclusion: The impact of COVID-19 and lockdowns police legitimacy

In 2021 and 2022, trust in the SAPS amongst ordinary South Africans remained relatively low, despite there being popular backing for President Cyril Ramaphosa's leadership of government's pandemic response and significant support for the security forces' use of aggressive tactics to enforce the COVID-19 regulations (Human Sciences Research Council, 2020). That is, a survey conducted by the University of Johannesburg and the HSRC, based on a nationally representative sample of 5,800 respondents indicated that less than 50% of the population trusted both the SAPS and the SANDF (Bohler-Muller et al., 2020). Furthermore, the study revealed that only 30% of respondents were of the view that the SAPS 'were doing a good job' (University of Johannesburg & Human Sciences Research Council, 2020).

Police legitimacy was further undermined by the National Coronavirus Command Council's requirement that the police enforce several unpopular regulations, especially the prohibition on the sale of tobacco products and alcohol. Public trust in the police was also diminished due to numerous reports about police corruption. The scandals relating to PPE corruption and lockdown bribe-taking within the SAPS further undermined police legitimacy. However, police legitimacy suffered the most damage during the July 2021 'riots' as the SAPS appeared largely powerless to contain the violence and looting, with the Minister of Police stating during his testimony to the Human Rights Commission hearing on the unrest that it was

> his observation and considered opinion that there was no concerted and/ or integrated effort from SAPS Crime Intelligence Division, policing divisions, and top management to properly plan for and to address the unrest that eventually led to a week-long destruction, looting, insurrection and loss of life.

(Cele, 2022)

This was reinforced by various reports that SAPS Crime Intelligence had failed to detect the July 2021 unrest before it began due to infighting, ineptitude, and corruption (AmaShabalala, 2022; Nair, 2021).

References

Africa, S., Sokupa, S., & Gumbi, M. 2021. *Report of the Expert Panel into the July 2021 Civil Unrest*. Pretoria: The Presidency.

AfroBarometer, & Transparency International. 2019. *2019 Global Corruption Barometer*. Retrieved from https://images.transparencycdn.org/images/2019_GCB_Africa3. pdf

Altbeker, A. 2007. *A Country at War with Itself*. Johannesburg and Cape Town: Jonathan Ball.

Altbeker, A. 2009. The building of the new South African Police Service. In M. S. Hinton & T. Newburn (Eds.), *Policing Developing Democracies* (pp. 260–279). Abingdon: Routledge.

AmaShabalala, M. 2022. Thrown to the wolves: How intelligence and police failed SA during July riots. *Times Live, 7 February 2022*. Retrieved from https://www. timeslive.co.za/sunday-times-daily/politics/2022-02-07-thrown-to-the-wolves-how-intelligence-and-police-failed-sa-during-july-riots/

Bayley, D. 1995. Getting serious about police brutality. In P. C. Stenning (Ed.), *Accountability for criminal justice: Selected essays* (pp. 93–109). Buffalo, NY: University of Toronto Press.

Benit-Gbaffou, C., Fourchard, L., & Wafer, A. 2012. Local politics and the circulation of community security initiatives in johannesburg. *International Journal of Urban and Regional Research, 36*(5), 936–957.

Bhengu, C. 2020. Mzansi reacts to police & army 'brutality' during lockdown - 'they must respect the law'. *HeraldLive, 31 March*. Retrieved from https://www. heraldlive.co.za/news/2020-03-31-mzansi-reacts-to-police-army-brutality-during-lockdown-they-must-respect-the-law/

Bohler-Muller, N., Davids, Y. D., Roberts, B., & Bekker, M. 2020. Human rights remain essential during the Covid-19 crisis. *Daily Maverick, 5 May*. Retrieved from https://www.dailymaverick.co.za/article/2020-05-05-human-rights-remain-essential-during-the-covid-19-crisis/

Bradford, B., Jackson, J., & Hough, M. 2013. Police Legitimacy in Action: Lessons from Theory and Practice. In M. Reisig & R. Kane (Eds.), *The Oxford Handbook of Police and Policing*. Oxford: Oxford University Press.

Burke, J. 2020. South African police fire rubber bullets at shoppers amid lockdown. *The Guardian, 28 March*. Retrieved from https://www.theguardian.com/world/2020/ mar/28/south-africa-police-rubber-bullets-shoppers-covid-19-lockdown

BusinessTech. 2020. Hundreds of crooked cops in South Africa under investigation for corruption. *BusinessTech, 4 November*. Retrieved from https://businesstech.co.za/news/government/445728/ hundreds-of-crooked-cops-in-south-africa-under-investigation-for-corruption/

Cele, B. 2020a. *Minister of Police, General Bheki Cele address to SAPS members in Pretoria* Retrieved from https://www.saps.gov.za/newsroom/msspeechdetail.php?nid=26726

Cele, B. 2020b. Written Reply to Question 1928. *Internal Question Paper, No. 32–2020*.

Cele, B. 2022. *Minister of Police, General Bheki Cele's testimony to the Human Rights Commission hearings on the July 2021 civil unrest* (Vol. 21 February 2022). Retrieved from https://www.youtube.com/watch?v=HCfLPbAZ_z4

Cele, B. & Lamola, R. 2020. *Ministers Bheki Cele and Ronald Lamola on implementation of Coronavirus COVID-19 disaster management regulations.* Retrieved from https://www.gov.za/speeches/joint-statement-ministers-bheki-cele-and-ronald-lamola-occasion-implementation-coronavirus

Corruption Watch. 2020. *Analysis of Corruption Trends Report 2020.*

Corruption Watch. 2021. *Annual Report 2020.* Retrieved from https://www.corruptionwatch.org.za/wp-content/uploads/2021/05/Corruption-Watch-AR-2020-DBL-PG-20210324.pdf

Daily Maverick. 2020. South Africa: Be aware and beware of the rise of the securocrats. *Daily Maverick, 13 May.* Retrieved from https://www.dailymaverick.co.za/article/2020-05-13-south-africa-be-aware-and-beware-of-the-rise-of-the-securocrats/

Deckert, A., Long, N. J., Aikman, P. J., Appleton, N. S., Davies, S. G., Trnka, S.,... Tunufa'i, L. 2021. 'Safer communities... together'? Plural policing and COVID-19 public health interventions in Aotearoa New Zealand. *Policing and Society, 31*(5), 621–637.

Duval, M. 2020. Cops jumped on my head. *Daily Voice, 7 May.* Retrieved from https://www.dailyvoice.co.za/news/cops-jumped-on-my-head-47651487

Eastwood, J. 2018. Rethinking militarism as ideology: The critique of violence after security. *Security dialogue, 49*(1–2), 44–56.

Eckhardt, W. 1969. The factor of militarism. *Journal of Peace Research, 6*(2), 123–132.

eNCA. 2020a. Cele: Push them if they don't listen. *7 April.* Retrieved from https://www.enca.com/news/cele-push-them-if-they-dont-listen

eNCA. 2020b. *National Command Council give update on COVID-19 lockdown, 27 March.* Retrieved from https://www.youtube.com/watch?v=YLRCsndfpHg

Evans, J. 2020. 'That's when I realised I was going to get a hiding' - journalist on alleged ordeal with FS police. *News24, 17 May.* Retrieved from https://www.news24.com/news24/SouthAfrica/News/thats-when-i-realised-i-was-going-to-get-a-hiding-journalist-on-alleged-ordeal-with-fs-police-20200517

Eyewitness News. 2021. SAPS duo arrested after demanding bribes during a roadblock. *Eyewitness News, 21 July 2021.* Retrieved from https://ewn.co.za/2021/07/21/saps-duo-arrested-after-demanding-bribes-during-a-roadblock

Farzanegan, M. R. 2021. The effect of public corruption on COVID-19 fatality rate: A cross-country examination. *CESifo Working Paper.* Retrieved from https://ssrn.com/abstract=3805464

Farzanegan, M. R., & Hofmann, H. P. 2021. Effect of public corruption on the COVID-19 immunization progress. *Scientific Reports, 11*(1), 23423.

Faull, A. 2007. Corruption and the South African Police Service. A Review and Its Implications. *ISS occasional Papers, 150.*

Goldsmith, A. 2005. Police reform and the problem of trust. *Theoretical Criminology, 9*(4), 443–470.

Herbert, S. 2006. Tangled up in blue: Conflicting paths to police legitimacy. *Theoretical Criminology, 10*(4), 481–504.

Heywood, M. 2021a. Covid-19 corruption tops R14-billion but to bust criminals we need to drastically boost prosecution services and courts. *Daily Maverick,*

21 September 2021. Retrieved from https://www.dailymaverick.co.za/article/2021-09-21-covid-19-corruption-tops-r14-billion-but-to-bust-criminals-we-need-to-drastically-boost-prosecution-services-and-courts/

Heywood, M. 2021b. La Vie en Rose: A single Mpumalanga company robbed SAPS of hundreds of millions in Covid-19 PPE tender. *Daily Maverick, 20 September 2021.* Retrieved from https://www.dailymaverick.co.za/article/2021-09-20-la-vie-en-rose-a-single-mpumalanga-company-robbed-saps-of-hundreds-of-millions-in-covid-19-ppe-tender/

Hornberger, J. 2013. From general to commissioner to general—on the popular state of policing in South Africa. *Law & Social Inquiry, 38*(3), 598–614.

Human Sciences Research Council. 2020. *Preliminary Results of Lockdown Survey: 8–24 April 2020.* Retrieved from http://www.hsrc.ac.za/uploads/pageContent/11529/COVID-19%20MASTER%20SLIDES%2026%20APRIL%202020%20FOR%20MEDIA%20BRIEFING%20FINAL.pdf

Independent Police Investigative Directorate. 2020. *Presentation to the Joint Meeting of the PCP and SCSJ on Police Misconduct Cases, 8 May 2020.* Cape Town: Independent Police Investigative Directorate.

IPSOS. 2021. *IPSOS Government Performance Barometer.* Johannesburg: IPSOS.

Jackson, J., Asif, M., Bradford, B., & Zakria Zakar, M. 2014. Corruption and police legitimacy in Lahore, Pakistan. *The British Journal of Criminology, 54*(6), 1067–1088.

Jones, D. J. 2020. The potential impacts of pandemic policing on police legitimacy: Planning past the COVID-19 crisis. *Policing: A Journal of Policy and Practice, 14*(3), 579–586.

Kääriäinen, J., & Sirén, R. 2011. Trust in the police, generalized trust and reporting crime. *European Journal of Criminology, 8*(1), 65–81.

Karrim, A. 2020. UN Human Rights Office highlights 'toxic lockdown culture' in SA. *News24, 28 April.* Retrieved from https://www.news24.com/news24/SouthAfrica/News/un-human-rights-office-highlights-toxic-lockdown-culture-in-sa-20200428

Khumalo, J. 2020. South Africans are now gatvol of lockdown. *City Press, 26 April.* Retrieved from https://www.news24.com/citypress/special-report/covid-19_survey/support-for-lockdown-plummets-20200426

Kiewit, L. 2020. 'Frustrated' police resort to force. *Mail & Guardian Online, 2 April.* Retrieved from https://mg.co.za/news/2020-04-02-frustrated-police-resort-to-force/

Knoetze, D. 2020. Covid-19: Lockdown creates ripe pickings for corrupt police. *GroundUp, 15 APRIL 2020.* Retrieved from https://www.groundup.org.za/article/covid-19-lockdown-creates-ripe-pickings-corrupt-police/

Kochel, T. R., & Skogan, W. G. 2021. Accountability and transparency as levers to promote public trust and police legitimacy: Findings from a natural experiment. *Policing: An International Journal, 44*(6), 1046–1059.

Kraska, P. B. 2007. Militarization and policing—Its relevance to 21st century police. *Policing: A Journal of Policy and Practice, 1*(4), 501–513.

Kutnjak Ivković, S., & Sauerman, A. 2015. Threading the thin blue line: transition towards democratic policing and the integrity of the South African police service. *Policing and Society, 25*(1), 25–52.

Lamb, G. 2018. Police militarisation and the 'war on crime' in South Africa. *Journal of Southern African Studies, 44*(5), 933–949.

Lamb, G. 2021a. Safeguarding the republic? The South African police service, legitimacy and the tribulations of policing a violent democracy. *Journal of Asian and African Studies, 56*(1), 92–108.

Lamb, G. 2021b. Why have South Africans been on a looting rampage? Research offers insights. *The Conversation, 16 July 2021.* Retrieved from https://theconversation.com/why-have-south-africans-been-on-a-looting-rampage-research-offers-insights-164571

Lamb, G. 2022. *Policing and Boundaries in a Violent Society: A South African Case Study.* London: Routledge.

Langa, M., & Leopeng, B. B. 2020. COVID-19: Violent policing of black men during lockdown regulations in South Africa. *African Safety Promotion: A Journal of Injury and Violence Prevention, 18*(2), 116–126.

Laufs, J., & Waseem, Z. 2020. Policing in pandemics: A systematic review and best practices for police response to COVID-19. *International Journal of Disaster Risk Reduction, 51*, 101812.

Lessler, J., Azman, A. S., McKay, H. S., & Moore, S. M. 2017. What is a Hotspot Anyway? *The American Journal of Tropical Medicine and Hygiene, 96*(6), 1270–1273.

Macdonald, J., & Stokes, R. J. 2006. Race, social capital, and trust in the police. *Urban Affairs Review, 41*(3), 358–375.

Maskály, J., Ivković, S. K., & Neyroud, P. 2021. Policing the COVID-19 Pandemic: Exploratory study of the types of organizational changes and police activities across the globe. *International Criminal Justice Review, 31*(3), 266–285.

Mazerolle, L., & Ransley, J. 2021. Policing health regulations in democratic societies: A focus on COVID-19 challenges and opportunities in Australia. *International Journal of Comparative and Applied Criminal Justice, 45*(3), 315–327.

Mbovane, T. 2020. Resident alleges police beat and shot him for filming lockdown operation. *GroundUp, 17 April.* Retrieved from https://www.groundup.org.za/article/resident-plans-court-bid-against-police-he-alleges-assaulted-and-shot-him-filming-them/

McBride, R. 2018. IPID briefing to the parliamentary portfolio committee on police. *29 March.* Retrieved from https://pmg.org.za/committee-meeting/26095/

Meyer, D. 2020. Ramaphosa: 'Africa, world leaders united in war against coronavirus'. *The South African, 26 March 2020.* Retrieved from https://www.thesouthafrican.com/news/ramaphosa-coronavirus-african-union-g-20-lockdown-2020/

Meyer, D. 2021. Hungry, unemployed, and without hope: How corruption and COVID launched South Africa's riots. *Fortune, 14 July 2021.* Retrieved from https://fortune.com/2021/07/14/how-corruption-covid-launched-south-africa-riots-zuma-ramaphosa-rand/

Mlambo, V. H., & Masuku, M. M. 2020. Governance, corruption and COVID-19: he final nail in the coffin for South Africa's dwindling public finances. *Journal of Public Administration, 55*(3-1), 549–565.

Mlamla, S. 2020. Western Cape most plagued by protests since start of lockdown. *Cape Argus, 11 August.* Retrieved from https://www.iol.co.za/capeargus/news/western-cape-most-plagued-by-protests-since-start-of-lockdown-e95c5ec9-690e-4e7f-a3d7-78d9c7b04e2f

Morgan, R., & Newburn, T. 1997. *The Future of Policing.* New York: Oxford University Press.

Mummolo, J. 2018. Militarization fails to enhance police safety or reduce crime but may harm police reputation. *Proceedings of the National Academy of Sciences, 115*(37), 9181–9186.

Nair, N. 2021. SAPS had no intelligence of July unrest before violence erupted: Sitole. *HeraldLive, 30 November 2021.* Retrieved from https://www.herald-live.co.za/news/2021-11-30-saps-had-no-intelligence-of-july-unrest-before-violence-erupted-sitole/

National Treasury. 2021. *Adjusted Estimates of National Expenditure 2021.* Pretoria: National Trreasury.

Newham, G. 2002. *Tackling Police Corruption in South Africa.* Retrieved from http://www.csvr.org.za/docs/policing/tacklingpolicecorruption.pdf

Newham, G., & Faull, A. 2011. Protector or predator? Tackling police corruption in South Africa. *Institute for Security Studies Monographs, 182,* 1–64.

Nyembezi, N. 2020. 11 police officers in Eastern Cape fired for smuggling alcohol during Level 5 lockdown. *SABC News, 17 November 2020.* Retrieved from https://www.sabcnews.com/11-police-officers-in-eastern-cape-fired-for-smuggling-alcohol-during-level-5-lockdown/

Onuoha, F. C., Ezirim, G. E., & Onuh, P. A. 2021. Extortionate policing and the futility of COVID-19 pandemic nationwide lockdown in Nigeria: Insights from the South East Zone. *African Security Review, 30*(4), 451–472.

Pelser, E. 2000. An overview of community policing in South Africa. In I. Clegg, R. Hunt, & J. Whetton (Eds.), *Policy Guidance on Support to Policing in Developing Countries* (pp. 102–121). Swansea: Centre for Development Studies, University of Wales.

Pijoos, I. 2020. Police pounce as toddler runs on beach - family arrested and charged. *Times Live, 5 May.* Retrieved from https://www.timeslive.co.za/news/south-africa/2020-05-05-police-pounce-as-toddler-runs-on-beach-family-arrested-and-charged/

Rall, M. 2020. 89 police officers arrested for selling booze confiscated during lockdown raids. *The Mercury, 22 April.* Retrieved from https://www.iol.co.za/mercury/news/watch-89-police-officers-arrested-for-selling-booze-confiscated-during-lockdown-raids-47037261

Reddy, M. 2020. Police use sjamboks and rubber bullets to enforce Hillbrow lockdown. *Mail & Guardian Online, 31 March.* Retrieved from https://mg.co.za/article/2020-03-31-police-use-sjamboks-and-rubber-bullets-to-enforce-hill-brow-lockdown/

Redpath, J., & Nagla-Luddy, F. 2015. 'Unconscionable and irrational' SAPS human resource allocation. *South African Crime Quarterly, 53*(1), 15–26.

Reisig, M. D., & Lloyd, C. 2009. Procedural justice, police legitimacy, and help-ing the police fight crime: Results from a survey of Jamaican adolescents. *Police Quarterly, 12*(1), 42–62.

Republic of South Africa. 1995. *South African Police Service Act, 1995 (Act 68 of 1995).* Cape Town: Government Printer.

SABC. 2020. Almost 300 000 arrested for contravening lockdown regulations: Crime Stats. *SABC News, 14 August.* Retrieved from https://www.sabcnews.com/sabcnews/almost-300-000-arrested-for-contravening-lockdown-regulations-crime-stats/

Samara, T. R. 2003. State security in transition: The war on crime in post apartheid South Africa. *Social Identities, 9*(2), 277–312.

Sherman, L. W., Williams, S., Ariel, B., Strang, L. R., Wain, N., Slothower, M., & Norton, A. 2014. An integrated theory of hot spots patrol strategy: Implementing prevention by scaling up and feeding back. *Journal of Contemporary Criminal Justice, 30*(2), 95–122.

Singh, O. 2020. Durban cops use sjamboks and plastic pipes to enforce lockdown. *Times Live, 29 April*. Retrieved from https://www.timeslive.co.za/news/south-africa/2020-04-29-in-pics-durban-cops-use-sjamboks-and-plastic-pipes-to-enforce-lockdown/

Skjelsbaek, K. 1979. Militarism, its dimensions and corollaries: An attempt at conceptual clarification. *Journal of Peace Research, 16*(3), 213–229.

South African Police Service. 2020a. *Media Statement: Police on High Alert in Anticipation of Planned Public Violence Action*. Retrieved from https://www.saps.gov.za/newsroom/msspeechdetail.php?nid=27094

South African Police Service. 2020b. *Police Management of the National State of Disaster Lockdown. Presentation to the Parliamentary Portfolio Committee on Police, 29 April*. Retrieved from https://static.pmg.org.za/200429Presentation-_PCoP_COVID-19_Operational-_29_April_2020.pdf

South African Police Service. 2021a. *Annual Crime Statistics 2020/21*. Pretoria: South African Police Service.

South African Police Service. 2021b. *Briefing on the Extent of the Recent Civil Unrest in South Africa and Efforts to Mitigate the Impact of the COVID-19 Pandemic within the Department to the Select Committee on Security and Justice, 13 August 2021*.

South African Police Service. 2022. *South African Police Service Annual Report 2020/21*. Pretoria: South African Police Service.

Steinberg, J. 2014. Policing, state power, and the transition from apartheid to democracy: A new perspective. *African Affairs, 113*(451), 173–191.

Steingrüber, S., Kirya, M., Jackson, D., & Mullard, S. 2020. Corruption in the time of COVID-19: A double-threat for low income countries. *U4 Anticorruption Resource Center. U4 Brief, 6*. Retrieved from https://www.u4.no/publications/corruption-in-the-time-of-covid-19-a-double-threat-for-low-income-countries

Steinhauser, G., & Aaisha Dadi Patel, A. D. 2021. South Africa's Looting, Violence Reflect Inequalities Exacerbated by Covid-19 Pandemic. *Wall Street Journal, 13 July 2021*. Retrieved from https://www.wsj.com/articles/south-africas-looting-violence-reflect-inequalities-exacerbated-by-covid-19-pandemic-11626189253

Stiegler, N., & Bouchard, J.-P. 2020. South Africa: Challenges and successes of the COVID-19 lockdown. *Annales Médico-psychologiques, Revue Psychiatrique, 178*(7), 695–698.

Stone, J. 2020. Push Ups And Squats – Soweto Residents Punished For Ignoring Lockdown. *2OceansVibe, 30 March*. Retrieved from https://www.2oceansvibe.com/2020/03/30/push-ups-and-squats-soweto-residents-punished-for-ignoring-lockdown-videos/#ixzz6fvd73S61

Tankebe, J. 2013. Viewing things differently: The dimensions of public perceptions of police legitimacy. *Criminology, 51*(1), 103–135.

Terrill, W., Paoline, E. A., & Gau, J. M. 2016. Three pillars of police legitimacy: Procedural justice, use of force, and occupational culture. In M. Deflem (Ed.), *The Politics Of Policing: Between Force And Legitimacy* (pp. 59–76). Bingley: Emerald Group Publishing Limited.

Times Live. 2020. 'Nothing wrong' with Cyril Ramaphosa wearing military uniform: Defence minister. *Times Live, 27 March*. Retrieved from https://www.

timeslive.co.za/news/south-africa/2020-03-27-nothing-wrong-with-cyril-ramaphosa-wearing-military-uniform-defence-minister/

Tyler, T. R. 2004. Enhancing police legitimacy. *The Annals of the American Academy of Political and Social Science, 593*(1), 84–99.

Tyler, T. R., Jackson, J., & Mentovich, A. 2015. The consequences of being an object of suspicion: Potential pitfalls of proactive police contact. *Journal of Empirical Legal Studies, 12*(4), 602–636.

University of Johannesburg, & Human Sciences Research Council. 2020. *UJ-HSRC Covid-19 Democracy Survey Summary Findings Wave 2, 19 August.* Retrieved from https://www.uj.ac.za/newandevents/Documents/2020-08-19%201300pm%20 Coronavirus%20Impact%20Survey%20Round%202%20summary%20 national%20results%20v4.pdf

Waseem, Z. 2021. Policing COVID-19 through procedural informality in Pakistan. *Policing and Society, 31*(5), 583–600.

Waterworth, T., & Chemaly, F. 2020. 'Crime holiday' in lockdown as Cele guns for booze. *The Independent on Saturday, 15 August.* Retrived from https://www.iol.co.za/ios/news/crime-holiday-in-lockdown-as-cele-guns-for-booze-5009670a-11f4-4fda-9e4f-e372baa8e652

Williams, M. 2020. SA's rotten cops among most crooked during Covid-19, finds Corruption Watch report. *News24, 22 September 2020.* Retrieved from https://www.news24.com/news24/SouthAfrica/News/sas-rotten-cops-among-most-crooked-during-covid-19-finds-corruption-watch-report-20200922

Yamen, A. E. 2021. Tax evasion, corruption and COVID-19 health risk exposure: A cross country analysis. *Journal of Financial Crime, 28*(4), 995–1007.

Zoorob, M. 2020. Do police brutality stories reduce 911 calls? Reassessing an important criminological finding. *American Sociological Review, 85*(1), 176–183.

9 The role of temporary social grants in mitigating the poverty impact of COVID-19 in South Africa

Eldridge Moses and Ingrid Woolard

Introduction

As COVID-19 spread across the globe in early 2020, national governments closed their borders and imposed economic and social lockdowns in an attempt to curb the spread of the virus. South Africa was one of the first countries in the global South to institute a lockdown and the severity of the restrictions was much harsher than in most other countries. The South African economy was already weak prior to the pandemic, with inequality and unemployment rates amongst the highest in the world. The unexpected shock of the lockdown resulted in large numbers of workers temporarily or permanently losing their jobs with a devastating impact on large numbers of households, especially the poor.

In anticipation of the crippling economic effects of the lockdowns, international organisations called on national governments to expand their social assistance safety nets to cushion the devastating impact on the poor and vulnerable. The World Bank reports that by the end of May 2020, most countries around the world had planned, introduced or adapted social protection measures. Reforms to social assistance measures alone benefitted almost 1.8 billion people (Gentilini *et al.*, 2020).

South Africa's social protection reforms, announced in two stages by the Minister of Employment and Labour on 25 March 2020 and by President Cyril Ramaphosa a month later, were among the boldest in the world (Seekings, 2020). The government speedily rolled out new forms of cash assistance in the forms of the Temporary Employer-Employee Relief Scheme (TERS), the Special COVID-19 Social Relief of Distress Grant (SRD) grant and 'top up' grants to the 18 million people already receiving grants. This was possible because of the well-developed and extensive system of social assistance already in place in the country.

In this chapter, we describe the extensive system of support that was already in place, analyse the efficacy of the COVID-19 response and reflect on what a post-pandemic social assistance system might look like. We make use of five waves of survey data from the National Income Dynamics Study Coronavirus Rapid Mobile Survey (NIDS-CRAM). This data was collected

DOI: 10.4324/9781003294931-9

telephonically during the time period April 2020 to May 2021 by a consortium of researchers at the University of Cape Town, the University of the Witwatersrand and Stellenbosch University (Ingle, Brophy, & Daniels, 2021). The sample for this data was drawn from the National Income Dynamics Study, a longitudinal study of 28 000 people spanning the period from 2007 to 2017. Therefore, we have rich background information on our respondents and are able to situate these individuals within the income distribution prior to the pandemic. We are thus able to describe the heterogeneous effects of the pandemic on the poor versus the non-poor.

We find that the TERS, SRD and top-up grants assisted many vulnerable households to stave off the worst of the impact of the pandemic. However, the relatively loose criteria for SRD grant receipt and administrative inefficiencies contributed to less-than-ideal targeting of the vulnerable, previously uncovered working-aged population. We also find that although the social assistance interventions assisted many households in enduring the pandemic-induced economic slowdown, there were also many households whose incomes were still below the poverty line after receiving these new grants. Given South Africa's fragile fiscal outlook, we therefore suggest that without strong complementary labour market interventions, the extension of a universal basic income is likely to be fiscally unsustainable.

The initial impact of the pandemic on households in South Africa

Before the hard lockdown in South Africa in March 2020, approximately two-thirds of South Africans were already living in poverty, or at risk of falling into poverty (Schotte, Zizzamia & Leibbrandt, 2018). The economic shock of the pandemic and initial lockdown introduced additional risks of severe economic strain, because of reduced working hours or job losses amongst those employed prior to the pandemic. While the initial impact on poverty is difficult to calculate due to the absence of February 2020 income in South African survey data, Jain *et al.* (2020) provide rough estimates of the impact on poverty through job losses. They posit that approximately 20% of the 5 million workers who lost jobs between February and April 2020 fell into poverty. When the dependants of these workers are accounted for, the estimated increase in poverty through job losses alone between February and April 2020 would be an additional 3 million people.

The ravages of the pandemic and economic slowdown on vulnerable households were reflected in reported food security and hunger indicators. April 2020 estimates from the NIDS-CRAM survey show that 47% of respondents reported that they lived in a household that had run out of money to buy food in the last month (Van der Berg, Patel, & Bridgman, 2021). When asked about hunger in the last week, 23% of respondents reported living in a household where at least one person had gone hungry. In contrast, 15% of respondents reported living in a household where at least one child had gone hungry in the last week, which when combined with the higher levels of adult hunger, suggest that children may have benefitted from 'shielding' from hunger.

The economic contraction experienced because of the pandemic and lockdown conditions are likely to have long-lasting impacts on South Africa's already fragile economic, fiscal and political landscapes. Central to South Africa's economic and fiscal recovery in the immediate future is the recovery of employment losses and growth of employment on the back of economic growth. Labour market success in the medium to long run is crucially dependent on human capital generated partly through the South African school system, where learning outcomes were affected profoundly and unequally by pandemic-related factors. Given their potential roles in poverty and inequality reduction, and their pivotal roles as sites of inequality generation or perpetuation in times of crisis, this section therefore focuses on the initial impacts of the COVID-19 pandemic on labour market and schooling outcomes.

The labour market impact of the pandemic in South Africa

The labour market impact of the pandemic was profound in South Africa. World Bank (2020) estimates suggest that by the end of December 2020, the number of employed in South Africa had decreased by approximately 1.5 million, and wages for those who were still employed, had fallen on average by 10%–15%.

Early evidence from the NIDS-CRAM survey in 2020 suggest that the initial impact of the hard lockdown in South Africa was disproportionately borne by women (Casale & Posel, 2020). Labour market outcomes prior to the pandemic, in terms of average wages earned, employment rates and representation in skilled occupations, were in favour of men. In addition, sectors that are dominated by women, such as the domestic services sector, were also more likely to be affected negatively by the hard lockdown. Unsurprisingly then, the labour market income gap between woman-headed and male-headed households widened as a result of the pandemic but not uniformly so. Hill and Köhler (2020) find that the gender wage gap increased significantly for earners within the bottom 40% of the wage distribution, possibly because women earners at the bottom of the distribution are more likely to be employed in occupations that do not lend themselves to allow working from home. The resultant reduction in work hours, along with increased childcare burdens during lockdown periods (particularly for women who could not afford paid childcare), is likely to result in much of the labour market impact being concentrated amongst women for some time to come.

Existing inequalities across space were exacerbated by the initial impact of the pandemic-related economic slowdown (Visagie & Turok, 2021). The labour market impact of the crisis was particularly severe for individuals residing outside of metropolitan areas, so the gap between metro and rural unemployment rose from 10 to 18 percentage points between April and June 2020, while the gap between metro resident unemployment and unemployment of city/town residents remained stable at approximately 8 percentage points. However, some individuals who reported that they were not employed prior to wave 1 and wave 2 of CRAM reported had gained employment by June 2020, which is indicative of some churning amongst the employed and unemployed. These employment gains were highest amongst metro and city/town dwellers and lowest amongst rural dwellers, so the net employment losses in rural areas were much larger than in urban areas.

Using NIDS-CRAM data, Daniels, Ingle and Brophy (2021) find that the South African labour market between March 2020 and March 2021 was quite responsive to lockdown severity, with the largest losses in employment occurring when lockdown levels are strictest, and employment recoveries occurring when lockdown restrictions are relaxed. The authors also find that furloughing (workers being placed on unpaid leave) was highest in quarter 2 of 2020, when lockdown conditions were strictest, and lowest when lockdown conditions were relaxed in subsequent periods.

Estimates from the Quarterly Labour Force Survey show that narrow unemployment[1] increased to 34.4% in quarter 2 of 2021, while the expanded unemployment rate was 44.4% in the same period (Daniels, Ingle, & Brophy, 2021). While these headline figures are staggering, they do not fully convey the precarity of employment and wages that was exacerbated by the pandemic, nor the substantially higher hurdles that new labour market entrants and the previously unemployed face going forward. Vulnerability to depression was significantly higher for individuals who were furloughed or lost employment in the first five months of the lockdown, relative to workers who remained in employment during the same period (Posel, Oyenubi, & Kollamparambil, 2021). This finding underscores the need for mental health support services to assist the newly unemployed or furloughed with coping strategies as they navigate an increasingly precarious labour market environment. The impact on household income and mental health is likely to be severe for some time to come, underlining the need for government assistance so that at the very least households are able to meet their basic nutritional and shelter needs.

The impact of the pandemic on children's education and nutrition

South Africa's Department of Basic Education[2] (2021) estimates that learning losses (school days lost) in 2020 amounted to anywhere between 50% and 75% of a normal year's learning. This is in line with simulation estimates from the World Bank, which estimates that learning losses could be as much as 0.6 schooling years (Azevedo *et al.*, 2020). But learning losses estimated in lost school days may underestimate the learning that is truly lost. Long disruptions in learning may in fact lead to some loss of prior learning as well (Gustafsson & Nuga, 2020), so that actual learning losses are 25% greater than a lost-days measure would imply. Therefore, if eight weeks of school days were lost, the actual learning loss is likely to be approximately equivalent to ten weeks.

But in terms of immediate physical needs during the hard lockdown periods, it was the loss of school-provided nutrition that was likely to place severe strain on vulnerable households with school-going children. Learner absences from school also place vulnerable households under increased nutritional and economic strain, as absences from school also mean not having access to the school meals provided by South Africa's National School Nutrition Programme (NSNP), nor the health support services that children sometimes have access to through schools. The potential welfare loss in terms of nutrition is tremendous, as 82% of learners in South Africa are in schools serviced by the NSNP (Department of Basic Education, 2019). In addition, the impact of lost nutrition or nutrition insecurity is likely to be long-lasting, particularly for children of younger ages who may suffer from stunting as a result. Shepherd and Mohohlwane (2021) estimate that between 55 and 133 days of school-feeding days were missed between March 2020 and the NIDS-CRAM Wave 4 reporting period.

Cross-country simulations suggest that schooling outcomes are also negatively affected in more permanent ways through extremely poor rates of return to school and higher than usual levels of permanent dropout (Azevedo *et al.*, 2020, UNESCO, 2020). Data from the final wave of NIDS-CRAM collected in April and May 2021 suggest that 10% of households in South Africa contained at least one learner who had not returned to school (Shepherd & Mohohlwane, 2021). The factors linked to school non-attendance in pre-pandemic South Africa, such as household economic strain and poor performance at school (Casale & Shepherd, 2020), are likely to feature even more prominently as reasons for school non-attendance during the pandemic, and after it has passed.

School closures and uneven returns to school are likely to exacerbate inequalities between poor and affluent children. While learning losses are likely to expect throughout the entire learner distribution in South Africa, the impact is likely to be largest amongst learners in no-fee paying schools (Reddy, Soudien, & Winnaar, 2021). The household equipment required for remote learning and teaching to be successful differs vastly between children from affluent and non-affluent households. Remote learning content provided via various television and radio channels only amounts to 5% of the instructional time that is provided during contact teaching (Van der Berg & Spaull, 2020).

The COVID-19 pandemic is without a doubt the largest exogenous labour market demand shock in international and South African recent history. It exposed and exacerbated the structural inequalities in South Africa's economy, which even before the pandemic were characterised by extremely low levels of employment and economic growth, as well as poor education outcomes for much of its population. The structural weaknesses within, and the fragility of the South African economy, are likely to contribute to an economic and labour market recovery that falls far short of the contraction that befell the country in 2020. In such an environment, the need for well-targeted social assistance is of utmost importance in assisting households to survive and recover from the effects of the pandemic.

Social assistance in South Africa prior to the pandemic

At the time of the transition to democracy in 1994, the South African social security system was already notably well developed for a middle-income country (Van der Berg, 1997). This fact can be ascribed to how the system developed under apartheid as a welfare state for whites which was then incrementally expanded under social and political pressure to incorporate other groups. Thus, at the advent of the new post-apartheid society, some important planks for a social assistance system were in place, namely a means-tested non-contributory pension for older adults and a disability grant for working-age adults that were unable to participate in the labour market. Post-apartheid, the Child Support Grant was introduced and has been expanded over time to include children up until the time they turn 18.

At 3.5% of GDP in 2019/2020 (National Treasury, 2020), spending on social assistance in South Africa is more than double the median spending of 1.5% of GDP across developing and transition economies (World Bank, 2018:16). The prioritisation of social assistance in the national budget is in line with Section 27(1) of the Constitution which states that 'everyone has the right to have access to … social security, including, if they are unable to support themselves and their dependants, appropriate social assistance'. This Constitutional framework has given rise to a system of social grants that are provided primarily for categories of individuals who are considered most likely to be unable to provide for their own needs, namely the elderly, people living with disabilities and children.

Of the approximately 5 million South Africans over the age of 60, three-quarters receive the Old Age Pension. At a value of R1 890 per month, the grant is about half what a person working full-time at the minimum wage would receive. The disability grant (of the same value) goes to 1 million people of working age that are unable to work because of chronic illness or disability.

The grant system includes three child grants. The Child Support Grant (CSG) is the main poverty-oriented child grant. It is available to all primary caregivers who pass a simple means test that is set at 10 times the value of the grant (or double this amount for the spouses' combined income if the caregiver is married). The Care Dependency Grant (CDG) is provided to caregivers of severely disabled children on the basis that these caregivers will have limited opportunity to earn money given the intensive care needs of these children. The Foster Child Grant (FCG) is provided to foster parents of children who are placed in foster care because they are considered by the courts to be in need of 'care and protection' in terms of the Children's Act. As of February 2020, the CSG was provided to 12.8 million children, the CDG to 155,000 children and the FCG to 350,000 children (National Treasury, 2020). The value of the CSG is much lower than the other child grants. At the time of writing (September 2021), the value of the CSG was R445 per month, as against R1 040 for the FCG and R1 860 for the Care Dependency Grant.

Social assistance grants in South Africa play an important role in reducing poverty. Prior to the pandemic, almost half (47%) of households received at least one cash transfer. Given their wide coverage, it is not surprising that cash transfers have far-reaching (immediate, short-run) poverty-alleviating implications. Goldman, Woolard and Jellema (2020) find that in 2015 cash transfers lifted about 6 million people above the food poverty line of R417 per person per month.

The inability of poorer households to invest in the productive capacity of their members, especially the education and health of children, has implications for the persistence of poverty. Cash transfer programmes provide a predictable and reliable source of income which can have significant effects upon the capacity of households to invest in human and physical capital, and thus break the intergenerational transmission of poverty. There is now a well-developed literature showing that household receipt of the Old Age Pension has a positive effect on child nutrition (Hamoudi & Thomas, 2005) despite the grant being intended to support the older adult. This supports the idea of income pooling which is an important aspect when we consider the impact of the grants – just because they are aimed at one group does not pre-suppose that they do not have positive impacts on others.

The evidence on the labour market effects of grant receipt is more mixed. Early research on the Old Age Pension suggested that it had substantial negative effects on the adult labour supply. Bertrand, Mullainathan and Miller (2003) found a reduction in working hours of members of working age when another member of the household reaches pension age, suggesting that pension receipt represents an income shock on the household level. However, the reduction in hours is highest when the pensioner is a woman. Posel, Fairburn and Lund (2006) followed the same methodology but expanded the definition of the household to include non-resident members. They found that African women were significantly more likely to be migrant workers when they were members of a household in receipt of a pension, especially when the pension recipient is female. The authors hypothesised that the reasons for the relationship between pension income and migration could be that the pension provides the means to migrate, and/or that the pension provides the means for the older person to care for the children of the migrant, freeing the migrant to seek work. The work of Ardington, Case and Hosegood (2009) also disputed the earlier findings of Bertrand, Mullainathan and Miller (2003). This study made use of data on non-resident (migrant) household members and panel data which allowed the authors to control for time-invariant differences between pension recipients and non-recipients. Their results suggested that the Old Age Pension had a positive effect on adult labour supply – the probability that prime-age adults are employed is approximately 3 percentage points higher in households with at least one pension recipient. Similar to Posel, Fairburn and Lund (2006), they argued that the Old Age Pension relieved financial and childcare constraints, which were short-run impediments to migrating.

More recently, Ranchhod (2017) has used panel data from the national Labour Force Survey to look at the impact of the cessation of the pension (either due to a pensioner dying or out-migrating) on household formation and labour supply. For people who maintained their residency status across waves, he found large and statistically significant increases in employment rates for middle-aged females and males (9.3 and 8.1 percentage points in each case), as well as for older adult females and males (10.3 percentage points in each case). These findings are consistent with those of Bertrand, Mullainathan and Miller (2003) and not necessarily inconsistent with the findings of Posel, Fairburn and Lund (2006) and Ardington, Case and Hosegood (2009) who broadened their definition of household membership to include migrants.

Agüero, Carter and Woolard (2007) used data from the KwaZulu-Natal Income Dynamics Study (KIDS) to test whether receipt of the Child Support Grant (CSG) during the first 36 months of a child's life had an impact on child nutrition as measured by height-for-age. The paper was conditioned on a measure of 'eagerness' of the mother in an attempt to capture the true causal effect of the CSG. The authors found that children who received the CSG during the first three years of their life (that is, within the so-called 'nutritional window' during which adult height is largely determined) had significantly higher height-for-age scores than those who did not. More recently, Eyal, Woolard and Burns (2018) finds that the CSG has a positive effect on keeping adolescents in school. They find that current CSG receipt in older teens has a positive and large impact on school enrolment, as does the cumulative duration of receipt. CSG beneficiaries have enrolment rates about ten percentage points higher than non-beneficiaries, which is a substantial increase given the overall high rates of enrolment. An extra ten years of receipt can raise enrolment rates by more than fifteen percentage points.

Given the evidence presented here, there is no doubt that the social assistance system that existed prior to the pandemic was channelling grant income into deprived South African households and that this income can and does change the behaviour of members of such households. Nonetheless, the existing system which focused on children, the disabled and the elderly was something of an artefact of history, rather than a reflection of a coherently designed system. Implicit in the design was that able-bodied people of working age would fall outside of the system of social support on the assumption that they should be able to earn income in the labour market. Even prior to the pandemic, this assumption was not well-grounded on empirical evidence. According to our analysis of NIDS Wave 5 (conducted in 2017), fewer than one in three adults of working age in the poorest decile was in fact employed.

Social assistance and insurance in South Africa during the pandemic

Early indicators of the impending possible humanitarian crisis came from the NIDS-CRAM Wave 1 survey (conducted in April 2020), when 53% of adult respondents reported that they were living in a household where they had run out of money to buy food in the current month (Wills *et al.*, 2020). Four out of every ten respondents reported that their household had lost its main source of income between the beginning of the strict lockdown conditions in late March and April 2020. GHS 2018 data indicate that 80% of non-grant-receiving households and 46% of grant-receiving households in South Africa report labour market incomes as their main income source. Given the importance of labour market incomes for both non-grant-receiving and grant-receiving households, the impact of job losses and reductions in hours worked due to the economic slowdown was likely to have profoundly negative impacts in terms of pushing a number of previously non-poor households into poverty and pushing the existing poor even further below the poverty line if no additional social assistance was provided.

The main income losses mentioned earlier were particularly devastating for poor households who were not receiving grants of any kind, highlighting the need for social assistance interventions that reached beyond the existing social assistance net and mitigated some of the economic losses felt by households because of unemployment or reduced working hours.

In response to reduced economic activity as well as employment losses, the South African government announced a fiscal stimulus package of R502 billion (National Treasury, 2020) on 21 April 2020. Approximately R40 billion was earmarked for wage protection through the Unemployment Insurance Fund (UIF) system, while R50 billion of the package was dedicated to social assistance in the form of the Social Relief from Distress (SRD) grant and top-ups to the existing grants paid by the Department of Social Development.

Social insurance

TERS was a key plank of the R500 billion package of support announced by President Ramaphosa on 21 April 2020. Although financed by the reserves accumulated by the Unemployment Insurance Fund, the TERS was in fact a wage subsidy aimed at avoiding retrenchments and stemming unemployment. TERS provided income support to employers who had fully or partially closed their operations in response to the pandemic. By subsidising incomes and firm liquidity, the goal of the intervention was to help employees to weather the shock of temporary firm closures and to assist firms in retaining workers and thereby avoiding the costly process of hiring and training new workers once economic activity recovered (Keenan & Lydon, 2020).

TERS reached the highest number of workers during the beginning of the national lockdown, with relatively few benefiting in 2021. On aggregate, we estimate that over 4 million individuals received TERS at least once over the period. We find that the number of recipients was highest during the most stringent lockdown level 5 in April 2020 (1.8 million) and level 3 in June 2020 (2 million), representing about 13.5% of all workers. Although many workers continued to benefit throughout the year as the economy re-opened, the number of active recipients had fallen to less than 1 million by March 2021.

Initially, TERS was limited to workers in firms that had paid contributions to the UIF but this was later expanded to any worker that could demonstrate an employment relationship. The TERS was rolled out rapidly and achieved significant coverage and scale. By March 2021, nearly R59 billion had been disbursed (Köhler & Hill, 2021). The size of the TERS benefit depended on the (previous) salary/wage of the individual employee with the income replacement rate ranging from 60% for the lowest-earning workers to 38% for the highest earning. In addition, the benefit had a floor of R3,500 per month and a ceiling of R6,730 per month. In other words, everyone with pre-pandemic earnings of more than R17,710 received R6,730 from TERS, regardless of how much above this limit they had been earning. Capping the benefit enhanced the progressivity of the scheme while also helping to keep down overall programme costs.

The TERS benefit was thus carefully designed to ensure that the income support to the most vulnerable was at a higher-income replacement level than for higher-income workers. This did, however, have a rather unexpected outcome. Because the 'floor' was set at R3,500 to coincide with the national minimum wage this meant that many workers actually received more under TERS than they had been earning pre-pandemic. This is because the national minimum wage of R3,500 per month is only slightly lower than the median wage of R4,000 (Bhorat, Lilenstein, & Stanwix, 2021). In Table 9.1, we show that the median earnings for the bottom half of the income distribution were less than the 'floor' of R3,500. The majority of these workers would have

Table 9.1 Receipt of TERS by decile

Household income decile (based on NIDS Wave 5)	% of adults accessing TERS in any wave of CRAM	Average pre-pandemic salary/ wage (per month in 2020 prices)
1	15.7	R1 065
2	12.6	R1 474
3	10.9	R1 460
4	15.2	R2 401
5	14.7	R2 456
6	27.5	R3 560
7	23.0	R4 492
8	23.2	R5 190
9	19.7	R8 691
10	18.7	R24 487
All	19.0	R8 340

Source: Author calculations based on NIDS Wave 5 and NIDS–CRAM, Waves 1–5.

received a TERS benefit of at least double what they would have earned had they not become (temporarily) unemployed.

Unfortunately, the Auditor-General's report of December 2020 revealed that TERS disbursements were also plagued by large-scale fraud and other irregularities, facilitated in large part by various government information systems that were not integrated well and 'a weak control environment' (Auditor-General South Africa, 2020a). Both problems, along with a rapid change in UIF processes, contributed to increased risk of fraud, overpayment, underpayment, rejection of genuinely eligible applications and payment to ineligible applicants (which included, amongst others, government employees, deceased persons, people already receiving social grants and students already receiving financial aid). The Auditor-General reported that by October 2020, R3.4 billion that had been paid incorrectly was recovered by the UIF (Auditor-General South Africa, 2020b). Investigations into TERS fraud and irregularities are still ongoing at the time of writing.

The social relief from distress grant and grant top-ups

As mentioned before, the South African government launched a series of social assistance interventions aimed at mitigating the possible economic and humanitarian impacts of pandemic-induced economic slowdown. In addition to the TERS job/wage security intervention, a commitment was made to increase the monthly child support grant by R300 per child beneficiary in May 2020, and all other existing grants by R250. From June to October 2020 the child support grant top-up was extended to *recipients only*, with eligible carers of children receiving a fixed amount of R500, irrespective of how many children were being cared for by the recipient. The other grant top-ups remained at R250 per beneficiary, while the COVID-19 grant was eventually extended to end in May 2021.

The coverage of the social assistance package was unprecedented, as a Special COVID-19 Social Relief of Distress Grant (SRD) grant was also introduced that now also included vulnerable working-aged adults who were not already recipients of government assistance, and who had traditionally been excluded from the social assistance net (Seekings, 2020). Bhorat, Oosthuizen and Stanwix (2020) estimated that approximately 10 million individuals would have been eligible for this grant at the time of its take-up in May 2020, which at a cost of R350 per payment, would have cost R3.5 billion per month if 100% of the eligible population was paid. According to our estimates using the NIDS-CRAM data, approximately 4.3 million applications for the SRD grant had been approved by June 2020. By March 2021, that number had risen to 6.1 million.

Figure 9.1 shows the June 2020 shares of SRD grant receipt by decile for broadly unemployed[3] adults over the age of 18 years, who report that they were not receiving a grant in April 2020. On the face of it, SRD grant receipts appear to be relatively poorly targeted, but this may be so for a number of reasons.

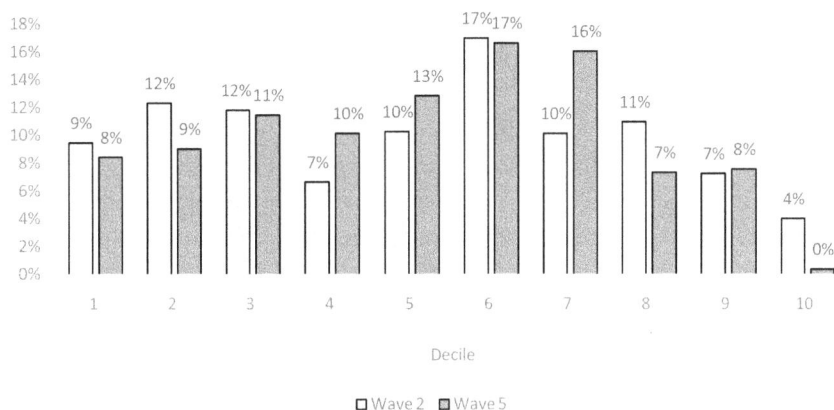

Figure 9.1 Social Relief of Distress ('COVID-19') Grant receipt by decile.
Source: Author calculations based on NIDS Wave 5 and NIDS-CRAM, Waves 2 and 5.

Firstly, the means criteria for SRD grant receipt are simply that individuals should not be earning any income, should not be employed, should not be students and should not be receiving any other form of government financial assistance. These relatively loose conditions for grant receipt allow for receipt of the SRD grant, regardless of the *household* income that individuals may benefit from. A second reason for the broad-ranging incidence of the SRD may be the fact that individuals could only apply for the grant through electronic channels such as WhatsApp, email or via cell phone USSD code. It may therefore be reasonable to expect that more educated individuals, both in terms of educational attainment and education about the grant, were more likely to apply for the grant first. The relatively small amount of R350 per month may have discouraged individuals at the very top end of the income distribution from applying, leading to the receipt incidence by decile in Waves 2 and 5.

Nevertheless, given that SRD grant receipt appears to be relatively evenly spread across the bottom and top half of the income distribution, it may be useful to consider how the *monetary values* of the SRD grant and grant top-ups affected household income distributions, and whether there was some sort of poverty alleviation effect.

The impact of the top-ups and SRD grant on poverty and inequality

The second wave of the NIDS-CRAM survey is the only survey-round in which we can observe whether individuals and households received both the SRD grant and the top-ups to all other grants. It, therefore, provides an opportunity for us to examine the combined impact of these interventions on poverty and inequality. The approach in this section is simply to compare what household incomes would have been in the absence of grant top-ups and the SRD grant. While the exercise does not control for household composition changes in response to receiving a grant, or in anticipation of receiving a grant,[4] it does provide some indication of which parts of the income distribution are affected most by the incomes from the grant top-ups and SRD grant. The NIDS-CRAM survey asks respondents how many child support, old age pension and COVID-19 grants were received by the household. This allows for a calculation of the additional income received by the household due to the grant top-ups and COVID-19 grants. The respondent is also asked whether they personally receive other grants, in addition to the CSG, OAP and COVID-19 grants. This allows for a conservative estimation of the total income received from grant top-ups and the COVID-19 grant.

Figure 9.2 shows the Lorenz curves[5] for the total household per capita incomes reported by NIDS-CRAM respondents in June 2020, as well as estimated household per capita incomes in the absence of grant top-ups and the SRD grant in the same month.

The Lorenz curves in Figure 9.2 show that much of the proportional income gains from the top-up grants and the SRD grant are concentrated in the middle of the income distribution, rather than at the lower end. But again, it should be borne in mind that South African incomes below the 90th percentile are low by international standards, so the middle of the income distribution still represents low per capita incomes on average. There is however

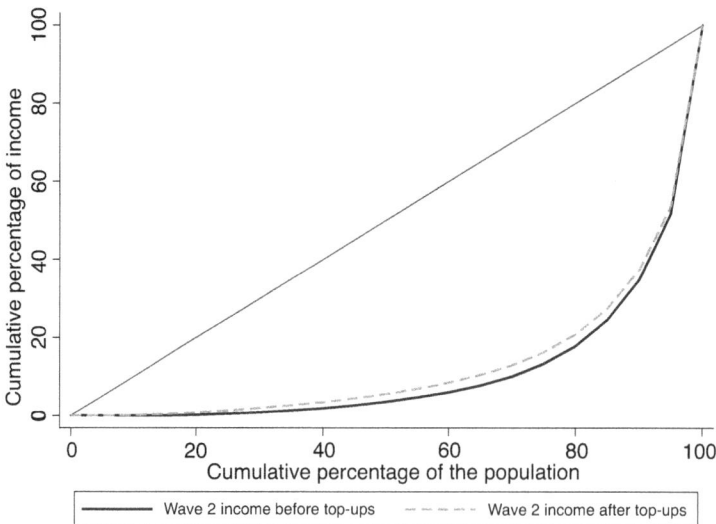

Figure 9.2 Lorenz curves with and without grant top-ups.
Source: Author calculations based on NIDS Wave 5 and NIDS-CRAM, Wave 2.

a slight reduction in inequality due to the top-ups and SRD grants. The Gini coefficient[6] is 0.72 before the additional social assistance, and 0.69 once the additional social assistance is accounted for.

The food poverty[7] headcount rate (the number of poor divided by the total population) based on the reported household income in June 2020 was 48.4%, while the average normalised poverty gap was 0.25. In the absence of the grant top-ups, and the SRD grant, the poverty headcount rate would have been 55.1%, and the normalised poverty gap[8] would have been 0.35. In other words, in the absence of the grant top-ups and the SRD grant, it would have taken R205 per poor person for them to meet their minimum nutritional needs. That average distance from the poverty line was reduced to R146, which represents a substantial gain for poor households as a result of the grant top-ups.

While the absolute magnitudes of the impact are likely to be estimated with some error, it is encouraging that the direction of the overall impact of the social security interventions is in favour of individuals in poorer households. An alternative approach to viewing the shares of top-up and SRD expenditure received by households is shown in Figure 9.2. The incidence of grant top-up and SRD grant expenditure appears to be somewhat pro-poor. As Figure 9.3 shows, individuals in the poorest 40% of households (as measured in April 2020 in NIDS-CRAM data) in South Africa benefitted from 48% of grant top-ups.

The findings above are somewhat encouraging from a monetary poverty or temporary economic strain alleviation perspective but the overall impact of the top-ups was inadequate to shield many already-vulnerable South Africans

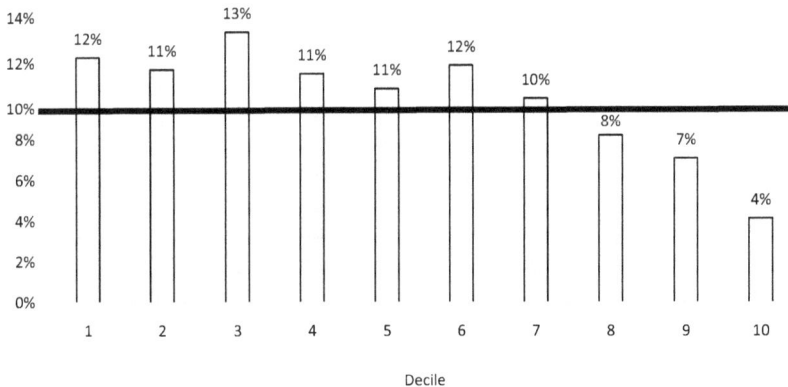

Figure 9.3 Share of grant top-up and COVID-19 expenditure by household income decile, June 2020.

Source: Author calculations based on NIDS Wave 5 and NIDS-CRAM, Wave 2.

Note:
The bold black line indicates the level of spending per income decile, had the social assistance payments been spread equally across income deciles.

from the increased pressure of the pandemic. Van der Berg, Patel and Bridgman (2021) show that although there were decreases in household hunger after the introduction of the social assistance interventions, by March 2021, there was still a third of households who ran out of money to buy food. This was despite the labour market recovering to some degree, and the COVID-19 grant still being paid until May 2021. Given this finding and the overwhelming contribution of labour market income inequality to overall inequality, the national focus should therefore be on job-creating economic growth to alleviate both poverty and inequality. The targeting success and lessons learned from the pandemic social assistance interventions also present an opportunity for policymakers to reimagine the South African social assistance environment.

Reimagining social assistance after the pandemic

South Africa's already weak economic situation has been exacerbated by the COVID-19 pandemic, exposing the precarity and poverty many households face. The levels of inequality and unemployment were already among the highest in the world and the latest employment statistics show 1.4 million fewer employed workers than pre-COVID-19. The looting and violence experienced in July 2021 served to further highlight the desperation of many. For people with no connection to the economy through jobs or other livelihoods, the economic cost of the riots would have seemed largely irrelevant to their own lived experience. The persistently high levels of poverty, unemployment and inequality pose pressing questions about what the state's post-COVID-19 response should be.

At the time of writing, the SRD grant had been extended for a fourth time (until March 2023), leading many to wonder whether the grant will be extended indefinitely. If the grant were to become permanent, the eligibility rules would need to be clarified and real-time assessment methods would need to be put in place. The key constraint to the effective implementation of the SRD grant has been the availability of data to verify information of claimants, particularly in the South African context of high labour market churn, and it seems likely that lags in data have incorrectly excluded high numbers of applicants in the existing implementation of the SRD grant.

Currently, the grant is beleaguered by both errors of inclusion and errors of exclusion. The grant is intended for unemployed persons living in poor households. However, it is assessed based on individual income leading to errors of inclusion. For example, a non-working person such as a stay-at-home mom or student (not receiving financial aid) is eligible for SRD even if they live in a middle-class or rich household. Additional errors of inclusion result from the fact that only formal sector employment is properly captured in administrative systems, meaning that all informal sector workers are potentially able to claim SRD. We estimate that as many as 21 million working-age adults could apply for SRD; this is more than double the number currently budgeted for.

Errors of exclusion arise when the state utilises out-of-date data to make an assessment of eligibility. The employment status of an individual is currently inferred from two imperfect databases derived from records of the Unemployment Insurance Fund (UIF) and employee tax records (i.e., IRP5 certificates). UIF contributions records are available for the most recent month, however, they are often incorrect: companies may fail to update the identity information when they replace employees, which can result in a previous employee with a false employment status, and a new employee with a false unemployment status. Tax certificates are available for the previous tax year (which runs from 1 March to 28 February) and indicate whether someone was employed at any point over the 12-month period. If an applicant was formally employed in, say, March 2020 and retrenched in April 2020, they will nonetheless have a tax certificate indicating employment and will be excluded from receiving the SRD (unless they appeal) until February 2021. The impact of outdated employment data is exacerbated by a context of high job turnover in the South African labour market.

The imperfections of the SRD might suggest that a Universal Basic Income Grant (UBIG) is preferable. The UBIG is certainly administratively simpler and has the additional benefit of promoting social cohesion by virtue of its universality. The obvious disadvantage of UBIG is that it is more costly since it goes to everyone, not just those in greatest need. While many commentators glibly talk of 'clawing back' through the personal income tax system this is not particularly effective given the narrowness of the tax base and the high threshold at which a person becomes liable for tax.

Various UBIG designs have been proposed, with price tags of between R194 and R256 billion per year. To put this into context, this would entail more than doubling the existing expenditure of South Africa's already-expansive social grant system. Given the other fiscal priorities such as infrastructure deficits and the long-awaited National Health Insurance, it seems unlikely that there will be the fiscal space to extend social assistance to this extent. It seems more likely that a means-tested version of the SRD will be put in place. For example, if the SRD of R350 per month were limited to individuals living in households with an income below the Food Poverty Line (of R624 per person per month), it would go to 16.8 million adults at a cost of R56 bn per annum (Goldman *et al.,* 2021). While still a significant cost, this seems within the realm of the feasible.

Concerns have been raised about the labour supply effects of either extending the SRD or implementing UBIG. The literature which we reviewed earlier in this chapter was inconclusive, with some authors finding positive effects and others finding negative effects on labour supply. In any event, given the extremely high levels of unemployment, these labour supply effects are possibly not all that important, especially if the value of the grant is small.

Nonetheless, labour market interventions are important complementary policies to cash transfers given that economic growth and job creation are central to fiscal sustainability. The state must renew its efforts in both active and passive labour market policies. Young people in particular need support in job search and job skills. In addition, the state has a role to play in directly creating job opportunities. Public employment programmes are complex to roll out at large-scale but have merit in our view. There is economic and social value in work such as caring for the elderly and young, teaching assistance in schools and maintaining infrastructure. In addition, these programmes provide some training and work experience to participants which can assist in some participants transitioning into regular employment.

Conclusion

The South African policy response to the COVID-19 pandemic was swift and substantial. While we find that the response was imperfect – with many individuals unable to access any additional support and some 'leakage' to non-poor households – the overall response was fairly well targeted towards the poor. The grant top-ups went to households in need, given the progressive structure of the existing grant system. This was easy to do, given the well-functioning grant system that was already in place. TERS was quickly put in place by the Unemployment Insurance Fund and served to cushion workers that were temporarily furloughed during the strictest lockdowns. These measures were supplemented by the Social Relief of Distress grant which targeted the unemployed in a break from the conventional thinking about which individuals are vulnerable. Overall, these complementary measures reduced poverty by about seven percentage points and increased the incomes of many more households even if they remained below the poverty line.

It is clear that the need for social insurance and enhanced social assistance will not evaporate post-pandemic. The groundwork has been laid for additional support to people of working age that are unable to find work or create a livelihood for themselves. It is evident that despite the constrained fiscal space and commitment of the National Treasury to fiscal consolidation, some form of continued support will be required for the unemployed. Researchers, commentators and policymakers will continue to grapple with these difficult choices over the months to come.

Notes

1 Narrow unemployment refers to unemployed individuals between the ages of 15 and 64 years old who are available to work, unemployed and actively seeking work. Expanded (or broad) unemployment includes the narrowly unemployed and individuals within the same group who are available to work but are not taking active steps to find work.
2 https://www.gov.za/speeches/basic-education-concerned-level-learning-losses-suffered-due-covid-19-19-aug-2021-0000.

3 The broad definition of unemployment includes all adults who were unemployed and were either looking for work or had stopped looking for work.
4 It is possible that households could change their composition if individuals or households respond to the announcement of grant conditions.
5 Lorenz curves are a graphical depiction of inequality within a population. To construct the curve, incomes are first ranked from poorest to richest. The cumulative proportion of the population is then plotted on the horizontal axis, while the cumulative share of income is plotted on the vertical axis. The red 45-degree line represents perfect equality (for example, the poorest 40% of the population earns 40% of the total income, or the poorest 80% of the population earns 80% of the income). The more space there is between the red diagonal line and the income distribution curve, the more unequal that country is.
6 The Gini coefficient is a measure of inequality that can range in value from 0 (perfect equality) to 1 (perfect inequality).
7 South Africa's national food poverty line in April 2020 prices was set at R585 per month, which is the amount of money considered to be just adequate for minimum nutritional needs to be met.
8 The normalised poverty gap measures the average gap between the incomes of the poor and the poverty line, expressed as a proportion of the poverty line.

References

Agüero, J., Carter, M., & Woolard, I. (2007). *The Impact of Unconditional Cash Transfers on Nutrition: The South African Child Support Grant.* International Policy Centre for Inclusive Growth working paper number 39. Brasília, Brazil: International Policy Centre for Inclusive Growth.

Auditor-General South Africa. (2020a). *COVID-19 Audit Report. Media Release 2 September 2020.* Retrieved from https://www.agsa.co.za/Portals/0/Reports/Special%20Reports/Covid-19%20Special%20report/2020%20Covid-19%20Media%20Release%20FINALISED.pdf. [Accessed 1 February 2022].

Auditor General South Africa. (2020b). *First Special Report on the Financial Management of government's Covid-19 Initiatives.* Retrieved from https://www.agsa.co.za/Reporting/SpecialAuditReports/COVID-19AuditReport.aspx. [Accessed 1 February 2022].

Azevedo, J., Hasan, A., Goldemberg, D., Iqbal, S., & Geven, K. (2020). *Simulating the Potential Impacts of COVID-19 School Closures on Schooling and Learning Outcomes: A Set of Global Estimates.* Policy Research Working Paper; No. 9284. Washington DC, United States: World Bank.

Ardington, C., Case, A., & Hosegood, V. (2009). Labor supply responses to large social transfers: Longitudinal evidence from South Africa. *American Economic Journal: Applied Economics, 1*(1), 22–48.

Bertrand, M., Mullainathan, S., & Miller, D. (2003). Public policy and extended families: Evidence from pensions in South Africa. *World Bank Economic Review, 17*(1), 27–50.

Bhorat, H., Oosthuizen, M., & Stanwix, B. (2020). *Social Assistance Amidst the Covid-19 Pandemic in South Africa: An Impact Assessment.* DPRU Working Paper 2020/06. Cape Town, South Africa: University of Cape Town Development Policy Research Unit.

Bhorat, H., Lilenstein, A., & Stanwix, B. (2021). *The Impact of the National Minimum Wage in South Africa: Early Quantitative Evidence.* DPRU Working Paper 2021/04.

Cape Town, South Africa: University of Cape Town, Development Policy Research Unit.

Casale, D., & Shepherd, D. (2020). *The Gendered Effects of the Ongoing Lockdown and School Closures in South Africa: Evidence from NIDS-CRAM Waves 1 and 2*. National Income Dynamics (NIDS)-Coronavirus Rapid Mobile Survey (CRAM) Wave 2 Working Paper No. 5. Cape Town, South Africa: National Income Dynamics Study– Coronavirus Rapid Mobile Survey.

Casale, D., & Posel, D. (2020). *Gender and the Early Effects of the COVID-19 Crisis in the Paid and Unpaid Economies in South Africa*. National Income Dynamics (NIDS)-Coronavirus Rapid Mobile Survey (CRAM) Wave 1 Working Paper No. 4. Cape Town, South Africa: National Income Dynamics Study– Coronavirus Rapid Mobile Survey.

Daniels, R., Ingle, K., & Brophy, T. (2021). *Labour Market Uncertainty & Dynamics in the Era of Covid-19: What We've Learnt from NIDS-CRAM & the Quarterly Labour Force Surveys* (QLFS). National Income Dynamics (NIDS)-Coronavirus Rapid Mobile Survey (CRAM) Wave 5 Working Paper No. 4. Cape Town, South Africa: National Income Dynamics Study– Coronavirus Rapid Mobile Survey.

Department of Basic Education. (2019). *General Household Survey (GHS): Focus on Schooling 2017*. Pretoria, South Africa: Department of Basic Education.

Department of Basic Education. (2021). *Basic Education Concerned at Level of Learning Losses Suffered Due to COVID-19*. Pretoria, South Africa: Department of Basic Education.

Eyal, K., Woolard, I., & Burns, J. (2018). *More than Just a Black-board: Cash Transfers and Adolescent Education in South Africa*. SALDRU Working Paper Number 125, Version 2. Cape Town, South Africa: Southern Africa Labour and Development Research Unit, University of Cape Town.

Gentilini, U., Almenfi, M., Dale, P., Blomquist, J., Natarajan, H., Galicia, G., Palacios, R., & Desai, V. (2020). *Social Protection and Jobs Responses to COVID-19: A Real-time Review of Country Measures*. Living Paper version 10 (May 22, 2020). Washington DC, United States: World Bank.

Goldman, M., Woolard, I., & Jellema, J. (2020). *The Impact of Taxes and Transfers on Poverty and Income Distribution in South Africa 2014/2015*. Research Paper No. 198. Paris, France: French Development Agency.

Goldman, M., Bassier, I., Budlender, J., Mzankomo, L., Woolard, I., & Leibbrandt, M. (2021). *Simulation of Options to Replace the Special COVID-19 Social Relief of Distress Grant and Close the Poverty Gap at the Food Poverty Line*. WIDER Working Paper 2021/165. Helsinki, Finland: United Nations University World Institute for Development Economics Research.

Gustafsson, M., & Nuga, C. (2020). *How Is the COVID-19 Pandemic Affecting Educational Quality in South Africa? Evidence to Date and Future Risk*. National Income Dynamics (NIDS)-Coronavirus Rapid Mobile Survey (CRAM) Wave 2 Insight Brief. Retrieved from https://cramsurvey.org/wp-content/uploads/2020/07/Gustafsson.-Nuga.-How-is-the-COVID-19-pandemic–affecting-educational-quality-in-South-Africa_-1.pdf [Accessed 1 February 2022].

Hamoudi, A., & Thomas, D. (2005). *Pension Income and the Well-Being of Children and Grandchildren: New Evidence from South Africa*. California Center for Population Research On-Line Working Paper Series number 043-05. Los Angeles, United States: University of California.

Hill, R., & Köhler, T. (2020). Mind the gap: *Analysing the Effects of South Africa's National Lockdown on Gender Wage Inequality.* National Income Dynamics (NIDS)-Coronavirus Rapid Mobile Survey (CRAM) Wave 2 Working Paper No. 7. Cape Town, South Africa: National Income Dynamics Study– Coronavirus Rapid Mobile Survey.

Ingle, K., Brophy, T., & Daniels, R.C. (2021). *National Income Dynamics Study – Coronavirus Rapid Mobile Survey (NIDS-CRAM) 2020 - 2021 Panel User Manual.* Release July 2021. Version 1. Cape Town, South Africa: Southern Africa Labour and Development Research Unit.

Jain, R., Budlender, J., Zizzamia, R., & Bassier, S. (2020). *The Labour Market and Poverty Impacts of COVID-19 in South Africa.* National Income Dynamics (NIDS)-Coronavirus Rapid Mobile Survey (CRAM) Wave 1 Working Paper No. 5. Cape Town, South Africa: National Income Dynamics Study– Coronavirus Rapid Mobile Survey.

Keenan, E., & Lydon, R. (2020). Wage subsidies and job retention. *Central Bank of Ireland Economic Letter*, 2020(11), 1–12.

Köhler, T., & Hill, R. (2021). *The Distribution and Dynamics of South Africa's TERS Policy: Results from NIDS-CRAM Waves 1 to 5.* National Income Dynamics (NIDS)-Coronavirus Rapid Mobile Survey (CRAM) Wave 5 Working Paper No. 7. Cape Town, South Africa: National Income Dynamics Study– Coronavirus Rapid Mobile Survey.

National Income Dynamics Study-Coronavirus Rapid Mobile Survey (NIDS-CRAM). (2020). *Wave 1* [dataset]. Version 3.0.0. Cape Town: Allan Gray Orbis Foundation [funding agency]. Cape Town: Southern Africa Labour and Development Research Unit [implementer], 2020. Cape Town: DataFirst [distributor], 2020. DOI: https://doi.org/10.25828/7tn9-1998

National Income Dynamics Study-Coronavirus Rapid Mobile Survey (NIDS-CRAM). (2020). *Wave 2* [dataset]. Version 3.0.0. Cape Town: Allan Gray Orbis Foundation [funding agency]. Cape Town: Southern Africa Labour and Development Research Unit [implementer], 2020. Cape Town: DataFirst [distributor], 2020. DOI: https://doi.org/10.25828/5z2w-7678

National Income Dynamics Study-Coronavirus Rapid Mobile Survey (NIDS-CRAM). (2020). *Wave 3* [dataset]. Version 3.0.0. Cape Town: Allan Gray Orbis Foundation [funding agency]. Cape Town: Southern Africa Labour and Development Research Unit [implementer], 2021. DOI: https://doi.org/10.25828/s82x-nx07

National Income Dynamics Study-Coronavirus Rapid Mobile Survey (NIDS-CRAM). (2021). *Wave 4* [dataset]. Version 2.0.0. Cape Town: FEM Education Foundation and Michael and Susan Dell Foundation [funding agencies]. Cape Town: Southern Africa Labour and Development Research Unit [implementer], 2021. Cape Town: DataFirst [distributor], 2021. DOI: https://doi.org/10.25828/y5qj-x095

National Income Dynamics Study-Coronavirus Rapid Mobile Survey (NIDS-CRAM). (2021). *Wave 5* [dataset]. Version 1.0.0. Cape Town: FEM Education Foundation and Michael and Susan Dell Foundation [funding agencies]. Cape Town: Southern Africa Labour and Development Research Unit [implementer], 2021. Cape Town: DataFirst [distributor], 2021. DOI: https://doi.org/10.25828/awhe-t852

National Treasury. (2020). *Budget Review 2020*. Retrieved from http://www. treasury.gov.za/documents/national%20budget/2020/review/fullbr.pdf. [Accessed 1 February 2022].

Posel, D., Fairburn, J., & Lund, F. (2006). Labour migration and households: A reconsideration of the effects of the social pension on labour supply in South Africa. *Economic Modelling,* 23(5), 836–853.

Posel, D., Oyenubi, A., & Kollamparambil, U. (2021). Job loss and mental health during the COVID-19 lockdown: Evidence from South Africa. *PLoS ONE,* 16(3), e0249352, https://doi.org/10.1371/journal.pone.0249352.

Ranchhod, V. (2017). *Household Responses to the Cessation of Grant Income: The Case of South Africa's Old Age Pension*. SALDRU Working Paper Number 213. Cape Town, South Africa: Southern Africa Labour and Development Research Unit, University of Cape Town.

Reddy, V., Soudien, C., & Winnaar, L. (2020). *Disrupted Learning during COVID-19: The Impact of School Closures on Education Outcomes in South Africa*. Retrieved from: https://repository.hsrc.ac.za/handle/20.500.11910/15402. [Accessed 13 September 2021].

Schotte, S., Zizzamia, R., & Leibbrandt, M. (2018). A poverty dynamics approach to social stratification: The South African case. *World Development,* 110(C), 88–103.

Seekings, J. (2020). *Bold Promises, Constrained Capacity, Stumbling Delivery: The Expansion of Social Protection in Response to the Covid-19 Lockdown in South Africa*. CSSR Working Paper 456. Cape Town, South Africa: Centre for Social Science Research, University of Cape Town.

Shepherd, D., & Mohohlwane, N. (2021). *The Impact of COVID-19 in Education – more than a Year of Disruption*. National Income Dynamics (NIDS)–Coronavirus Rapid Mobile Survey (CRAM) Wave 5 Working Paper No. 11. Cape Town, South Africa: National Income Dynamics Study– Coronavirus Rapid Mobile Survey.

Turok, I., & Visagie, J. (2021). *Driven Further Apart by the Pandemic? Contrasting Impacts of COVID-19 on People and Places*. National Income Dynamics (NIDS)–Coronavirus Rapid Mobile Survey (CRAM) Wave 5 Working Paper No. 12. Cape Town, South Africa: National Income Dynamics Study– Coronavirus Rapid Mobile Survey.

United Nations Educational, Scientific and Cultural Organization. (2020). *UNESCO COVID-19 Education Response: How Many Students Are At Risk of Not Returning to School? Advocacy Paper*. Retrieved from https://unesdoc.unesco.org/ark:/48223/pf0000373992. [Accessed 13 September 2021].

Van der Berg, S. (1997). South African social security under apartheid and beyond. *Development South Africa*, 14(4), 481–503.

Van der Berg, S., & Spaull, N. (2020). *Counting the Cost: COVID-19 School Closures in South Africa & Its Impact on Children*. Research on Socioeconomic Policy (RESEP) Working Paper. Stellenbosch, South Africa: Stellenbosch University.

Van der Berg, S., Patel, L., & Bridgman, G. (2021). *Hunger in South Africa- Results from Wave 4 of NIDS-CRAM*. National Income Dynamics (NIDS)–Coronavirus Rapid Mobile Survey (CRAM) Wave 4 Working Paper No. 11. Cape Town, South Africa: National Income Dynamics Study– Coronavirus Rapid Mobile Survey.

Wills, G., Patel, L., Van der Berg, S., & Mpeta, B. (2020). *Household Resource Flows and Food Poverty during South Africa's Lockdown: Short-term Policy implications for Three Channels of Social Protection*. National Income Dynamics (NIDS)-Coronavirus

Rapid Mobile Survey (CRAM) Wave 1 Working Paper No. 12. Cape Town, South Africa: National Income Dynamics Study– Coronavirus Rapid Mobile Survey.

World Bank. (2018). *The State of Social Safety Nets 2018*. Washington DC, United States: World Bank.

World Bank. (2020). *Building Back Better from COVID-19, with a Special Focus on Jobs*. Washington, DC, United States: World Bank.

10 COVID-19 and mental health well-being in South Africa

Impact, responses, and recommendations

André Janse van Rensburg, Arvin Bhana, and Inge Petersen

Introduction

Events of significant crisis have long been known to cause mental distress. This has been the case in major economic recessions (for instance, the 2008 Global Recession), where associations with higher prevalence rates of common mental disorders, substance use disorders, and suicidal behaviour have been suggested (Frasquilho et al., 2016). During periods of war, terrorism, and conflict, significant increases in the prevalence of mental disorders have been found (Murthy and Lakshminarayana, 2006, Musisi and Kinyanda, 2020), and similar psychological responses have been noted in the wake of environmental disasters (Morganstein and Ursano, 2020). Infectious disease outbreaks – particularly the post-2000 outbreaks of SARS-CoV-1, swine flu (H1N1), Middle East respiratory syndrome coronavirus (MERS-CoV), avian influenza (H7N9), Ebolavirus, and, more recently, the SARS-CoV-2 (COVID-19) pandemic – have highlighted the critical impact of such events on population mental health (Zürcher et al., 2020). The academic community seemingly realised the importance of this relationship, particularly in the context of decades of negligence of mental health in global health agendas. In this chapter, we summarise the main trends in the literature describing the impact of the pandemic – both direct and indirect – on mental health outcomes, particularly in South Africa. We also describe how governments, the private sector, and civil society responded to mental distress in the context of the pandemic, by paying particular attention to responses in South Africa that focused on different population groups.

The effects of COVID-19 on population mental health

Broadly speaking, research has generated foci on the mental health of the general population, and on specific populations that had a particular high risk of experiencing mental distress. This included occupations such as frontline healthcare workers (HCWs); people living with certain conditions that elevate their risk of worsening mental health outcomes; people living in socioeconomic disadvantage; and vulnerable age groups such as elderly

DOI: 10.4324/9781003294931-10

people, children, and adolescents. The mental health impact on these groups is described further below, globally and in South Africa.

The general population

During the first months of the pandemic's spread, papers emerged from China – the country of origin – detailing both the impact of COVID-19 on the mental well-being of HCWs and the general population (Kang et al., 2020, Lai et al., 2020, Qiu et al., 2020), as well as the mental health system's response to this burden (Li et al., 2020). Subsequently, several studies have emerged which together provide a global view of the mental health effects of COVID-19. An analysis of survey data from 18 Middle Eastern and North African countries suggested 30.9% of participants suffered from severe psychological impact, with most reporting feelings of horror, apprehension, and helplessness, as well as work-related and financial-related stress, due to COVID-19 (Al Dhaheri et al., 2021). In the USA, four in ten people reported suffering from mental and substance use disorders during the pandemic's first stages, up from one in ten reported the previous year – this emerged alongside suggestions that many adults reported negative impacts on sleeping, substance use, worry, and stress (Panchal et al., 2020).

Systematic reviews and meta-analyses suggested relatively high rates of mental ill-health. One report suggested a relatively high prevalence of symptoms of anxiety (between 6.33% and 50.9%); depression (between 14.6% and 48.3%); post-traumatic stress disorder (PTSD; between 7% and 53.8%); psychological distress (between 34.43% and 38%); and stress (between 8.1% and 81.9%) (Xiong et al., 2020). In an analysis that included 60 studies, global rates of depression and anxiety were estimated at 24% and 21.3%, respectively, with high variation across countries and regions (Castaldelli-Maia et al., 2021). A systematic review of 107 studies on mental health prevalence rates from January to July 2020 suggested pooled global prevalence rates of 28.6% for depression, 27.4% for anxiety, 30.2% for PTSD, 40.1% for stress, 45.4% for psychological distress, and 27.7% for sleep problems (Nochaiwong et al., 2021). An analysis from the Organisation for Economic Co-operation and Development (OECD) highlighted that mental health prevalence rates have been relatively stable up until 2020, when (especially) depressive and anxiety symptoms increased in a number of countries – in countries like Belgium, France, Italy, Mexico, and New Zealand, rates doubled at the beginning of 2020 (Organisation for Economic Co-operation and Development, 2021).

This trend was further supported by the 2020 Global Burden of Disease study, which estimated a global increase in the prevalence of depressive disorders of 27.6%, and an increase of 25.6% in anxiety disorders, which translates into an increase of estimated disability-adjusted life years (DALYs) of 137.1 per 100 000 and 116.1 per 100 000, respectively. Further, women and younger people were suggested to be more affected than men and older people (Santomauro et al.). An umbrella review of the global evidence of the effects of COVID-19 on mental health by the WHO suggested statistically signifi-cant increases in pooled effect sizes of depression, anxiety, and general mental health problems in the first year of the pandemic compared to pre-pandemic measures. Younger people, women, and people having pre-existing health conditions were particularly at risk, with little evidence from low-to-middle-income countries (LMICs) (World Health Organization, 2022).

Several datasets describing mental health trends emerged from South Africa as well (though none were nationally representative). One survey (957 adults living in Soweto) suggested that 14.5% of adults were at risk for developing depression, which was also positively correlated with a higher perception of COVID-19 risk (Kim et al., 2020). An online survey (1214 respondents) by the South African Depression and Anxiety Group (SADAG) showed that 65% of participants felt stressed or very stressed during the first lockdown. Fifty-five percent experienced anxiety and panic, 46% felt the financial pres-sure, 40% reported feeling depressed, 30% reported worsening family rela-tions, and 12% contemplated suicide (South African Depression and Anxiety Group, 2021). A survey among 860 people conducted in the Western Cape during the same period suggested that a substantial proportion of participants met the diagnostic threshold for mental disorders (46% for anxiety and 47.2% for depression) – particularly among younger people, women, and people liv-ing in urban areas. Importantly, less than 20% of these participants consulted a healthcare practitioner (De Man et al., 2021).

The UJ-HSRC COVID-19 Democracy Survey asked respondents to list emotions experienced regularly during the week preceding the inter-views, the most common response being stress (57%), followed by fear (42%), frustration/irritability (39%), depression (36%), boredom (30%), sadness (27%), loneliness (27%), and anger (24%). Only 17% reported feel-ing regularly happy (University of Johannesburg (UJ) and Human Sciences Research Council (HSRC), 2020). Data from the National Income Dynamics-Coronavirus Rapid Mobile Survey (NIDS-CRAM), suggested that depressive symptoms doubled from 12% to 24% between 2017 and June 2020 (Spaull et al., 2020). In another poll, survey results from more than 1200 adults suggested that 49% of respondents felt anxious, 48% felt frus-trated, 31% felt depressed, and 6% have contemplated suicide. More than half (56%) reported higher levels of psychological and emotional distress compared to before the pandemic. Almost two-thirds (65%) neglected their health, and 52% had trouble sleeping. This survey further illuminated how people dealt with elevated distress levels, with 81% using unhealthy food, 20% using alcohol, 18% using cigarettes, and 6% using cannabis to cope – only 22% cited psychopharmaceutical support (Pharma Dynamics, 2021). The aforementioned global analysis of the impact of COVID-19 on mental health suggested that, during 2020, there was a 42.7% and 39.9% increase in depressive and anxiety disorders, respectively – translating into 148 and 181.3 additional DALYs for depressive disorders and for anxiety disorders, respectively (Santomauro et al.).

Vulnerable groups

During the course of the pandemic, it became apparent that a number of groups were particularly vulnerable to negative mental health outcomes. HCWs, many of whom, were thrust into challenging, demanding, and chaotic situations with much uncertainty and a lack of clinical guidance on treatment and prevention protocols, particularly suffered (and still do). Six months after the initial outbreak in Wuhan, 20.87% of HCWs in the Central Hospital experienced probable PTSD, which was further associated with higher levels of psychiatric and somatic illness and insomnia (Zhang et al., 2020). One-quarter (23%–27%) of HCWs in a study in Saudi Arabia showed significant levels of anxiety and depression during a period of lockdown (Fageera et al., 2021). An evidence synthesis of the effects of COVID-19 on HCWs during the pandemic suggested that at least one in five reported depressive and anxiety symptoms (higher amongst women), while two in five reported insomnia (Pappa et al., 2020). A South African study suggested that during the first wave of COVID-19, HCWs experienced substantial mental health challenges, which were significantly associated with having been infected with COVID-19, and having had to quarantine as a close contact of someone who was infected. Worryingly, being a manager was also associated with worse mental health outcomes (Curran et al., 2021). Previous outbreaks suggest that the impact on HCWs mental health outcomes did not vary greatly (Preti et al., 2020).

In addition to HCWs, several vulnerable groups have been identified that could suffer from disproportionate negative mental health outcomes. As the literature thus far has already noted, women have been repeatedly highlighted as being particularly vulnerable to depressive and anxiety-related symptoms. Groups that have been socially disadvantaged – for instance people of colour, and members of the LGBTQI+ community, have been rendered vulnerable to mental distress by the conditions imposed by the pandemic (Dawson et al., 2021, Wang et al., 2021). Children and adolescents – despite having less risk of contracting COVID-19 – have been impacted by disruptions in school routines, as well as by increased isolation and other related impacts of strict lockdown measures (Golberstein et al., 2020). Elderly people, the homeless population, people with pre-existing, and comorbid health conditions are all more exposed to mental distress brought on by the conditions of the pandemic (Khan et al., 2020). People who have had COVID-19 disease have been suggested to have high levels of PTSD and depressive symptoms, as well as people with pre-existing serious psychological disorder (Vindegaard and Benros, 2020). This population has been particularly vulnerable to worsening symptoms, especially during strict periods of lockdown. One study suggested significantly high levels of PTSD, depression, anxiety, stress, and insomnia, possibly aggravated by disruptions in care and rapid de-prioritising of non-COVID-19 health programmes (Hao et al., 2020). Increased self-isolation and service disruption have also had detrimental mental health effects on people living with neurocognitive disorders (Dellazizzo et al., 2021).

Causal pathways between COVID-19 pandemic contexts and mental distress

The psychological responses summarised above are the result of a myriad of direct and indirect causal pathways. In terms of HCWs, reviews from previous epidemics and pandemics indicate that almost all healthcare providers will experience elevated levels of stress, anxiety, and fatigue due to exposure to extraordinary high workload, alterations to tasks and responsibilities, risk of infection, more difficult working conditions that include wearing protective clothing and procedures, as well as exposure to emotional events and trauma due to higher rates of patient deaths (Magill et al., 2020, Rieckert et al., 2021). Elevated stress levels and sleep deprivation can lead to workplace errors, as well as long-term burn-out, depression, anxiety, and PTSDs (Rieckert et al., 2021). As for communities, lockdowns promoted fear, loneliness, and uncertainty (Yao et al., 2020), while rumours and misinformation in the era of social media have driven fear, anxiety, and stress via a constant stream of information (much of it unverified) (Kumar and Nayar, 2021). Exposure to COVID-19-related traumatic events – death, illness, poverty, etc. – has been a strong predictor of PTSD and depressive symptoms (Nearchou and Douglas, 2021).

Lockdowns have also led to a rise in domestic violence, further aggravated by a decrease in victims' mobility and accessing support services (Kumar and Nayar, 2021). Disruptions in health service access have affected many with pre-existing conditions (Yao et al., 2020), and, while the evidence described thus far has shown a substantial increase in need for mental health services during the pandemic, there was also a concomitant reduction in resources and investment in mental health systems – particularly in African countries (World Health Organization, 2020). A global recession and its associated knock-on effects, including rapidly increasing food prices and job loss, further aggravated mental distress (Spaull et al., 2021). It is important to keep in mind that, while much of mental symptomology resides on an individual level, the pandemic has substantially elevated structural drivers (Hunt et al., 2021). The aforementioned SADAG survey showed that 16% of respondents lived alone, a recurring theme in their helpline conversations. Even if there are multiple people living in a household, family dynamics will be put under strain should one member fall ill, and increase fears of infection spread among family members (South African Depression and Anxiety Group, 2021). An additional impact has been a substantial curb on movement and access to vital services, particularly for victims of sexual and gender-based violence who were more exposed to victimisation and less able to seek help (Médecins Sans Frontières, 2020).

It is almost impossible to isolate mental distress prevalence trends from South Africa's socioeconomic make-up. The UJ-HSRC COVID-19 Democracy Survey produced the unexpected finding that these feelings reduced after two months of lockdown (e.g. feelings of stress reduced from

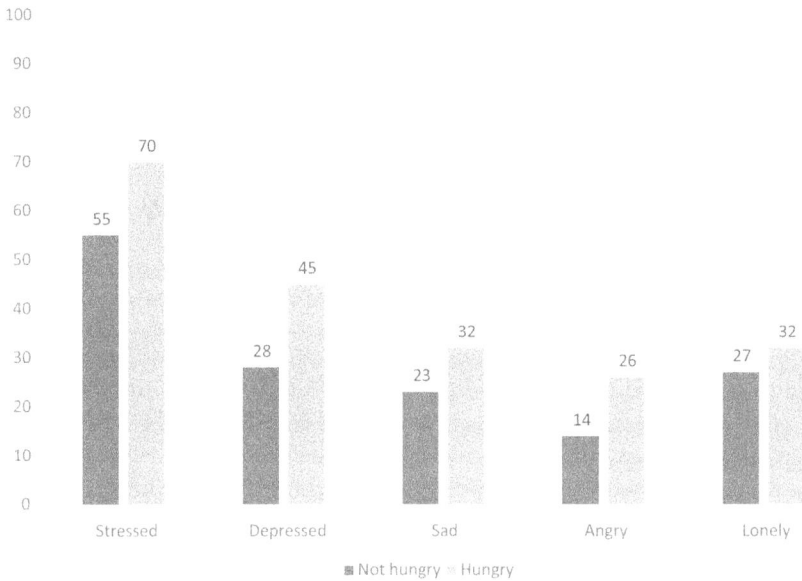

Figure 10.1 Influences of hunger on psychological responses to COVID-19 during lockdown (University of Johannesburg (UJ) and Human Sciences Research Council (HSRC), 2020).

58% to 36%). Further analysis suggested that this reduction can be ascribed to substantial variation among racial groups – while statistically significant decreases in psychosocial distress occurred among Black, Indian, and Coloured populations, high proportions of fear, stress, frustration, depressed emotions, and sadness remained among White participants. Further, while anger remained stable among Black participants, it increased substantially among White participants. The result was an overall decrease despite proportional differences across racial groups (University of Johannesburg (UJ) and Human Sciences Research Council (HSRC), 2020). Increases in depressive symptoms from pre-COVID-19 to COVID-19 lockdown eras from NIDS-CRAM data were especially large among men, non-Black population groups, people with tertiary education, and those within the top 20% income bracket. Pre-existing gaps in depressive symptoms in terms of rich and poor, men, and women, higher and lower education levels, were substantially reduced and in some cases even reversed (Spaull et al., 2020).

As depicted in Figure 10.1, food insecurity was a particularly central influence in determining psychological response. Feelings of stress, depressed mood, sadness, anger, and loneliness were all more likely among people who reported regular hunger (University of Johannesburg (UJ) and Human Sciences Research Council (HSRC), 2020). This trend was mirrored by NIDS-CRAM, where those who reported experiencing hunger 'Every day' or 'Almost every day' were twice as likely to exhibit depressive symptoms. People who experienced perpetual hunger were also twice as likely to report depressive symptoms than those experiencing less often (Spaull et al., 2020).

Further analysis from NIDS-CRAM revealed that in 40% of food-insecure households adults exhibited depressed symptoms one year after the height of the first hard lockdown (April 2020), compared to 26% of food-secure households. When considering children having a lack of access to school (and school meals), the 40% rises to 51%. Analysis of NIDS-CRAM Waves 2, 3, and 4 highlighted inconsistent access to school meals even when schools were still open (Spaull et al., 2021).

Adults with above-average levels of depressive symptoms and living in large households have been shown to be more likely to exhibit high levels of worry, while those in large households with regular access to government grants were less worried (Spaull et al., 2021). Ultimately, the perception of risk increased depressive symptoms among those with higher incomes, while the less affluent received a degree of protection from depressive symptoms from the social grant (Oyenubi and Kollamparambil, 2020). Unemployment has emerged as a key challenge in current and future mental distress, elevating the importance of the COVID-19 Relief Grant. Based on the Quarterly Labour Force Survey (QLFS) for the second quarter of 2021, unemployed people increased by more than a half million to 7.8 million in total. This resulted in an unemployment rate of 34.4%, its highest level since its inception in 2008 (applying an expanded definition of unemployment results in a rate of 44.4% in the second quarter) (Statistics South Africa, 2021).

Responses to mental health effects of COVID-19

Global

While many countries formulated COVID-19 mental health response plans, a survey of 28 African countries suggested that less than one-third was fully funded (World Health Organization, 2020). Nevertheless, mental health resources and responses came from many sources – government, civil society, private and corporate sectors, grassroots community mobilisation, and professional organisations. The International Society for Traumatic Stress Studies curates a body of COVID-19 mental health resources,[1] including webinars, informational posters and website, and videos. These are categorised for Mental Health Professionals, Healthcare Workers, Parents and Caregivers, Teachers and School Staff, Business and Community Leaders, and for anyone else (International Society for Traumatic Stress Studies, 2021).

Low-to-middle-income countries

There have also been promising examples of mental health user organisation involvement in rendering support in LMICs. Kola et al. (2021) provide

China
- Online mental health education materials produced and disseminated through WeChat, Weibo, and TikTok
- Artificial intelligence programmes used for the detection of psychological crises during the pandemic
- WeChat also used for the delivery of cognitive behavioural therapy for depression, anxiety, and insomnia

Philippines
- National Center for Mental Health toll-free crisis hotline, which has had a four times increase in the number of calls

India
- Toll-free mental health helpline number
- Kerala state Government has established a multidisciplinary team
- 1140 psychiatrists, counsellors, and social workers trained to assess the psychological health of people with COVID-19, older people living alone, and children
- 1-3 million calls to people in quarantine and other vulnerable individuals
- Opioid drug replacement therapy dispensed fortnightly to more than 500 000 patients

Turkey
- Apps built to allow access to mental health specialists online
- Fairy tale reading project for children

Lebanon
- COVID-19 call centre operators trained in psychological first aid
- Social media campaign targeting young people
- Development of child-friendly quarantine protocols

Maldives
- Psychological first aid via hotlines for front-line workers and other populations at risk of COVID-19 to provide support and identify potential severe mental health issues that would benefit from referral
- Hotlines to migrant workers

Pakistan
- Trained 3610 community members to provide mental health first aid for health-care workers
- Aga Khan University, Karachi, has launched a nationwide child and adolescent mental health response by providing online training in parent-mediated therapy

Serbia
- National line for psychosocial support during COVID-19
- 3556 hotline calls for mental health
- Mobile teams of health professionals located at quarantine points

Liberia
- MHPSS training and law enforcement
- Community healing dialogues

Suriname
- Helpline 123
- Social workers refer to specialists for support with people in quarantine and other populations

Uganda
- Training of staff in all regional referral hospitals on MHPSS
- Home outreach programmes for people with severe mental illness

South Africa
- Programmes encouraging front-line workers to call hotlines
- Specific hotlines set-up for front-line workers

Nicaragua
- The Nicaraguan Association for the Development of Psychology offers virtual online resources for educational, informative, and reflective material, and tools to train professionals

Honduras
- Médecins Sans Frontières offers phone-based psychosocial care to hospitalised patients and care to survivors of violence, and has established a mental health phone helpline

Costa Rica
- The Costa Rican Social Security Fund has established a virtual visit system using tablets, phones, etc, for patients to engage with relatives to enhance mood

Brazil
- Academic recommendations for delirium management in patients with obsessive compulsive disorder or those in intensive care units
- Outreach programmes for people with severe mental illness

Peru
- Patient Health Questionnaire-9 chatbot to screen for individuals with depression in affected communities
- Remote delivery of the Thinking Health Programme and Problem Management Plus via phone

- Low-income
- Lower-middle income
- Upper-middle income
- High-income

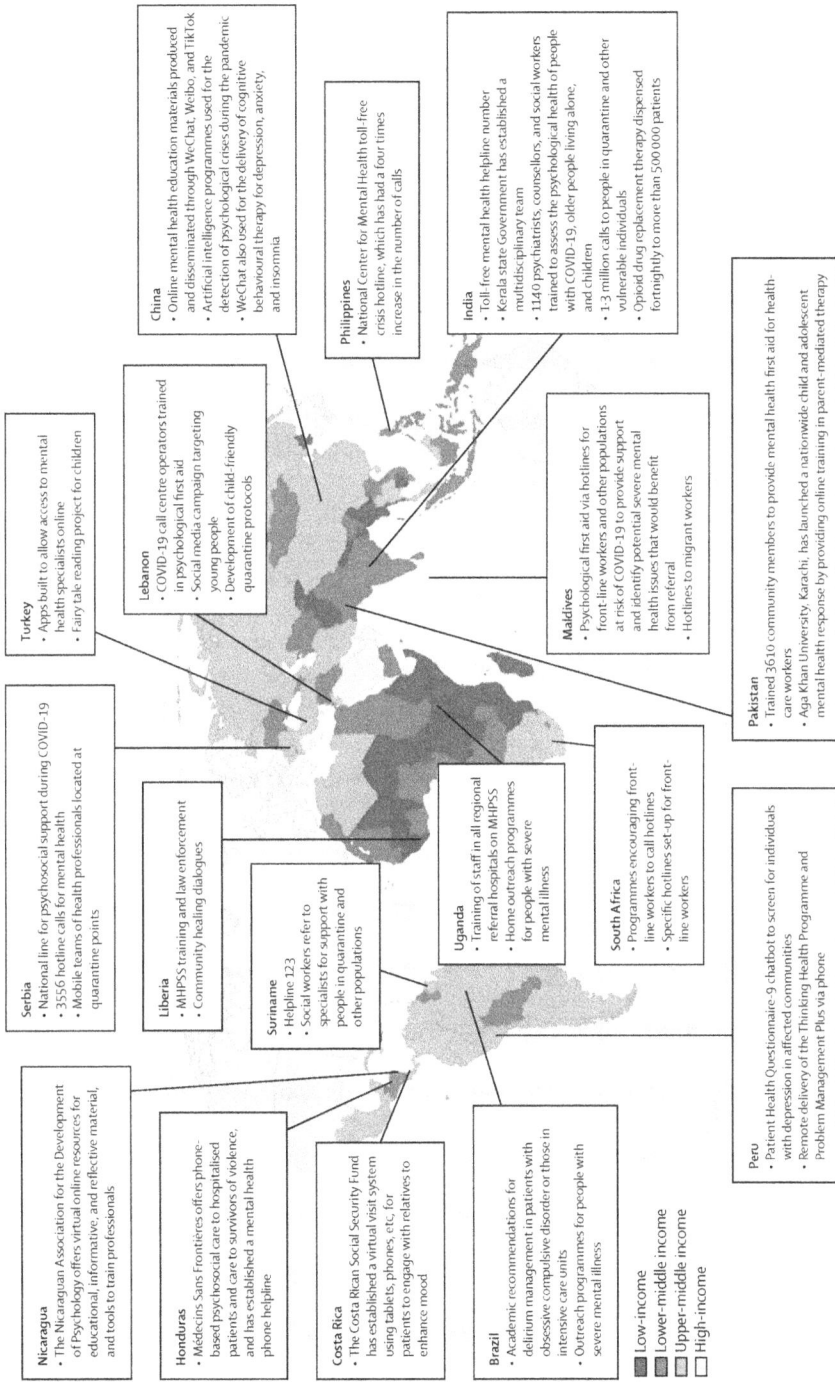

Figure 10.2 LMIC responses to COVID-19 mental health impacts (Kola et al., 2021).

an overview of responses by LMICs to COVID-19 mental health impacts, summarised in Figure 10.2. In terms of population initiatives, many LMICs have built up substantial expertise in addressing mental health needs during humanitarian emergencies, and this capacity was applied to COVID-19 as well. This was reflected in the relative rapid development of national mental health response plans and included strategies developed and endorsed in Lebanon, South Africa, Kenya, Uganda, the Maldives, and India.

Many information, education, and communication material have been generated by governments, multilateral, humanitarian, and development organisations. In particular, the International Federation of Red Cross and Red Crescent Societies Reference Centre for Psychosocial Support has amassed a wealth of mental health resources aimed at constrained contexts during COVID-19 (IFRC Reference Centre for Psychosocial Support, 2022). The Inter-Agency Standing Committee launched a briefing note 'Addressing Mental Health and Psychosocial Aspects of COVID-19 Outbreak', in multiple languages and in easy-to-read and Braille formats (IASC Reference Group on Mental Health and Psychosocial Support, 2020) and the Africa Centres for Disease Control and Prevention released 'Guidance for mental health and psychosocial support for COVID-19' (Africa Centres for Disease Control and Prevention, 2020). The Mental Health Innovation Network and WHO jointly launched 'Stories from the field: Providing mental health and psychosocial support during the COVID-19 pandemic', a guidance aiming to share innovation and best practice through personal narratives (Mental Health Information Network and World Health Organization, 2020).

In Pakistan, the NGO Basic Needs Pakistan established 60 mental health first aid instructors and trained thousands of community members as 'mental health first aiders', offered online and phone counselling and consultation, promoted social media awareness about COVID-19's impact on mental health, as well as creating rapid mental health response teams to provide community-based psychological support (BasicNeeds Pakistan (BNPAK), 2020). A social media campaign in India, #sparkthejoy, encouraged acts of kindness in relation to mental health issues during COVID-19 (Firework, 2020), while the Luchando contra el COVID-19 programme was launched in Trinidad and Tobago to support the mental health needs of Venezuelan migrants through videos in Spanish on coping with stress and protecting vulnerable groups, a toll-free helpline, and online counselling services (Nakhid-Chatoor, 2020). Further, Psychiatric Disability Organisation Kenya provided psychosocial support to prison staff in Nakuru; the Zimbabwe Obsessive Compulsive Disorder Trust provided peer-based support to help address COVID-19-related anxiety; and the Global Mental Health Peer Network instituted bimonthly online COVID-19 and mental health virtual support groups (Kola et al., 2021). There are also many examples of mental health services being maintained under pandemic contexts, such as Socios en Salud in Peru that provides automated, chatbot depression screening and referral, and hybrid systems of in-person and remote services (including antipsychotic injections and food security monitoring) for people living with psychotic disorders in Brazil and Uganda (Kola et al., 2021).

South Africa

Below, following a brief overview of South Africa's mental health system contexts, selected dimensions of the country's mental health response to the impact of COVID-19 are described – the development, collation, and dissemination of mental health resources; collaboration between academia and government to develop and disseminate an online wellness resource; and the potential of community mobilisation to ameliorate some of the more pressing determinants of mental distress in the contexts of the pandemic.

South Africa's mental health system in context

Both prior to and following the introduction of the country's Mental Health Care Act (17 of 2002) and National Mental Health Policy Framework and Strategic Plan 2013–2020 (Department of Health, 2012), much has been written about South Africa's mental health system. In the period following the introduction of these two key documents, the mental health system was highlighted as having substantial variation in the distribution of mental health resources between provinces, between urban and rural areas, and between public and private sectors of care – central features of South Africa's post-apartheid legacy (Janse van Rensburg et al., 2018). The system is also very much hospital-centric, with a heavy reliance on very limited numbers of mental healthcare specialists, despite fractional instances of integration with PHC in some areas. Services in communities were fragmented and uncoordinated, with several NGOs and different government departments providing largely responsive care without appropriate oversight and intersectoral governance. Very few mental health indicators feature in district health information systems (Flisher et al., 2007, Lund et al., 2010, Petersen et al., 2009, Petersen and Lund, 2011, Janse van Rensburg et al., 2018).

Although the National Policy has now lapsed, an evaluation of its performance is yet to be carried out. However, there have been indications that the implementation of the policy remains far removed from its admirable ideals. The most vivid example here is the failure to establish a community-based system of care for people who live with severe mental and neurological conditions. Despite progress in the availability of psychotropic medications, and an apparent acceptance among PHC staff to help manage long-term psychiatric conditions, there has been a persistent lack of investment in community-based psychosocial rehabilitation and long-term support, which, in parallel with decreasing psychiatric hospital beds, mimics failed deinstitutionalisation strategies in other parts of the world (Petersen and Lund, 2011). The Life Esidimeni tragedy, where, during 2015–2016, 144 people with severe mental illness died due to neglect following a disastrous state-driven deinstitutionalisation project that involved moving patients from hospital settings to unregistered, unregulated NGOs, along with similar, smaller scale failures, have illustrated the dire consequences of poor mental health systems with inadequate community investment, and underlined an urgency for ambitious, evidence-based reform (Robertson et al., 2018, Janse van Rensburg, 2021, Janse van Rensburg et al., 2019).

Failures in progress in terms of the ideals of South Africa's policy and legislation have further been highlighted in a recent national survey (Docrat et al., 2019). It found that South Africa's mental health expenditure is significantly focused on specialised in-patient psychiatric care (45%), with only 7.9% being spent in PHC mental health services – community-level investment is unknown due to the involvement of a variety of sectors, service providers, and types of care offered. Mental health readmissions put enormous strain on the mental health budget – it is estimated that 24.2% of those discharged into community settings following psychiatric hospitalisation are readmitted within three months. This translates to an annual cost of USD112.6 million, 18.2% of total mental health care expenditure. Worryingly, the current prevalence estimates are for adults, and not for child mental health. With only 6.8% of mental health service users aged under 18 accounted for, a coordinated, intersectoral response to child and adolescent mental health challenges remains almost completely absent (this was also supported by recent studies (Babatunde et al., 2020a, Babatunde et al., 2020b, Babatunde et al., 2021, Mokitimi et al., 2018). Taken as a whole, South Africa faces a mental health treatment gap for mental, developmental, and neurological conditions of 92% (Docrat et al., 2019).

Psychoeducation and counselling support

South African academic, government, and civil society bodies have generated online information pages, many of which have been zero rated by the Internet Service Providers' Association of South Africa (ISPA). This means that, as long as the country's State of Disaster continues, access to online content that offers COVID-19 information, education, and support will be free of data charges (both fixed and mobile) for the public. Selected examples are provided in Table 10.1.

South Africa's very limited supply of mental health professionals, as well as its notorious public-private divide, meant that many people in need simply could not access mental health services. There were, however, instances of private and academic actors who offered free services during this time. SADAG's 24-hour counselling helpline was overburdened during times of lockdown, especially given that mobility was limited during the lockdown. Nonetheless, the organisation initiated free online support groups, run by trained volunteers, for people whose regular face-to-face support groups were suspended. As part of the Mental Health Toolkit made available by the KZNDoH, a list of registered mental health professionals was provided who provided free

Table 10.1 Online resources for COVID-19-related mental health in South Africa

Details of online resource	Weblink
The KwaZulu-Natal Department of Health's (KZNDoH) Mental Health and Substance Use Directorate provides a range of mental health-related resources on a page aimed at both the general public and HCWs	http://www.kznhealth.gov. za/mental/covid19.htm
The Centre for Rural Health, University of KwaZulu-Natal, developed psychosocial well-being support materials to different groups, offered data-free on a dedicated COVID-19 Hub. These materials have also been adopted by the KZNDoH and hosted on their page.	https://crh.ukzn.ac.za/ covid-19-hub/
Stellenbosch University's Department of Psychiatry provides a curated list of resources (General resources, Mental health resources, Resources for adults, Resources for children and their carers, COVID-19 in the elderly, Resources for health care workers) on a dedicated page	http://www.sun.ac.za/ english/faculty/ healthsciences/psychiatry/ covid-19-resources
University of Cape Town's Department of Psychiatry and Mental Health COVID-19 Resources page (Managing Mental Health; Managing Mental Health during the COVID-19 Pandemic: Resources from the WHO; Children, Adolescents and Parenting; Credible Updated Information sources for COVID-19; Resources for healthcare workers)	http://www.psychiatry. uct.ac.za/news/ covid-19-resources-0
The South African Depression and Anxiety Group (SADAG) hosts pages with links related to information about Covid19 And Lockdown, Covid-19 Helpful Tips, and Covid-19 Reliable Resources	https://bit.ly/3CxutfF
CIPLA pharmaceuticals hosts a COVID-19 information page, that includes information on mental health	https://www.cipla. co.za/our-medicine/ therapeutic-areas/ covid-19
The Regional Psychosocial Support Initiative developed a series of videos on grief and mental health for children and adolescents in South Africa	https://repssi.org/

counselling services to those who couldn't afford private care. The University of KwaZulu-Natal's Centre for Applied Psychology offered three free online sessions for anyone suffering from mental health difficulties during the COVID-19 period. The Psychological Society of South Africa (PsySSA) coordinated a national list of psychologists, psychiatrists, and social workers who offered free support during the pandemic. Several psychiatrists further offered pro bono support to HCWs struggling with mental health issues (Exec Committee: Durban Practising Psychologists' Group (DPPG), 2020). The Foundation for

Professional Development offered a free online 7-Day Mental Health Survival Kit for Lockdown Course (Foundation for Professional Development, 2021), while the Healthcare Workers Care Network (HWCN) offered free support, pro bono therapy, resources, training, and psychoeducation to all HCWs (HealthCare Workers Care Network, 2021).

Addressing the mental health of children and adolescents

A particularly pressing concern, one that arguably merits a section on its own, is the impacts of and responses to children's mental health during COVID-19. The disruptions of infection containment strategies and strict lockdowns severely disrupted schooling, which, on top of education, is a major provider of social welfare in the form of meals and facilitating access to social security structures. Lockdowns and their associated social isolation meant that little access to peers was possible and that a substantial number of vulnerable children went hungry and was exposed to home environments with increased stress and uncertainty. Though comprehensive research exploring how these factors have affected children's mental health, it is assumed, based on previous effects of large-scale disasters, that increases in post-traumatic stress, anxiety, and depressive disorders will emerge, as well as increases in substance abuse (Spaull and van der Berg, 2020).

The school system largely focused on throughput, with rapidly compressed timelines to complete curricula. This undoubtedly increased pressure felt by both educators and learners. A school readiness survey conducted by the Department of Basic Education (DoBE) suggested that more than 50% of principals believe that learners and teachers need psychosocial support, that 49% had arrangements in place with social service agencies to provide psychosocial support in their schools, and that 44% had staff available in their schools to provide learner psychosocial support (Department of Basic Education, 2020). Within these contexts, partnerships between schools and the education sector in broad, and NGOs, universities and community resources were (and remain) particularly important. An example is resources developed by the University of Cape Town's (UCT) Schools Development Unit (SDU). The Unit launched a certified short course for educators and learning support assistants, 'Psychological First Aid for Educators (PFA) in the COVID-19 Context', aimed to empower the application of basic psychological first aid in the school context (Swingler, 2021). Another initiative, also produced by the Unit, is the 'My South African Pandemic Story' programme, which is a series of workbooks based on the principle of 'giving children psychological hands' (H.A.N.D.S: Honestly communicate, Actively cope, Network with peers and adults, in a Developmentally Specific way). The workbooks encourage an active facing of difficulties posed by the pandemic, supported by educators and parents (The Schools Development Unit, 2020).

Collaboration between academia and government: The APC wellness resource

Building on existing project relationships, a collaboration between the Centre for Rural Health (UKZN), the Knowledge Translation Unit (UCT), and the Department of Health resulted in the development of a psychosocial wellness resource for HCWs, presented as a free online course within the nationally adopted Adult Primary Care (APC) platform and the Mental Health Integration (MhINT) programme in KwaZulu-Natal (Knowledge Translation Unit, 2021). This initiative arose from the pressing need to offer support to overburdened and overstretched HCWs and in the context of alarming reports that highlighted elevated levels of mental distress. The programme was informed by evidence that suggests the need for a multi-pronged approach that includes (i) Enhancing health care provider resilience through ensuring that health care providers are equipped with accurate information about the disease outbreak, infection prevention and control measures including the use of PPE, and self-care strategies and skills to cope with associated stress of pandemics; and (ii) Organisational interventions such as ensuring reasonable provider-patient ratios commensurate with care provider capabilities, reasonable work shift hours that include provision for adequate breaks during shifts, ensuring adequate resources including access to PPE, as well as referral resources for psychosocial support (Rieckert et al., 2021). This resource helps to address the first issue of promoting resilience amongst healthcare providers and should be accompanied by organisational interventions to address these other aspects. The resource follows the APC case format, grounding the learning in case studies of different health care provider characters in the tea room. It uses short narrative vignettes to introduce characters in the tea room who are faced with common stressors experienced by health care providers during the COVID-19 pandemic. These common stressors were identified through a review of the literature (locally and internationally), an online survey of over 400 providers during the first COVID-19 wave (Curran et al., 2021), as well as interviews with frontline staff.

While most health care providers have been found to experience adverse psychological outcomes during epidemics and pandemics, a small percentage have been found to require specialised mental health services (Magill et al., 2020). A stepped mental health response is recommended to protect the limited mental health specialist resources available, which is especially the case in LMICs. This wellness resource adopts such an approach, providing strategies and self-help skills to strengthen self-care, starting with lifestyle strategies that have been proven to assist in coping with stress and promoting psychological well-being (Velten et al., 2014). The next step assists providers to cope through capacitating themselves in self-help skills that draw on evidence-based psychological interventions, including cognitive behavioural techniques of healthy thinking, problem management, and mindfulness that have been shown to be effectively delivered through online applications

(Linardon et al., 2019, Hwang et al., 2021). Should providers still require additional support, the resource provides contact details of counselling hotlines and referral pathways to mental health specialists. A description of the course is provided in Box 10.2.

Community-driven initiatives

There are many examples of community initiatives that emerged during the pandemic in South Africa. During the first lockdown in Durban, the Denis

---

Box 10.2: APC wellness resource modules

Given international and local literature that indicates that the majority of health care providers experience extraordinary levels of stress and burn-out during pandemics, including during the COVID-19 pandemic, the wellness resource begins with a module that addresses this general concern of stress and burnout amongst healthcare providers and is the only module that is compulsory, with health care providers being able to choose other issues that address their particular needs. This initial module suggests lifestyle behaviours that have been shown to reduce stress and promote psychological wellbeing such as exercise, health eating, adequate sleep and social engagement (Velten et al., 2014).

The second module is directed at operational managers, but is also useful for all health care providers. It provides information and self-help skills on the use of problem management to empower managers to deal with day to day problems in the workplace as well as containing leadership skills which have been shown to be crucial during times of crisis to promote a sense of safety, calming, a sense of self- and community efficacy, connectedness, and hope (Hobfoll et al., 2007).

The third module is for health care providers dealing with burnout and the emotional impact of breaking bad news. This module provides information and self-help skills to calm oneself using mindfulness techniques that have been shown to be particularly useful in reducing stress and improving provider wellbeing (Gilmartin et al., 2017). The third module deals with managing anxiety in the face of having to provide healthcare in the context of a highly infectious disease pandemic. The module draws on self-help cognitive behavioural therapy (CBT) techniques which have been shown to have equivalence to face to face CBT be effective (Carlbring et al., 2018) to help providers to assess whether their negative thoughts are grounded in reality and to promote healthy thinking. In addition, and on the request of a group of nurses during a focus group, this module provides a checklist to assist nurses to contain their own anxiety when dealing with emotionally charged situations.

The fifth module helps providers cope with their own loss and bereavement. The module provides information on the stages of grief (Kübler-Ross and Kessler, 2005) as well as strategies for grieving within the context of COVID 19 where

people may not be able to perform certain rituals and activities that assist people through the grieving process.

To ensure that providers are adequately equipped with the necessary information and skills on how to protect themselves and their families from COVID-19 infection and transmission, an Infection, Prevention and Control (IPC) module is also included. This module provides up to date information of COVID-19 IPC protocols. Given that being vaccinated will also protect healthcare providers from infection, a module on vaccine hesitancy has also been included.

Hurley Centre collaborated with the local municipality to support approximately 1500 homeless people in several buildings and tented camps throughout the city. A militarised response to enforce lockdown regulations – a feature in many instances during this period – was therefore largely avoided. It allowed for trust to be built between the Centre and an expanding homeless community and to increase utilisation of the free clinic and its associated social welfare services (Broughton, 2020).

There are many examples, not formally described, of communities forming networks to identify and support vulnerable households through soup kitchens, food parcels, and other forms of support. The establishment of Community Action Networks (CANs) in the Western Cape, which branched out to areas in Gauteng and the Eastern Cape as well, is a fitting example of the activation of communities in the face of challenge. Started by a group of health professionals, educators, artists, and activists, CANs were formalised through WhatsApp groups and an array of other communication platforms. This includes food delivery to those in need, care for elderly community members, the dissemination of information resources, and promoting and coordinating advocacy efforts. This allowed for a decentralised, neighbourhood-driven needs assessment, autonomous problem-solving, and empowered communities to tap into local resources and self-organise in the face of overwhelmed public health and social services. Further, the digital platform allowed for a degree of collaboration across apartheid-era racial and spatial lines and could perhaps also be seen as an important tool for social solidarity (Odendaal, 2021). The impact of these initiatives, though not easily quantifiable nor well described, on mental health outcomes, would certainly yield important insights into the potential of community activation in health system resilience.

Recommendations for a better future response

Biological disasters bring about fear, uncertainty, stigmatisation, and severe strains on systems and routine services, resulting in elevated levels of mental distress among a variety of populations, the long-term effects of which are yet to be fully explored (Hsieh et al., 2021). Experiences of the chaos of COVID-19 in mental health systems, as well as earlier pandemic experiences, have provided valuable lessons on how to strengthen systems for a better response and, perhaps, for better routine outcomes outside of times of crisis. During disasters, responses such as psychological first aid, psychological debriefing, mental health intervention, and psychoeducation are critical to minimise short-, medium-, and long-term mental health damage (Hsieh et al., 2021). In South Africa, there were many instances of online psychoeducation, provided by government, for-profit, non-profit, academic and professional bodies, and free mental health services were made available to those in need. Though limited, these resources offer valuable buffers to vulnerable groups, especially to HCWs who offer suffer the brunt of trauma exposure during disasters.

In the absence of a comprehensive overview of South Africa's mental health response, it is difficult to gauge how people-centred it has been. It might be safe to assume that, given the substantial challenges that the country's mental health system faced pre-COVID-19, the response has been decidedly non-people-centred. The militarised response that South Africa adopted to enforce its extreme lockdown certainly did not aim to empower communities, and people were not 'participants as well as beneficiaries of trusted health systems that respond to their needs and preferences in humane and holistic ways' (World Health Organization, 2016).

More than ever, South Africa needs to explicitly adopt strategies that put people at the centre of services, towards building a system that (1) empowers and engages people and communities; (2) strengthens governance and accountability; (3) reorients the model of care to community-based services; (4) co-ordinates services within and across sectors; and (5) creates an enabling environment to achieve these goals (World Health Organization, 2016). The emergence of bottom-up, community-driven problem-solving has revealed a critical resource in mental health system reform, and policymakers should carefully consider how these networks can be used to develop community-focused systems of care. In terms of addressing the mental health plight of children and adolescents, the Human Sciences Research Council has published a policy brief outlining recommendations for the integration of psychosocial support in the recovery plans of the DoBE, which includes integrating psychosocial health and well-being support into the National Policy on HIV, STIs, and TB, decentralising psychosocial support programming to include district officials, by including psychosocial support specialists at the district level, and empowering educators in providing psychosocial support (Namome et al., 2021).

For a substantial period now, evidence has been building of the effectiveness and feasibility of using non-specialist workers, trained and supported by mental health professionals, to deliver basic mental health services (including symptom screening and referral, and basic counselling) in LMICs. Beyond 'task-shifting', this approach has developed to be more collaborative in nature and has more accurately been termed 'task-sharing'

(Patel, 2012, Petersen et al., 2011a). Task-sharing has been intensely studied in South Africa (Spedding et al., 2014), particularly to find practical ways in which mental health services can better be integrated into the PHC system, where trained and supervised lay workers can screen for depressive, anxiety and substance use symptoms, provide basic counselling, refer for specialist care, and in some cases even provide support for people living with severe mental illness. Initiatives include the Mental Health and Poverty Research Programme Consortium (Petersen et al., 2011b) and the pioneering Programme for Improving Mental Health Care (PRIME) (Hanlon et al., 2016, Petersen et al., 2016, Petersen et al., 2012), which provided a blueprint for additional studies exploring mental health integration through task-sharing (Fairall et al., 2018, Myers et al., 2019, Centre for Rural Health, 2021).

Many of these lessons are being scaled up and more firmly embedded in the health system, as demonstrated in the S-MhINT programme (Inge Petersen et al., 2021). Given the significant increases in mental health demands highlighted earlier in the chapter, it is critical to drive the scale-up of these evidence-based interventions and to create enabling health service environments for mental health to be delivered by lay health workers. Task-sharing should further not only be thought of as an intervention for clinical spaces, but should also be applied to schools and home outreach contexts, where child and youth care school assistants can be empowered to provide psychosocial services, and social auxiliary workers can support people with severe mental and neurodevelopmental conditions (a population particularly neglected in mainstream narratives of mental health needs during COVID-19).

In a roadmap to strengthen global mental health systems to tackle the impact of the COVID-19 pandemic, the authors provide comprehensive guidance for countries to help inform strategies during the pandemic (Maulik et al., 2020). The roadmap delineates strategies according to low, medium, and high resource availability, and here an overview is provided that is relevant to South Africa (Figure 10.3).

From these recommendations, a crucial recommendation is that mental is best tackled by not limiting the response to only overcome crisis but to integrate and embed mental health care within the broader health system in order to improve reach, effectiveness, and sustainability. This is further underlined by the WHO, which notes that in recovering from COVID-19, countries plan for long-term sustainability; address a broad range of population mental health needs; engage professional organisations; review mental health policies and plans as part of recovery and reform efforts; promote effective intersectoral coordination; drive whole-system strengthening; invest in HCWs' health; draw from key demonstration projects to generate funding for scale-up; and investing in advocacy to maintain change momentum (Ghebreyesus, 2020). A timeous policy window has opened up, with the lapsing of the National Policy and the impending National Health Insurance reforms, to 'build back

Mental health system specific recommendations	Recommendations relevant to service providers and other stakeholders	Recommendations relevant to researchers and research funders
Strengthen leadership and governance	Develop or strengthen equitable, accessible and appropriate community-based mental health services and clinic-based services for those needed special care	Develop research to improve information systems
Identify appropriate finance mechanism to support policies and programmes; develop schemes to cover longer term mental health care	Train adequate primary care staff to cater to the increased mental health needs at the community level	Develop research on epidemiology, neurobiological effects, community-based and special population-based interventions, linkages with environmental and social sciences
	Implement mental health promotion and prevention programmes	
Promote programmes specifically targeting vulnerable groups	Strengthen civil society	Develop innovative solutions to improve mental health systems; support technology enabled solutions to support service delivery; identify strategies to enable more efficient supply chain logistics models for medicines; use of social media to deliver interventions on mental health promotion
	Enable employers to manage stress at workplace	

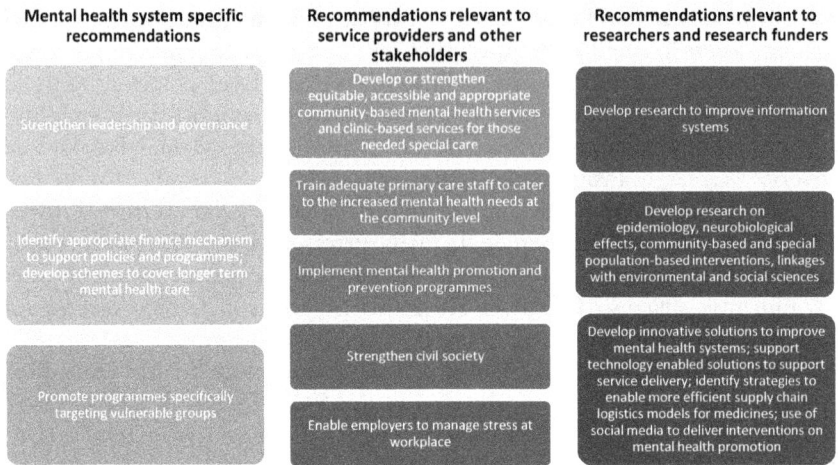

Figure 10.3 Roadmap to strengthen mental health systems (Maulik et al., 2020).

better', and bring service users and communities into the centre of overhauls to improve South Africa's mental health system.

Note

1 American Psychological Association, National Center for PTSD, Center for the Study of Traumatic Stress, The Schwartz Center for Compassionate Healthcare, American Medical Association, Mayo Clinic, Mental Health America, National Alliance for Caregiving, National Child Traumatic Stress Network, National Child Traumatic Stress Network, Stanford Medicine: Division of Child and Adolescent Psychiatry, Centers for Disease Control and Prevention, World Health Organization, University of Colorado Colorado Springs, Harvard TH Chan School of Public Health, Substance Abuse and Mental Health Services Administration, Medical University of South Carolina, European Society for Traumatic Stress Studies, Global Collaboration on Traumatic Stress, Korean Society for Traumatic Stress Studies, Japanese Society for Traumatic Stress Studies.

References

Africa Centres for Disease Control and Prevention (2020). Guidance for mental health and psychosocial support for covid-19. https://africacdc.org/download/guidance-for-mental-health-and-psychosocial-support-for-covid-19/.
Al Dhaheri, A. S., Bataineh, M. a. F., Mohamad, M. N., Ajab, A., Al Marzouqi, A., Jarrar, A. H., Habib-Mourad, C., Abu Jamous, D. O., Ali, H. I., Al Sabbah, H., Hasan, H., Stojanovska, L., Hashim, M., AbdElhameed, O. A., Shaker Obaid, R. R.,

Elfeky, S., Saleh, S. T., Osaili, T. M. & Cheikh Ismail, L. (2021). Impact of covid-19 on mental health and quality of life: Is there any effect? A cross-sectional study of the mena region. *PLOS One, 16*, e0249107.

Babatunde, G. B., Bhana, A. & Petersen, I. (2020a). Planning for child and adolescent mental health interventions in a rural district of South Africa: A situational analysis. *Journal of Child & Adolescent Mental Health, 32*, 45–65.

Babatunde, G. B., Van Rensburg, A. J., Bhana, A. & Petersen, I. (2020b). Stakeholders' perceptions of child and adolescent mental health services in a South African district: A qualitative study. *International Journal of Mental Health Systems, 14*, 1–12.

Babatunde, G. B., Van Rensburg, A. J., Bhana, A. & Petersen, I. (2021). Barriers and facilitators to child and adolescent mental health services in low-and-middle-income countries: A scoping review. *Global Social Welfare, 8*, 29–46.

Basicneeds Pakistan (Bnpak). (2020). *Basicneeds Pakistan: Supporting mental health in under-resourced communities during the covid-19 pandemic* [Online]. https://www.mhinnovation.net/blog/2020/may/12/basicneeds-pakistan-supporting-mental-health-under-resourced-communities-during. [Accessed].

Broughton, T. (2020). Covid-19 lockdown bridges social divide for durban's homeless. *GroundUp*. https://www.groundup.org.za/article/covid-19-lockdown-bridges-social-divide-durbans-homeless/.

Carlbring, P., Andersson, G., Cuijpers, P., Riper, H. & Hedman-Lagerlof, E. (2018). Internet-based vs. Face-to-face cognitive behavior therapy for psychiatric and somatic disorders: An updated systematic review and meta-analysis. *Cognition Behavior Therogy, 47*, 1–18.

Castaldelli-Maia, J. M., Marziali, M. E., Lu, Z. & Martins, S. S. (2021). Investigating the effect of national government physical distancing measures on depression and anxiety during the covid-19 pandemic through meta-analysis and meta-regression. *Psychological Medicine, 51*, 881–893.

Centre for Rural Health. (2021). *Mhint: Mental Health Integration into Primary Care* [Online]. Online webpage: https://crh.ukzn.ac.za/mhint-mental-health-integration-into-primary-care/. Available: https://crh.ukzn.ac.za/mhint-mental-health-integration-into-primary-care/ [Accessed].

Curran, R., Bachmann, M., Van Rensburg, A. J., Murdoch, J., Awotiwon, A., Ras, C.-J., Petersen, I. & Fairall, L. (2021). Personal and Occupational Experiences of Covid-19 and their Effects on South African Health Workers' Wellbeing. *South African Medical Journal, 111*(7), 607–608. doi: 10.7196/SAMJ.2021.v111i7.15733.

Dawson, L., Kirzinger, A. & Kates, J. (2021). *The Impact of the Covid-19 Pandemic on LGBT People*. San Francisco, CA: The Kaiser Family Foundation.

De Man, J., Smith, M. R., Schneider, M. & Tabana, H. (2021). An exploration of the impact of COVID-19 on mental health in South Africa. *Psychology, Health & Medicine, 27*(1), 120–130. doi: 10.1080/13548506.2021.1954671.

Dellazizzo, L., Léveillé, N., Landry, C. & Dumais, A. (2021). Systematic review on the mental health and treatment impacts of COVID-19 on neurocognitive disorders. *Journal Pers Medicine, 11*(8), 746. doi: 10.3390/jpm11080746.

Department of Basic Education (2020). *School Readiness Survey*. Pretoria: DBE.

Department of Health (2012). *National mental health policy framework and strategic plan 2013–2020*. Pretoria: DoH.

Docrat, S., Besada, D., Cleary, S., Daviaud, E. & Lund, C. (2019). Mental health system costs, resources and constraints in South Africa: A national survey. *Health Policy and Planning, 34*, 706–719.

Exec Committee: Durban Practising Psychologists' Group (Dppg) (2020). List of psychological support during covid-19. http://www.kznhealth.gov.za/mental/covid19/contacts/free-psychology-services.pdf.

Fageera, W., Babtain, F., Alzahrani, A. S. & Khrad, H. M. (2021). Lock-down effect on the mental health status of healthcare workers during covid-19 pandemic. *Frontiers in Psychiatry, 12*, 683603.

Fairall, L., Petersen, I., Zani, B., Folb, N., Georgeu-Pepper, D., Selohilwe, O., Petrus, R., Mntambo, N., Bhana, A., Lombard, C., Bachmann, M., Lund, C., Hanass-Hancock, J., Chisholm, D., Mccrone, P., Carmona, S., Gaziano, T., Levitt, N., Kathree, T. & Thornicroft, G. (2018). Collaborative care for the detection and management of depression among adults receiving antiretroviral therapy in South Africa: Study protocol for the cobalt randomised controlled trial. *Trials, 19*, 193.

Firework. (2020). *Covid-19: A little act of kindness can #sparkthejoy* [Online]. https://www.thehindu.com/society/little-act-of-kindness-can-sparkthejoy/article31430300.ece. [Accessed].

Flisher, A. J., Lund, C., Funk, M., Banda, M., Bhana, A., Doku, V., Drew, N., Kigozi, F. N., Knapp, M. & Omar, M. (2007). Mental health policy development and implementation in four African countries. *Journal of Health Psychology, 12*, 505–516.

Foundation for Professional Development. (2021). *7 day mental health survival kit for lockdown course* [Online]. https://student.foundation.co.za/course/readmore/moodle-35. [Accessed].

Frasquilho, D., Matos, M. G., Salonna, F., Guerreiro, D., Storti, C. C., Gaspar, T. & Caldas-De-Almeida, J. M. (2016). Mental health outcomes in times of economic recession: A systematic literature review. *BMC Public Health, 16*, 115.

Ghebreyesus, T. A. (2020). Addressing mental health needs: An integral part of covid-19 response. *World Psychiatry, 19*, 129.

Gilmartin, H., Goyal, A., Hamati, M. C., Mann, J., Saint, S. & Chopra, V. (2017). Brief mindfulness practices for healthcare providers - a systematic literature review. *American Journal Medicine, 130*, 1219 e1–1219 e17.

Golberstein, E., Wen, H. & Miller, B. F. (2020). Coronavirus disease 2019 (covid-19) and mental health for children and adolescents. *JAMA Pediatrics, 174*, 819–820.

Hanlon, C., Fekadu, A., Jordans, M., Kigozi, F., Petersen, I., Shidhaye, R., Honikman, S., Lund, C., Prince, M., Raja, S., Thornicroft, G., Tomlinson, M. & Patel, V. (2016). District mental healthcare plans for five low-and middle-income countries: Commonalities, variations and evidence gaps. *British Journal of Psychiatry, 208*, s47–s54.

Hao, F., Tan, W., Jiang, L., Zhang, L., Zhao, X., Zou, Y., Hu, Y., Luo, X., Jiang, X., Mcintyre, R. S., Tran, B., Sun, J., Zhang, Z., Ho, R., Ho, C. & Tam, W. (2020). Do psychiatric patients experience more psychiatric symptoms during covid-19 pandemic and lockdown? A case-control study with service and research implications for immunopsychiatry. *Brain, Behavior, and Immunity, 87*, 100–106.

Healthcare Workers Care Network. (2021). *Healthcare workers care network* [Online]. https://www.healthcareworkerscarenetwork.org.za/. [Accessed].

Hobfoll, S. E., Watson, P., Bell, C. C., Bryant, R. A., Brymer, M. J., Friedman, M. J., Friedman, M., Gersons, B. P., De Jong, J. T., Layne, C. M., Maguen, S., Neria, Y., Norwood, A. E., Pynoos, R. S., Reissman, D., Ruzek, J. I., Shalev, A. Y., Solomon, Z., Steinberg, A. M. & Ursano, R. J. (2007). Five essential elements of immediate and mid-term mass trauma intervention: Empirical evidence. *Psychiatry, 70*, 283–315; discussion 316–69.

Hsieh, K.-Y., Kao, W.-T., Li, D.-J., Lu, W.-C., Tsai, K.-Y., Chen, W.-J., Chou, L.-S., Huang, J.-J., Hsu, S.-T. & Chou, F. H.-C. (2021). Mental health in biological disasters: From sars to covid-19. *International Journal of Social Psychiatry, 67*, 576–586.

Hunt, X., Breet, E., Stein, D. & Tomlinson, M. (2021). *The covid-19 pandemic, hunger, and depressed mood among South Africans.* Johannesburg: National Income Dynamics Study (NIDS) & Coronavirus Rapid ….

Hwang, W. J., Ha, J. S. & Kim, M. J. (2021). Research trends on mobile mental health application for general population: A scoping review. *Intergrated Journal Environmental Residental Public Health, 18*(5), 2459.

Iasc Reference Group on Mental Health and Psychosocial Support (2020). Interim briefing note addressing mental health and psychosocial aspects of covid-19 outbreak. https://interagencystandingcommittee.org/iasc-reference-group-mental-health-and-psychosocial-support-emergency-settings/interim-briefing-note-addressing-mental-health-and-psychosocial-aspects-covid-19-outbreak.

Ifrc Reference Centre for Psychosocial Support (2022). Corona / covid-19 resource library. https://pscentre.org/resource-category/covid19/.

Inge Petersen, Ph.D., Christopher G. Kemp, Ph.D., Deepa Rao, Ph.D., Bradley H. Wagenaar, Ph.D., Kenneth Sherr, Ph.D., Merridy Grant, M.Soc.Sci., Max Bachmann, Ph.D., Ruanne V. Barnabas, D.Phil., Ntokozo Mntambo, M.Soc. Sci., Sithabisile Gigaba, M.Soc.Sci., André Van Rensburg, Ph.D., Zamasomi Luvuno, Ph.D., Ishmael Amarreh, Ph.D., Lara Fairall, Ph.D., Nikiwe N. Hongo, M.B.Ch.B., M. B. A., & Arvin Bhana, Ph.D. (2021). Implementation and scale-up of integrated depression care in South Africa: An observational implementation research protocol. *Psychiatric Services, 72*, 1065–1075.

International Society for Traumatic Stress Studies. (2021). *Covid-19 Resources* [Online]. https://istss.org/public-resources/covid-19-resources. [Accessed 19 September 2021].

Janse Van Rensburg, A. (2021). *The political economy of mental illness in South Africa.* London: Routledge.

Janse Van Rensburg, A., Khan, R., Fourie, P. & Bracke, P. (2019). Politics of mental healthcare in post-apartheid South Africa. *Politikon, 46*, 192–205.

Janse Van Rensburg, A., Wouters, E., Fourie, P., Van Rensburg, D. & Bracke, P. (2018). Collaborative mental health care in the bureaucratic field of post-apartheid South Africa. *Health Sociology Review, 27*, 279–293.

Kang, L., Li, Y., Hu, S., Chen, M., Yang, C., Yang, B. X., Wang, Y., Hu, J., Lai, J., Ma, X., Chen, J., Guan, L., Wang, G., Ma, H. & Liu, Z. (2020). The mental health of medical workers in wuhan, china dealing with the 2019 novel coronavirus. *Lancet Psychiatry, 7*, e14.

Khan, K. S., Mamun, M. A., Griffiths, M. D. & Ullah, I. (2020). The mental health impact of the covid-19 pandemic across different cohorts. *International Journal of Mental Health and Addiction, 20*(1), 380–386. doi: 10.1007/s11469-020-00367-0.

Kim, A. W., Nyengerai, T. & Mendenhall, E. (2020). Evaluating the mental health impacts of the covid-19 pandemic: Perceived risk of COVID-19 infection and childhood trauma predict adult depressive symptoms in urban South Africa. *Psychology Medicine, 52*(8), 1587–1599. doi: 10.1017/S0033291720003414.

Knowledge Translation Unit. (2021). *Adult primary care* [Online]. https://knowledgetranslation.co.za/pack/south-africa/. [Accessed 15 October 2021].

Kola, L., Kohrt, B. A., Hanlon, C., Naslund, J. A., Sikander, S., Balaji, M., Benjet, C., Cheung, E. Y. L., Eaton, J., Gonsalves, P., Hailemariam, M., Luitel, N. P.,

Machado, D. B., Misganaw, E., Omigbodun, O., Roberts, T., Salisbury, T. T., Shidhaye, R., Sunkel, C., Ugo, V., Van Rensburg, A. J., Gureje, O., Pathare, S., Saxena, S., Thornicroft, G. & Patel, V. (2021). Covid-19 mental health impact and responses in low-income and middle-income countries: Reimagining global mental health. *The Lancet Psychiatry, 8,* 535–550.

Kübler-Ross, E. & Kessler, D. N. Y. S., 2005. (2005). *On grief and grieving: Finding the meaning of grief through the five stages of loss,* New York: Scribner.

Kumar, A. & Nayar, K. R. (2021). Covid 19 and its mental health consequences. *Journal of Mental Health, 30,* 1–2.

Lai, J., Ma, S., Wang, Y., Cai, Z., Hu, J., Wei, N., Wu, J., Du, H., Chen, T., Li, R., Tan, H., Kang, L., Yao, L., Huang, M., Wang, H., Wang, G., Liu, Z. & Hu, S. (2020). Factors associated with mental health outcomes among health care workers exposed to coronavirus disease 2019. *JAMA Netw Open, 3,* e203976.

Li, W., Yang, Y., Liu, Z. H., Zhao, Y. J., Zhang, Q., Zhang, L., Cheung, T. & Xiang, Y. T. (2020). Progression of mental health services during the covid-19 outbreak in china. *Int J Biol Sci, 16,* 1732–1738.

Linardon, J., Cuijpers, P., Carlbring, P., Messer, M. & Fuller-Tyszkiewicz, M. (2019). The efficacy of app-supported smartphone interventions for mental health problems: A meta-analysis of randomized controlled trials. *World Psychiatry, 18,* 325–336.

Lund, C., Kleintjes, S., Kakuma, R. & Flisher, A. J. (2010). Public sector mental health systems in South Africa: Inter-provincial comparisons and policy implications. *Social Psychiatry Psychiatr Epidemiol, 45,* 393–404.

Magill, E., Siegel, Z. & Pike, K. M. (2020). The mental health of frontline health care providers during pandemics: A rapid review of the literature. *Psychiatr Serv, 71,* 1260–1269.

Maulik, P. K., Thornicroft, G. & Saxena, S. (2020). Roadmap to strengthen global mental health systems to tackle the impact of the covid-19 pandemic. *International Journal of Mental Health Systems, 14,* 1–13.

Médecins Sans Frontières. (2020). *Supporting mental health during a pandemic* [Online]. https://bit.ly/2XjFemm: MSF. [Accessed 16 September 2021].

Mental Health Information Network & World Health Organization (2020). Stories from the field: Providing mental health and psychosocial support during the covid-19 pandemic. https://www.mhinnovation.net/stories-field-providing-mental-health-and-psychosocial-support-during-covid-19-pandemic.

Mokitimi, S., Schneider, M. & De Vries, P. J. (2018). Child and adolescent mental health policy in South Africa: History, current policy development and implementation, and policy analysis. *International Journal of Mental Health Systems, 12,* 1–15.

Morganstein, J. C. & Ursano, R. J. (2020). Ecological disasters and mental health: Causes, consequences, and interventions. *Frontiers in Psychiatry, 11,* 1–15.

Murthy, R. S. & Lakshminarayana, R. (2006). Mental health consequences of war: A brief review of research findings. *World Psychiatry: Official Journal of the World Psychiatric Association (WPA), 5,* 25–30.

Musisi, S. & Kinyanda, E. (2020). Long-term impact of war, civil war, and persecution in civilian populations – conflict and post-traumatic stress in African communities. *Frontiers in Psychiatry, 11,* 1–12.

Myers, B., Petersen-Williams, P., Van Der Westhuizen, C., Lund, C., Lombard, C., Joska, J. A., Levitt, N. S., Butler, C., Naledi, T., Milligan, P., Stein, D. J. & Sorsdahl, K. (2019). Community health worker-delivered counselling for common mental disorders among chronic disease patients in South Africa: A feasibility study. *BMJ Open, 9*, e024277.

Nakhid-Chatoor, M. (2020). *Luchando contra el covid-19: Supporting the mental health of venezuelan migrants in trinidad and tobago* [Online]. https://www.mhinnovation. net/blog/2020/may/8/luchando-contra-el-covid-19-supporting-mental-health-venezuelan-migrants-trinidad. [Accessed].

Namome, C., Winnaar, L. & Arends, F. (2021). Improving psychosocial support in SA schools during and after covid-19 as part of a recovery plan. http://www.hsrc. ac.za/uploads/pageContent/1045497/HSRC%20Policy%20Brief%205%20-%20 Improving%20psychosocial%20support%20in%20SA_print-ready_25-2-2021. pdf: Human Sciences Research Council.

Nearchou, F. & Douglas, E. (2021). Traumatic distress of covid-19 and depression in the general population: Exploring the role of resilience, anxiety, and hope. *Integrated Journal Environment Res Public Health, 18*(16), 8485.

Nochaiwong, S., Ruengorn, C., Thavorn, K., Hutton, B., Awiphan, R., Phosuya, C., Ruanta, Y., Wongpakaran, N. & Wongpakaran, T. (2021). Global prevalence of mental health issues among the general population during the coronavirus disease-2019 pandemic: A systematic review and meta-analysis. *Scientific Reports, 11*, 10173.

Odendaal, N. (2021). Recombining place: Covid-19 and community action networks in South Africa. *International Journal of E-Planning Research (IJEPR), 10*, 124–131.

Organisation for Economic Co-Operation and Development (2021). Tackling the mental health impact of the covid-19 crisis: An integrated, whole-of-society response. *OECD Policy Responses to Coronavirus (COVID-19)*. Paris: Organisation for Economic Co-operation and Development.

Oyenubi, A. & Kollamparambil, U. (2020). *Covid-19 and depressive symptoms in South Africa*. Johannesburg: National Income Dynamics Study (NIDS) & Coronavirus Rapid ….

Panchal, N., Kamal, R., Orgera, K., Cox, C., Garfield, R., Hamel, L. & Chidambaram, P. (2020). The implications of covid-19 for mental health and substance use. *Kaiser Family Foundation, 21*, Online report, https://abtcounseling.com/wp-content/ uploads/2020/09/The-Implications-of-COVID-19-for-Mental-Health-and-Substance-Use-_-KFF.pdf.

Pappa, S., Ntella, V., Giannakas, T., Giannakoulis, V. G., Papoutsi, E. & Katsaounou, P. (2020). Prevalence of depression, anxiety, and insomnia among healthcare workers during the covid-19 pandemic: A systematic review and meta-analysis. *Brain, Behavior, and Immunity, 88*, 901–907.

Patel, V. (2012). Global mental health: From science to action. *Harvard Review of Psychiatry, 20*, 6–12.

Petersen, I., Bhana, A., Baillie, K. & Mha, P. P. R. P. C. (2012). The feasibility of adapted group-based interpersonal therapy (ipt) for the treatment of depression by community health workers within the context of task shifting in South Africa. *Community Mental Health Journal, 48*, 336–341.

Petersen, I., Bhana, A., Campbell-Hall, V., Mjadu, S., Lund, C., Kleintjies, S., Hosegood, V. & Flisher, A. J. (2009). Planning for district mental health services in South Africa: A situational analysis of a rural district site. *Health Policy Plan, 24*, 140–150.

Petersen, I., Fairall, L., Bhana, A., Kathree, T., Selohilwe, O., Brooke-Sumner, C., Faris, G., Breuer, E., Sibanyoni, N., Lund, C. & Patel, V. (2016). Integrating mental health into chronic care in South Africa: The development of a district mental healthcare plan. *British Journal of Psychiatry, 208*, s29–s39.

Petersen, I. & Lund, C. (2011). Mental health service delivery in South Africa from 2000 to 2010: One step forward, one step back. *South African Medical Journal, 101*, 751–757.

Petersen, I., Lund, C. & Stein, D. J. (2011a). Optimizing mental health services in low-income and middle-income countries. *Current Opinion in Psychiatry, 24*, 318–323.

Petersen, I., Ssebunnya, J., Bhana, A., Baillie, K. & Mha, P. P. R. P. C. (2011b). Lessons from case studies of integrating mental health into primary health care in South Africa and uganda. *International Journal of Mental Health Systems, 5*, 8.

Pharma Dynamics. (2021). *South Africans' stress levels have shot up by 56% since start of pandemic according to survey* [Online]. https://pharmadynamics.co.za/south-africans-stress-levels-have-shot-up-by-56-since-start-of-pandemic-according-to-survey/. [Accessed 16 September 2021].

Preti, E., Di Mattei, V., Perego, G., Ferrari, F., Mazzetti, M., Taranto, P., Di Pierro, R., Madeddu, F. & Calati, R. (2020). The psychological impact of epidemic and pandemic outbreaks on healthcare workers: Rapid review of the evidence. *Curr Psychiatry Rep, 22*, 43.

Qiu, J., Shen, B., Zhao, M., Wang, Z., Xie, B. & Xu, Y. (2020). A nationwide survey of psychological distress among Chinese people in the covid-19 epidemic: Implications and policy recommendations. *Gen Psychiatr, 33*, e100213.

Rieckert, A., Schuit, E., Bleijenberg, N., Ten Cate, D., De Lange, W., De Man-Van Ginkel, J. M., Mathijssen, E., Smit, L. C., Stalpers, D., Schoonhoven, L., Veldhuizen, J. D. & Trappenburg, J. C. (2021). How can we build and maintain the resilience of our health care professionals during covid-19? Recommendations based on a scoping review. *BMJ Open, 11*, e043718.

Robertson, L. J., Janse Van Rensburg, B., Talatala, M., Chambers, C., Sunkel, C., Patel, B. & Stevenson, S. (2018). Unpacking Recommendation 16 of the Health Ombud's Report on the Life Esidimeni Tragedy. *South African Medical Journal, 108*(5), 362–363. doi: 10.7196/SAMJ.2018.v108i5.13223.

Santomauro, D. F., Mantilla Herrera, A. M., Shadid, J., Zheng, P., Ashbaugh, C., Pigott, D. M., Abbafati, C., Adolph, C., Amlag, J. O., Aravkin, A. Y., Bang-Jensen, B. L., Bertolacci, G. J., Bloom, S. S., Castellano, R., Castro, E., Chakrabarti, S., Chattopadhyay, J., Cogen, R. M., Collins, J. K., Dai, X., Dangel, W. J., Dapper, C., Deen, A., Erickson, M., Ewald, S. B., Flaxman, A. D., Frostad, J. J., Fullman, N., Giles, J. R., Giref, A. Z., Guo, G., He, J., Helak, M., Hulland, E. N., Idrisov, B., Lindstrom, A., Linebarger, E., Lotufo, P. A., Lozano, R., Magistro, B., Malta, D. C., Månsson, J. C., Marinho, F., Mokdad, A. H., Monasta, L., Naik, P., Nomura, S., O'halloran, J. K., Ostroff, S. M., Pasovic, M., Penberthy, L., Reiner Jr, R. C., Reinke, G., Ribeiro, A. L. P., Sholokhov, A., Sorensen, R. J. D., Varavikova, E., Vo, A. T., Walcott, R., Watson, S., Wiysonge, C. S., Zigler, B., Hay, S. I., Vos, T., Murray, C. J. L., Whiteford, H. A. & Ferrari, A. J. Global prevalence and burden of depressive and anxiety disorders in 204 countries and territories in 2020 due to the covid-19 pandemic. *The Lancet*.

South African Depression and Anxiety Group. (2021). *Sadag's online survey findings on covid-19 and mental health* [Online]. https://bit.ly/3EneiTD. Available: https://bit.ly/3EneiTD [Accessed 16 September 2021].

Spaull, N. & Al., E. (2020). Nids-cram wave 2 synthesis report. https://cramsurvey.org/reports/#: The National Income Dynamics Study Coronavirus Rapid Mobile Survey (NIDS-CRAM)

Spaull, N., Daniels, R. & Al., E. (2021). Nids-cram wave 5 synthesis report. https://cramsurvey.org/reports/#: The National Income Dynamics Study Coronavirus Rapid Mobile Survey (NIDS-CRAM)

Spaull, N. & Van Der Berg, S. (2020). Counting the cost: Covid-19 school closures in South Africa and its impact on children. *South African Journal of Childhood Education, 10*, 1–13.

Spedding, M. F., Stein, D. J. & Sorsdahl, K. (2014). Task-shifting psychosocial interventions in public mental health: A review of the evidence in the South African context. *South African Health Review, 2014*, 73–87.

Statistics South Africa. (2021). *Quarterly labour force survey (qlfs), 2nd quarter 2021* [Online]. http://www.statssa.gov.za/?page_id=1856&PPN=P0211&SCH=72944: StatsSA. [Accessed 16 September].

Swingler, H. (2021). *Mental health awareness month: Psychosocial skills injection for teachers* [Online]. https://www.news.uct.ac.za/article/-2021-10-22-mental-health-awareness-month-psychosocial-skills-injection-for-teachers: University of Cape Town. [Accessed 2022 09 March].

The Schools Development Unit (2020). *My South African Pandemic Story*. Cape Town: University of Cape Town.

University of Johannesburg (UJ) and Human Sciences Research Council (HSRC) (2020). UJ-HSRC COVID-19 democracy survey. Pretoria: University of Johannesburg and the Human Sciences Research Council.

Velten, J., Lavallee, K. L., Scholten, S., Meyer, A. H., Zhang, X. C., Schneider, S. & Margraf, J. (2014). Lifestyle choices and mental health: A representative population survey. *BMC Psychol, 2*, 58.

Vindegaard, N. & Benros, M. E. (2020). Covid-19 pandemic and mental health consequences: Systematic review of the current evidence. *Brain, Behavior, and Immunity, 89*, 531–542.

Wang, Q., Xu, R. & Volkow, N. D. (2021). Increased risk of covid-19 infection and mortality in people with mental disorders: Analysis from electronic health records in the united states. *World Psychiatry, 20*, 124–130.

World Health Organization (2016). Framework on integrated, people-centred health services. *Geneva: World Health Organization*, 2019.

World Health Organization. (2020). *Covid-19 halting crucial mental health services in Africa, who survey* [Online]. https://www.afro.who.int/news/covid-19-halting-crucial-mental-health-services-africa-who-survey: WHO. [Accessed 20 September 2021].

World Health Organization (2022). Mental health and covid-19: Early evidence of the pandemic's impact. *Scientific Brief 2 March*. Geneva.

Xiong, J., Lipsitz, O., Nasri, F., Lui, L. M. W., Gill, H., Phan, L., Chen-Li, D., Iacobucci, M., Ho, R., Majeed, A. & Mcintyre, R. S. (2020). Impact of covid-19 pandemic on mental health in the general population: A systematic review. *Journal of Affective Disorders, 277*, 55–64.

Yao, H., Chen, J.-H. & Xu, Y.-F. (2020). Patients with mental health disorders in the covid-19 epidemic. *The Lancet Psychiatry, 7*, e21.

Zhang, H., Shi, Y., Jing, P., Zhan, P., Fang, Y. & Wang, F. (2020). Posttraumatic stress disorder symptoms in healthcare workers after the peak of the covid-19 outbreak: A survey of a large tertiary care hospital in Wuhan. *Psychiatry Research, 294*, 113541.

Zürcher, S. J., Kerksieck, P., Adamus, C., Burr, C. M., Lehmann, A. I., Huber, F. K. & Richter, D. (2020). Prevalence of mental health problems during virus epidemics in the general public, health care workers and survivors: A rapid review of the evidence. *Frontiers in Public Health, 8*, 560389–560389.

11 New foundations

Strengthening early childhood care and education provisioning in South Africa after COVID-19[1]

Gabrielle Wills and Jesal Kika-Mistry

Introduction

There are significant returns to investing in the youngest segment of a population. Future life trajectories are better for children who access early childhood care and education (ECCE) programmes that contribute positively to their cognitive, linguistic, and socio-emotional development (Vegas & Santibanez, 2010; Naudeau et al., 2011; Richter et al., 2021). Over the longer term, ECCE offers a cost-effective mechanism to produce a well-trained and capable workforce (Lynch, 2005; Schweinhart et al., 2005). As a result, investments in ECCE can lead to improved economic growth and reduced reliance on social assistance programmes. Beyond economic arguments, children's access to quality care and education opportunities is a basic human right. Yet, for all the benefits of ECCE, it receives far less priority than schooling, higher education, or health in national budgets.

In many low-to-middle-income countries, limited public finance for ECCE and weak supporting systems hamper equitable access to quality ECCE programming (Richter et al., 2017). On the one hand, South Africa has made significant strides in government provisioning of one year of pre-school in the form of a reception year (grade R) (United Nations Chidlren's Fund, 2019). On the other hand, public funding to access ECCE services (excluding school-based grade R) for younger children has been very limited. Rising access to ECCE among 0 to four-year-olds has largely been provided through informal private sector operators, with slow expansion in subsidies aimed at these programmes. With limited public financing, children's access to quality non-grade R ECCE programmes ultimately depends on whether parents/caregivers can afford ECCE programme fees (Richter et al., 2012; Biersteker et al., 2016). Consequently, ECCE provisioning has been characterised by structural inequalities in programme access and quality. The sustainability of ECCE programmes serving those already attending has also been highly susceptible to economic shocks.

After recurrent calls for reform in the ECCE sector, there have been signals in recent years of increased prioritisation of ECCE for younger children in policy documents and political commitments. A renewed focus on early

DOI: 10.4324/9781003294931-11

childhood was expressed in national plans for a 'function shift' by April 2022, where the oversight of early childhood development has been transferred from the Department of Social Development (DSD) to the Department of Basic Education (DBE) (Department of Basic Education, 2021).[2] Events surrounding the COVID-19 pandemic, however, threatened to almost undo 20 years of growth in access to non-grade R ECCE and compromise sector reform in South Africa.

A series of policy papers were produced to track ECCE attendance trends since the onset of the pandemic in March 2020 using the National Income Dynamics Study – Coronavirus Rapid Mobile Survey (NIDS-CRAM) (Wills, Kotze & Kika-Mistry, 2020; Wills & Kika-Mistry, 2021a, 2022; Wills, Kika-Mistry & Kotze, 2021). The longitudinal NIDS-CRAM survey, a nationally representative survey of South African adults, was initiated at the start of the pandemic to track the socio-economic impacts of the pandemic and related lockdowns. In addition to tracking employment, hunger, and COVID-19 health-related behaviours, a module on ECCE was included from the second data collection period. Adult respondents were asked to identify whether any child in the household had attended an ECCE programme in the past seven days, and in February 2020 – before the onset of the pandemic.[3] The resulting data was used to map out how the attendance of children at ECCE programmes changed over the 2020–2021 period in relation to pre-pandemic levels. While the results communicated the devastating consequences of the pandemic on children's access to ECCE opportunities, a lot has been learnt about the sector from the pandemic experience. As government implements an early childhood development function shift, COVID-19 has reinforced what needs to be fixed and what needs to be financed in the ECCE system.

In this chapter, we explore the underlying structural weaknesses in the provisioning of non-grade R ECCE that were exposed through the pandemic, and the strengths that have surfaced. Through a lens of sustainability, capacity, and accountability, we consider what policy and civil society responses (and in some cases non-responses) to the resulting crisis reveal about how ECCE is viewed and prioritised by government. We also consider what can be learnt from the pandemic experience for the purpose of system reform. We then discuss key reforms to promote increased sustainability, build capacity, and improve accountability for a stronger ECCE system for future generations.

As a point of clarification, much of what is discussed in this chapter focuses on the provisioning of ECCE. This is one subcomponent of the multisectoral definition of early childhood development which also includes antenatal support, health and nutrition interventions, water and sanitation, child protection, and parent and family-based support programmes (Richter et al., 2017). Within the broader concept of early childhood development, we focus on ECCE that excludes school-based grade R.

Background

ECCE in South Africa before the pandemic

One of the most significant gains made in education service delivery in post-apartheid South Africa was the expansion of access to ECCE (Department of Basic Education, 2019). Part of the expansion was driven by the introduction of a formal reception class the year preceding grade 1, known as grade R (United Nations Children's Fund, 2019), which is predominately delivered through public provisioning in primary schools. However, access to privately provided non-grade R ECCE opportunities also expanded notably. In 1998, 18% of children aged 0–6 years were attending a pre-school, or a form of education and care at an institution outside a school. By 2017, this comparative estimate had reached 43% (Department of Basic Education, 2020). Expansion in ECCE attendance was observed among children aged 0–2, 3–4, and 5–6 years and occurred largely before 2012.

The provision of non-grade R ECCE in South Africa operates as a quasi-market, with a large composition of informal services provided by private providers such as non-profit organisations, subsistence entrepreneurs, or micro-social enterprises (Richter et al., 2012; BRIDGE et al., 2020). Although a small proportion of these informal ECCE operators benefit from state subsidies paid to registered providers on a per-child attending per-day basis, the majority of ECCE operators rely on fee collections from parents/caregivers as their primary income source (Wills & Kika-Mistry, 2021b). In this respect, South Africa's childcare market bares similarity to low-fee private schooling systems in developing countries. If one excludes grade R and the care of day-mothers, 'gogos' or childminders from definitions of ECCE enrolment, fees were charged for around 90% of children aged 0–5 years attending ECCE programmes in 2017/2018. Pre-pandemic, ECCE access and the quality of programming received were directly related to the ability to pay fees and fee amounts paid. This in turn resulted in inequalities in access (Richter et al., 2012). Major concerns were also regularly raised about the poor quality of ECCE programming. In a functional provincial context, Biersteker et al. (2016) observed that on average, ECCE programmes assessed on international quality scales were of minimal quality.

In the years preceding the onset of the pandemic, there were signals of structural reform in the ECCE sector. This was reflected in the increased political will to prioritise ECCE, aligning with goals expressed in the National Development Plan and strong international trends to raise the profile of early learning (Wotipka et al., 2017; South African Government News Agency, 2020). The National Integrated Early Childhood Development Policy (NIECDP) approved by Cabinet in 2015, recognised early childhood development as a universal right, a national priority, and public good to which all children are entitled. This was accompanied by the release of the National Curriculum Framework for children from Birth to Four (Department of Basic Education (DBE), 2015). To complement the new policies, the introduction of a conditional early childhood development grant in 2017/2018 for site infrastructure and maintenance, and some additional funding for subsidies, presented a 'ring-fenced' financial commitment to facilitate alignment with plans for implementation of the NIECDP (Ghordan, 2016). These developments should not be overlooked. However, significant shortcomings in ECCE public financing and administration systems were also evident pre-pandemic. In particular, the reach and depth of public ECCE finance were very limited (Desmond et al., 2019; Wills & Kika-Mistry, 2021b). With regards to the reach of public financing, possibly only a third of early learning programmes (excluding grade R) were receiving the state subsidy (Department of Basic Education & The Lego Foundation, 2022). Further, about a quarter of fully registered or conditionally registered programmes were not receiving the state subsidy (BRIDGE et al., 2020). The limited reach of subsidies is attributed to bottlenecks in ECCE programme registration – a consequence of onerous criteria to qualify for subsidies, significant costs of meeting such criteria, and administratively burdensome processes to apply (Giese & Budlender, 2011; Ilifa Labantwana, 2014; Kotze, 2015). The relatively low ratio of subsidised to non-subsidised programmes is also a function of the lack of allocated public finance to support a larger number of registered programmes.

In terms of the depth of financing, at R17 per-child per-day in 2022, the value of the subsidy is too low to support decent wages or quality programming (Desmond et al., 2019). Biersteker et al. (2016), for example, found no link between subsidy receipt and the quality of ECCE programmes in the Western Cape despite strong linkages between programme quality and user-fees paid. In the main, parents or caregivers are paying fees for children to attend programmes, even in under-resourced contexts. For example, of children aged 0–5 years attending non-grade R ECCE programmes in 2017/2018 and living in households whose main source of income is from social grants, over half were paying more than R100 per month and 17% were paying over R200 per month.[4] Relative to the R17 subsidy, it is further estimated that the state spends roughly six times more per child attending a public school compared to an ECCE programme (Wills, Kotze & Kika-Mistry, 2020).

This financing model, with low supply-side subsidies and significant parent co-payments, has over-exposed the ECCE sector to demand-side shocks, compromising the sustainability of programme offerings, and exacerbating inequalities in access. Before the pandemic, ECCE fee payments were already sporadic and sensitive to downturns in the economy (Carter & Barberton, 2014). This has presented a particular challenge for the sustainability of a sizeable proportion of unregistered programmes that are solely reliant on parent fees. In this context, children's access to ECCE opportunities was extremely vulnerable to the impacts of the COVID-19 pandemic.

Against this backdrop, we consider policy and civil society responses related to ECCE that emerged during the COVID-19 pandemic in South Africa. We also explore the strengths and weaknesses in the ECCE system that were brought to the fore.

ECCE attendance trends in South Africa during COVID-19

Following the South African declaration of a state of national disaster to contain the spread of COVID-19, all operators of ECCE programmes (and all schools) were instructed to close on 18 March 2020, nine days before a hard lockdown began. However, the reopening of ECCE programmes was delayed relative to the phased reopening of the economy and schools from 1 June 2020 – an issue which caused much contestation. Non-profit organisations approached the courts to fight for what they argued was government prejudice against privately owned ECCE programmes. Specifically, it was deemed prejudicial where grade Rs could go back to public schools, but private ECCE operators that also provide grade R were not allowed to open (an issue which pointed to misalignment in legislation). It was further argued that the closure of ECCE programmes was unconstitutional and unlawful, limiting children's access to education and not in their best interests (Ally, Parker & Peacock, 2022).

On 6 July 2020, a court judgement ruled that all privately operated ECCE programmes could open immediately but required that they follow COVID-19 guidelines and precautions (Skole-Ondersteuningsentrum NPC and Others v Minister of Social Development and Others, 2020). This is just one of a series of court cases, policy developments, and related events that would unfold.

Figure 11.1 presents a timeline depicting some key dates, policy developments, and the emergence of support for the ECCE sector from March 2020 to July 2021. We discuss specific events in Figure 11.1 in more detail throughout this chapter. What is useful to note now from the figure is the extent of developments in the ECCE sector over this period which occurred in addition to variations in lockdown levels and economic activity in South Africa. Over the same period, there were some dramatic changes in child attendance at ECCE programmes. This is seen in Figure 11.2 which shows South African ECCE attendance trends from the start of 2020 to the second quarter of 2021 using NIDS-CRAM data.

It is not possible to attribute changes in ECCE attendance levels in South Africa to any one of the specific events in Figure 11.1, but stark changes in attendance levels over the period are reflective of the sensitivity of ECCE access to the regulatory environment, school closures, and macro-events.

18 March 2020 — DSD instructs all ECCE programmes to close

1 June 2020 — Phased reopening of the economy

6 July 2020 — High Court Judgement ruled that ECCE programmes could reopen subject to meeting safety standards

15 October 2020 — President's economic stimulus package announced for sector

25 January 2021 — Initial school reopening data for new calendar year

16 April 2021 — DSD removed cap on number of employees per ECD programme that could receive funding from stimulus package

17 July 2021 — DSD announces vaccines for ECD workforce and social development sector from 19 July

11 May 2020 — DSD Minister directs all provincial DSDs to continue paying subsidies to registered programmes

29 June 2020 — DSD released guidelines and SOPs for reopening but no date announced

30 July 2020 — DSD announced R1.3 billion of country's stimulus package will go to youth compliance officers to collect data from ECCE programmes

20 October 2020 — North Gauteng High Court ruled that Minister and MECs must pay full subsidies for 2020/21 financial year

15 February 2021 — Schools reopen after delayed reopening

19 June 2021 — DBE announces vaccines for teachers and school support staff from 23 June

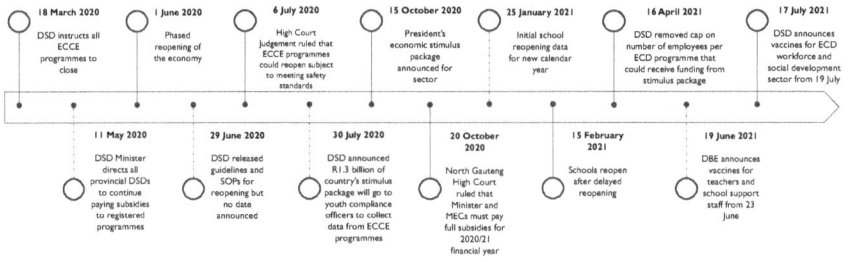

Figure 11.1 Key dates, policy changes, and support for ECCE sector in response to COVID-19.

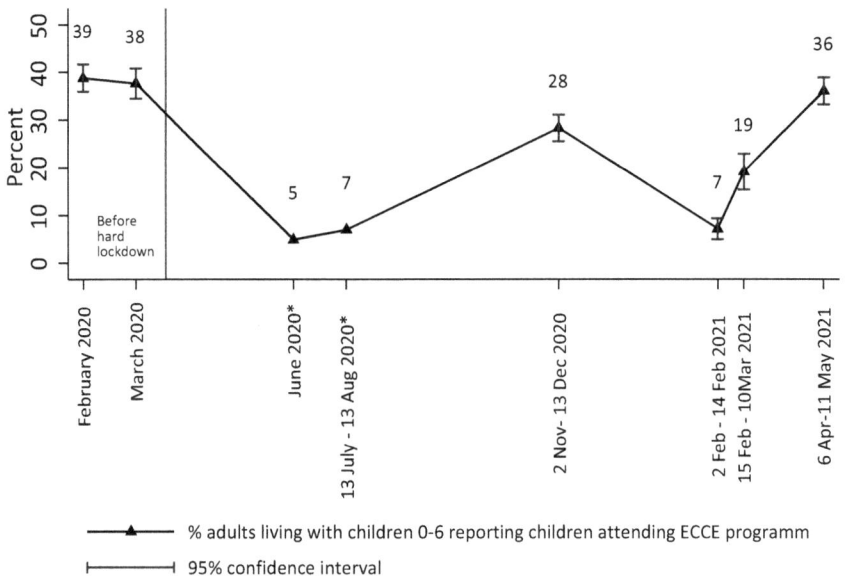

Percent (y-axis): 0, 10, 20, 30, 40, 50

Data points: 39, 38, 5, 7, 28, 7, 19, 36

Before hard lockdown

x-axis: February 2020, March 2020, June 2020*, 13 July - 13 Aug 2020*, 2 Nov - 13 Dec 2020, 2 Feb - 14 Feb 2021, 15 Feb - 10Mar 2021, 6 Apr-11 May 2021

— ▲ — % adults living with children 0-6 reporting children attending ECCE programm
├———┤ 95% confidence interval

Figure 11.2 ECCE attendance trends (excluding grade R) from 2020 to 2021. Percentage of adults living with children aged 0–6 years indicating that at least one child attended an ECCE programme.

Source: Wills and Kika-Mistry (2022) using NIDS-CRAM waves 2–5. Notes: Weighted, clustered, and stratified estimates. Sample includes respondents living with children 0–6 by wave. The 20- to 30-minute NIDS-CRAM telephonic survey is a broadly representative sample of persons 15 years or older in 2017 in South Africa, who were re-interviewed in 2020 for NIDS-CRAM (Kerr, Ardington & Burger, 2020). In waves 2–5 collected in July–August 2020, November–December 2020, February–March 2021, and April–May 2021 adults were asked whether any child in the household had attended an early child development programme (ECD) in the past seven days. Additionally, they were asked whether any child had attended an ECD programme in February 2020 (waves 3–5), in March 2020 (wave 2), and in June 2020 (wave 2).

Figure 11.2 shows that in February 2020, before the first case of COVID-19 was detected in South Africa, about 39% of NIDS-CRAM adult respondents living with children aged 0–6 years indicated that at least one child was attending an ECCE programme. In the weeks after ECCE programmes could reopen, not more than 7% of NIDS-CRAM respondents living with children aged 0–6 years and interviewed between mid-July and mid-August 2020 reported any child attending an ECCE programme in the past seven days. Towards the end of 2020, a partial recovery in ECCE attendance occurred, albeit nowhere near pre-pandemic levels. In November/December 2020, 28% of respondents living with children aged 0–6 years reported at least one child attending an ECCE programme in the past seven days (Wills & Kika-Mistry, 2022).

Unfortunately, the recovery in ECCE attendance observed in the fourth quarter of 2020 was short-lived. Even though ECCE programmes were allowed to operate when public schools were shut in early February 2021, and COVID-19 infections had subsided after a second peak, attendance plummeted to 7%. In the weeks following the delayed reopening of schools, more ECCE programmes opened again, and children started returning with about 19% of respondents living with children aged 0–6 years (and interviewed between 15 February and 11 March 2021) reporting at least one child attending an ECCE programme in the past seven days (Wills & Kika-Mistry, 2022).

The second fall in ECCE attendance in early 2021 was particularly concerning for the sector. After the first plunge in attendance in mid-2020, the permanent closure of ECCE programmes and the loss of tens of thousands of ECCE-related jobs were imminent concerns after sustained inactivity and non-payment of user fees. However, by April/May 2021, ECCE attendance rebounded again, edging towards pre-pandemic levels. Of respondents living with children aged 0–6 years in April/May 2021, 36% reported that at least one child had attended an ECCE programme in the past seven days.

Given the ever-changing policy environment we find ourselves in, it is important to clarify that our reflections and knowledge of sector trends during a pandemic is largely limited to the period between February 2020 to April 2021, the duration over which ECCE attendance trends were measured through the NIDS-CRAM surveys. The final (fifth) wave of NIDS-CRAM was followed by a severe third peak in COVID-19 infections in June/July 2021, and the reinstatement of stricter lockdown measures. There is no available data to identify how this third wave of infections impacted ECCE attendance trends.[5]

COVID-19 and the sustainability, capacity, and accountability of the ECCE system

Table 11.1 presents a summary of key policy messages and ECCE system strengths and weaknesses that emerged from our analysis of developments in the ECCE sector and attendance trends over the pandemic period. The findings are framed in relation to three system dimensions – sustainability, capacity, and accountability.

By sustainability, we refer broadly to resources enabling children's unhindered access to ECCE programmes and that limit the fragility of ECCE programmes, reflected in the extent to which they close on a temporary or permanent basis (Neuman, McConnell & Kholowa, 2014). By capacity, we refer to the systems, knowledge, human resources, and institutional structures to support ECCE service delivery (Nores & Fernandez, 2018). We refer to accountability as answerability and the expectation of account-giving in the ECCE system. This includes both formal and informal accountability – that in turn depend on capacities – such as monitoring, programme evaluation, legal mobilisation, and the use of data for continuous quality improvement (Couchenour & Chrisman, 2016).

We now provide a discussion of Table 11.1, focusing in turn on each dimension.

Sustainability

Conditions of fragility exposed through COVID-19

The troughs in ECCE attendance that emerged due to COVID-19-related events, and the patterns of recovery that were observed, highlight how children's access to quality ECCE programming is highly vulnerable to economic and health shocks. The July/August 2020 plunge in attendance implied that COVID-19 was a major threat to the sustainability of private ECCE provisioning and in turn, children's access to care and educational opportunities. It also brought to the fore two key conditions that lead to such fragility.

The primary condition is the overreliance of ECCE provisioning on private fee collection. The ability to pay fees over the pandemic period was the strongest determinant of whether children were attending ECCE programmes when periods of recovery were observed. For example, in November/December 2021, we found that respondents were four times as likely to report that a child was attending an ECCE programme in the past seven days if they could afford ECCE fees, even after controlling for prior attendance and individual or home background characteristics (Wills & Kika-Mistry, 2021c). The results also highlighted how households' ability to afford ECCE fees has been closely tied to structural inequalities. For example, compared to respondents who could afford ECCE fees in October 2020, respondents who report that they or someone in their household could not afford ECCE fees were more likely to be black, women, poorer, grant recipients, less likely to be employed and more likely to be unemployed but searching for work (Wills, Kika-Mistry & Kotze, 2021).

The highly decentralised nature of ECCE provisioning created a second condition for sector fragility. Compared to public schooling, where clear

Table 11.1 Strengths, weaknesses, and policy messaging in the ECCE sector as highlighted through the COVID-19 pandemic

	Strengths exposed	Weaknesses exposed	Positive policy messaging during the pandemic exhibited in state support	Negative policy messaging during the pandemic exhibited in state support
Sustainability	Entrepreneurial resilience (especially when uncertainty is reduced through a flow of public funding support)	A sector extremely vulnerable to economic shocks due to overreliance on private fee collection and decentralised nature of sector	The sustainability of ECCE programmes does matter to government as reflected in provision of a stimulus package and revised lockdown regulations that enable programmes to remain open	The slower response in allocating stimulus relief for ECCE relative to other sectors initially implied a disregard for sustaining jobs in the sector
Capacity	Effective NGOs to engage in crisis support	Weak communication from overseeing government department on regulations pertaining to ECCE exposed current leadership capacity constraints Absence of information systems to leverage for effective management and support in times of crisis	For the first time, 'illegal' unregistered programmes are implicitly viewed as offering valuable services Appetite and capacity exists to build information systems	Slow roll-out of stimulus package weakens perceptions about state capacity to support the sector Poor messaging about the value of ECCE practitioners relative to teachers through slow prioritisation in the vaccination roll-out
Accountability	Sector attracts generous philanthropic backing which could be leveraged for innovative financing and experimentation Significant advocacy capacity exists within the sector to lobby for support and engage in legal battles against unjust policies, implementation issues, or failure to exercise statutory obligations		Accountability for public spending on ECCE matters but government is willing to balance this need (given the informal context) against the need to provide timeous support	

operating directives are provided as to when to open and when to close, the private nature of ECCE provisioning means that the operational schedules of ECCE programmes are decided in a very decentralised manner. Further, in the face of financial constraints after months of not being able to collect fees, and additional costs of meeting COVID-19 safety protocols during the pandemic, this made it difficult for many programmes to reopen. This limited access to ECCE opportunities.

Policy messaging about the value of sustaining private ECCE provisioning

The delayed reopening of ECCE programmes relative to other sectors (and public schools with grade R) reflected poorly on government's regard for private provisioning of ECCE. Furthermore, the slower response in allocating sector-specific stimulus relief for ECCE, relative to some other sectors, initially implied a disregard from government for the need to protect jobs in private ECCE programmes. Due to the informal nature of ECCE provisioning, it was challenging for ECCE workers to access general social income protection such as Unemployment Insurance Fund (UIF) pay-outs or Temporary Employment Relief Scheme (TERS) payments.

However, government messaging took a turn in mid-October 2020. President Cyril Ramaphosa announced a stimulus package in the form of a 'Public investment in a mass employment strategy to build a new economy' on 15 October 2020. As strong concerns were expressed about the need for ECCE sector relief, a budget of R380 million was initially included in the larger package to support employees or sole practitioners of eligible early childhood development programmes (The Presidency, Republic of South Africa 2020). In addition, R116 million was earmarked for the DSD to provide top-up payments to 25,000 employees to help ECCE programmes meet COVID-19 regulations necessary for reopening (The Presidency Republic of South Africa, 2020).

This was arguably one of the most significant and ambitious initiatives that government had ever engaged in to provide financial support to South Africa's ECCE sector. Not only registered but unregistered providers were eligible to receive relief pay-outs. In April 2021, the DSD also removed the cap that was placed on the number of employees per ECCE programme that could receive a payment of R4 186 (Department of Social Development, 2021a). This meant that ECCE services meeting all the necessary requirements would receive funding for all the employees that they applied for.

The eventual outcome of ECCE policy developments communicated that sustaining private provisioning of ECCE, even of 'illegal' unregistered programmes, was now an imperative for government. This message was reinforced by explicitly allowing ECCE operators to remain open even when public schools were instructed to close from the second half of 2020 (Department of Co-operative Governance, 2021).

Entrepreneurial resilience

While the patterns of ECCE attendance pointed to the vulnerability of private ECCE operations to income shocks, it also highlighted the entrepreneurial resilience of ECCE operators. A significant recovery in ECCE attendance occurred by April–May 2021 even though most ECCE operators that applied for the Early Childhood Development-Employment Stimulus Relief Fund (ECD-ESRF) had not yet received payments (see Figure 11.2). A largely informal ECCE sector may have been able to bounce back, buoyed by concurrent recoveries in the labour market when lockdown restrictions were reduced (Bassier et al., 2021; Casale & Shepherd, 2022). Of course, the prospect of receiving relief government funds, which are sizable in relation to monthly ECCE practitioner salaries, may have also encouraged reopening efforts, particularly of lower fee programmes (Wills & Kika-Mistry, 2022). Relatedly, court cases which provided legal accountability for the payment of subsidies owed to registered programmes, unlocked some certainty in government funding flows.

As South Africa moves forward to secure ECCE opportunities for young children, it is necessary to address conditions in this quasi-market that leave it vulnerable to shocks. The COVID-19 crisis revealed that this requires increased government oversight and more public financing. For example, the April/May 2021 recovery in ECCE attendance may in part be attributable to the prospect of public stimulus relief, which contributed to conditions of improved financial certainty for ECCE entrepreneurs. The risk of suppressed ECCE access through individualised decisions of ECCE operators to reopen was also directly mitigated by government attaching a condition to receiving relief funds, namely, that ECCE programmes that were not yet fully operational due to COVID-19 had to be open within 60 days of receipt of relief funds (Department of Social Development, 2021b).

Capacity

Weak leadership, weak communication. and lack of information systems hindered sector recovery

It is in times of crisis that one becomes aware of the critical need for strong leadership, effective and clear communication, and efficient systems in government. The COVID-19 crisis exposed weakness on all three fronts in the ECCE sector.

Significant confusion marred the initial reopening of ECCE programmes and then whether they could stay open as the pandemic progressed. A key issue initially was the absence of clear operating directives and communication from the DSD on this matter. In mid-2020, the DSD directives on when ECCE programmes could reopen were delayed or contradictory in lieu of overriding regulations on the reopening of the economy or school reopening directives from the DBE (Ally, Parker & Peacock, 2022). In early 2021 when schools were directed to close again due to new COVID-19 surges, government gazettes made provision for ECCE programmes to remain open (Department of Co-operative Governance, 2021). The fact that ECCE programmes could stay open despite school closures was, however, not well communicated or understood by ECCE operators or parents. ECCE operators shut when they didn't need to. For parents of ECCE attendees, they likely took comfort in the safety of DBE notices on school closures which were communicated widely and informed by close deliberations with COVID-19-related national command councils. Consequently, a strong association between ECCE attendance and school reopening is observed in NIDS-CRAM data collected over February/March 2021 (Wills & Kika-Mistry, 2021a).

Weak communication from the DSD on this ECCE reopening was augmented by not having an information system, with clear records on ECCE operators, where they are situated and up-to-date contact details. The systems were simply not in place to effectively communicate to providers or to provide rapid transfer of funds to support the sector. Poor communication and limited dialogue with larger umbrella non-governmental organisations (NGOs) also fuelled virulent advocacy campaigns.

Policy messaging through COVID-19 response initiatives

Despite administrative weaknesses exposed through the COVID-19 crisis, policy actions eventually communicated a willingness and capacity to address glaring gaps in information systems. For example, the DSD and Nelson Mandela Foundation initiated the Vangasali Campaign, which seeks to collect information related to ECCE facilities, where they are and whether they are registered or not. The resulting database also supported recent initiatives by the DBE to run a Census of ECCE programmes across the country, identifying their location, enrolment numbers, and type of programme offered (Department of Basic Education & The Lego Foundation, 2022).

In the medium term, the intent of the Vangasali Campaign was also to facilitate support to identified unregistered ECCE programmes to help them meet necessary registration requirements (South African Government, 2020) (Albeit the reach of the campaign has likely been limited relative to the number of unregistered programmes.) In addition to the inclusion of unregistered programmes in the provision of relief funding, this has communicated that government acknowledges the value and potential of unregistered ECCE providers.

Despite many encouraging responses from government, policy messaging has not been positive in two key areas. First, the roll-out of relief support in the form of the ECD-ESRF has been much slower than anticipated, largely due to the lack of existing information systems and the informal nature in which programmes operate. The DSD identified and validated ECD-ESRF applications for nearly 120,000 employees from ECCE operator submissions. After indicating that payments would start from 31 March 2021, by mid-May 2021, delays in pay-outs were still being experienced with payments only covering about 20% of ECCE workers expecting a pay-out (Daniels, 2021; Dano, 2021). In March 2022, more than 50% of employee payments were still outstanding. This has been attributed to site, staff and Central Supplier Database Bank verifications, untraceable programmes, and programmes that have closed down (Parliamentary Monitoring Group, 2022).

ECCE practitioners were also not prioritised in the phased roll-out of vaccines (Motshekga, 2021), despite teachers in public and private institutions having been prioritised in June 2021. Vaccinating ECCE practitioners provides an important barrier to the spread of the virus and keeping ECCE sites open. It also allays parent/caregiver fears of children contracting the virus at ECCE programmes – these fears were a significant contributing factor to children not returning to ECCE programmes during the pandemic (Wills & Kika-Mistry, 2021c). However, the social development sector, which includes the ECCE workforce, was eventually prioritised in vaccine rollouts a month later in July 2021.

A system strengthened through effective NGOs and philanthropic support

The COVID-19 crisis demonstrated the effectiveness of large or umbrella NGOs in the ECCE sector to engage in crisis support, and to broadly advocate for sector reform. Varied and ongoing efforts by NGOs to provide ECCE programmes with practical support to facilitate reopening were initiated (DGMT, 2020; Brooks & Hartnack, 2021; SmartStart, 2021: 22). This included providing coaching and financial support to ECCE programmes in meeting necessary COVID-19 safety protocols, salary support through vouchers and the provision of food and food vouchers to feed children at programmes, which is a significant cost component of operating. NGO support was swift and quite widespread. This was enabled through generous philanthropic giving. Evidently, a strength of this sector is its ability to attract private donations.

Accountability

Advocacy for accountability as a strength of the ECCE sector

The COVID-19 pandemic also highlighted that significant capacity for advocacy and self-organisation exists within a largely informal ECCE sector (Ally, Parker & Peacock, 2022). NGOs representing thousands of ECCE providers campaigned for relief support and engaged in legal mobilisation against unjust policy, unconstitutional decisions, poor governance, and unmet statutory obligations on the part of actors in the DSD (Ally, Parker & Peacock, 2022) that were deepening the ECCE crisis.

NGOs were particularly successful in challenging unconstitutional decisions by provincial Departments of Social Development to withhold subsidies from ECCE operators. During the mandatory closure of programmes from March to June 2020, over 50% of the early childhood development subsidy was withheld from registered programmes on the basis that children were not attending and would have no need for the nutrition and stimulation components of the subsidy. The non-payment of owed subsidies was considered unconstitutional, furthering the plight of some registered ECCE programmes (Vorster 2020). On 20 October 2020, a court judgement against the Minister of Social Development and all Members of the Executive Council (MECs) (except the MEC in the Western Cape) ruled that the Minister and MECs must pay full subsidies to registered ECCE programmes for the duration of all lockdown alert levels, whether they are operational or not, for the entire 2020/21 financial year (SA Childcare (Pty) Ltd and seven others v Minister of Social Development and Others 2020). This was a significant win for advocacy groups and the sector. The payment of owed subsidies would significantly improve the financial position of registered programmes. Yet, these legal battles could have been avoided if provincial Social Development departments demonstrated capacity and transparency in executing their function to pay subsidies, demonstrated by exception in the Western Cape.

In the first 6–8 months of the pandemic, ECCE practitioners and advocacy groups strongly voiced their grievances and concerns about ECCE being overlooked in wider income protection packages that were proposed for different sectors. Concerns were backed by evidence of the devastating impacts on the ECCE sector, and the 'plight' of its workforce (BRIDGE et al., 2020). Civil society groups were eventually successful in securing relief support for the sector from government and shaped the nature of ECCE relief that would finally be provided. Rather than providing short-term relief, government initially proposed a medium-term solution to support unregistered programmes in accessing subsidies through ECCE registration campaigns. COVID-19 relief funds were initially going to be used to employ 'youth compliance officers' – unemployed youth that are not currently part of the ECCE workforce – to accelerate the registration of programmes (Nkgweng, 2020).[6] Historically, however, registration has been a slow process and limited in reach. Through the outcry of advocacy and early childhood development forums, this proposal was overturned on the logic that the ECCE workforce needed immediate income support.

Financial accountability displayed in government's relief response

The advocacy efforts of 2020/2021 reveal an existing capacity in the sector to hold government to account and advocate for ECCE improvements (particularly through legal mobilisation). It is important to recognise, though, that in the relief response, government also demonstrated a commitment to be accountable for public spending on ECCE. Due to the informal nature of the sector, and the absence of existing information systems, no clear platform or approaches existed to transparently distribute relief funds to ECCE providers and practitioners. In this context, the reasonable requests for quick government relief for the sector conflicted with the need to uphold accountable financial processes. National Treasury, working with the DSD, eventually reached a compromise in the design of an application process for relief funds that balanced the need for financial accountability with providing relief support to ECCE operators and their employees. The underlying reason behind the delayed provision of support, while frustrating, demonstrated a commitment to transparent public funding flows.

Reforming South Africa's ECCE sector

In a review of studies on systems and capacity in ECCE, Nores and Fernandez (2018) identify eight critical aspects for enabling systemic strength and support for early childhood services. These include strong collaboration arrangements and centralised leadership, vertical alignment, horizontal alignment, evidence-based programmes, and policies, linking programmes to programme outputs and outcomes, investing in the early childhood workforce, implementing continuous improvement cycles, and partnerships. The scope of our paper limits us from a detailed discussion of reforms in each of these eight areas. But the conceptual framework provides a tool to articulate key priority areas for increased sustainability, capacity, and accountability in South African ECCE provisioning.

Addressing financial sustainability through registration, increased subsidy amounts, and increased public spending on ECCE

Nores and Fernandez (2018) identify collaborative arrangements and centralised leadership as the first critical aspect of strong ECCE systems. The ECCE 'function shift' may serve to address the leadership vacuums in the current ECCE environment. Yet strong collaboration and centralised leadership requires the political prioritisation of ECCE, a national ECCE policy of co-responsibility and financing to match this (Neuman & Devercelli, 2013; Richter et al., 2017).

South Africa has made significant strides in developing ECCE policies, and political prioritisation has been demonstrated. However, without funding and appropriate systems aligned to these, ECCE policy has often been viewed as a symbolic commitment rather than something that was ever intended to be implemented. As Jansen and Sayed (2001, p196) reflect '… a consistent feature of educational policy is that symbolic commitments to overcome the legacy of apartheid inequities are not always realised in the crucible of practice'.

Funding

Effective finance strategies resulting in higher-performing ECCE systems are characterised by an appropriate balance of three dimensions: sustainability, equity in access, and administrative simplicity (Valerio & Garcia, 2013). However, the current financing system in South Africa has not been able to strike this balance.

The bulk of ECCE-related budget allocations in South Africa are made at the provincial level through the 'equitable share formula'. The equitable share is strongly weighted to education, but non-school-based ECCE has fallen under social services and welfare (prior to the function shift), which is accounted for under a broader poverty variable in the formula. Once provincial budget amounts are allocated, provinces are not obliged to follow the formula, resulting in inequalities in how funds are allocated across provinces. With medium-term plans for more ECCE programmes to be registered, it will be important for the DBE to safeguard budgets to accommodate newly registered ECCE programmes. Increasing the earmarked conditional grant for ECCE as determined by the national government could be one way of doing this.

There is also an inherent need to reconsider the value of the daily subsidy to ensure that ECCE programmes receive adequate and sustainable financing. Replicating a middle-income country programme of adequate quality, similar to Chilean pre-school programmes, the cost is estimated to be around R42 per child per day, or 2.5 times the current subsidy amount (Desmond et al., 2019). Extrapolating these costs, the Chilean model provides a coverage level of 80% of the targeted 65% of children between the ages of 3 and 4.5 years. This is estimated at R6.7 billion per year (USD 450 million). If fully funded, rather than partially subsidised, R13 billion annually would be required. By comparison, the planned national budget in 2023/2024 allocated for subsidies of children of a much wider aged group (0–5) is estimated at just R3.3 billion[7] (National Treasury, 2021: 328). There is also very little evidence to suggest that current budgets are being set with population growth planning in mind or in terms of the demand for services (Neuman & Devercelli, 2013) despite this being required in policy (Republic of South Africa, 2015).

Simplify registration criteria and streamline the registration process

Reports have been commissioned over the years to review practices related to ECCE programme registration and funding (Ilifa Labantwana, 2014). A recurring theme is the need to reduce onerous requirements for registration and to simplify complex and administratively burdensome processes (Giese & Budlender, 2011; Ilifa Labantwana, 2014). For example, to register as an ECCE provider, each service provider must submit multiple applications. Due to poorly aligned processes, duplication of effort and documentation occurs. Significant inconsistencies are also apparent across provinces in how registration criteria are applied. Reform has been slow despite calls for over a decade to address registration inefficiencies through more efficient information and work-flow management systems. A possible reason for this is that with insufficient budgets allocated to ECCE to expand subsidies through new programme registrations, the DSD was not actively identifying ECCE programmes requiring registration (despite it being illegal for unregistered programmes with more than six children to operate). By maintaining low volumes of registration requests, the system was able to cope and thus there was little pressure on the DSD to address system inefficiencies (Ilifa Labantwana, 2014). However, increasing children's access to ECCE programmes and the active identification of ECCE programmes in need of registration will require more efficient systems to handle higher application volumes.

It is necessary to streamline the registration process and reduce administrative complexity in the regulatory system through improved standard operating procedures and data systems. This could also free up capacity among existing government officials and social workers to focus on ECCE programme improvement rather than merely monitoring compliance.

Building capacity through training ECCE practitioners and expanding the ECCE workforce of government officials

A key component of ECCE capacity building, that is strongly linked to effective ECCE programming, is developing 'pedagogical leadership' (Fukkink & Lont, 2007; Nutbrown, 2018). This requires upskilling, training, and continuous professional development of ECCE practitioners (Cavallera et al., 2019). With a poorly trained ECCE workforce (Kotze, 2015), it will be incumbent upon the DBE to establish a core skills programme to upgrade qualifications while creating expectations for minimum qualifications of new entrants. It is also critical to increase human resources for oversight and administrative roles. A 2016 audit of human resource capacity in the early childhood development sector highlighted the enormous gaps in the number of government officials responsible for overseeing the management and implementation of ECCE programmes from birth to four years (Biersteker & Picken, 2016). A ratio of government officials to children in all ECCE facilities was estimated at about 1:2350 in 2015.[8] At this ratio, one cannot expect to implement a system of quality assurance in the sector, or a programme for upskilling ECCE practitioners.

Even before the COVID-19 pandemic which squeezed government budgets, unfilled and frozen posts for ECCE oversight roles had already been identified across national and provincial departments. Dedicated social workers appointed through the DSD already faced large caseloads, which impacted on being able to provide sufficient support for the quality implementation of programmes (Biersteker & Picken, 2016). Clarifying the role of social workers in the DSD, who are the dominant 'boots on the ground' in overseeing ECCE programmes, will be vital. The DBE will also need to engage in a significant drive to appoint and train individuals to evaluate and guide ECCE programmes on how to implement effective ECCE learning programmes. Biersteker and Picken (2016) articulate required areas of training and warn against shifting current DBE staff (with typically primary teaching qualifications) into ECCE positions without ensuring they have the content knowledge that fosters learning through play appropriate for 0–4-year-olds. It is also necessary to budget for resources to support the effective utilisation of personnel, such as ensuring access to vehicles to conduct ECCE site visits, and the presence of data systems, computers and internet access at DBE/DSD offices (Ilifa Labantwana, 2014).

However, human resource capacity development in the context of a function shift presents a political challenge if the bargaining power of private ECCE practitioners aligns more closely to that of teachers on the civil service payroll. If ECCE practitioners are challenged to upskill or are subject to increased accountability processes under the DBE, the influence of teacher unions, and particularly, the South African Democratic Teachers Union (SADTU), may become more prevalent in the ECCE landscape. This presents new challenges for managing expectations around pay, working conditions, and sustaining a system of private provisioning of ECCE. The need for strong government leadership at national, provincial, and district levels will become particularly important in navigating unionisation of the ECCE workforce (Taylor & Draper, 2014). Furthermore, vertical alignment with leadership structures that already exist in a well-organised system of informal ECCE forums will be necessary.

Data systems to support accountability for integrated service delivery and continuous improvement cycles

In most countries, including South Africa, the multi-faceted nature of early childhood development requires an integrated and cross-sectoral approach to service delivery (Richter et al., 2017). In addition to health, welfare and education departments, public works departments and municipalities play key roles in the registration of ECCE programmes and the provision of related infrastructure. Regardless of which department has overriding oversight for ECCE, 'horizontal alignment' across role players and departments is necessary to address fragmentation in service delivery (Nores & Fernandez, 2018). This necessitates proper planning, the establishment of structures for integrated ECCE leadership and coordination, and articulated roles and responsibilities as expressed in policy and legal frameworks.[9] Data systems can also support sustained and effective intersectoral coordination and collaboration. For example, under Rwanda's National Early Development Program, seven ministries or agencies contribute data to an ECCE dashboard (Raikes, Sayre & Davis, 2021: 4). The dashboard provides visibility of real-time indicators of progress against agreed goals or actions, promoting accountability across different departments responsible for ECCE service delivery improvements.

The availability of comprehensive data systems can also strengthen monitoring, support continuous quality improvement, and promote timely interventions (Neuman & Devercelli, 2013). For example, in Chile, an electronic database of all pregnant women and children entering the health system can be accessed by health, education, and social development authorities to update information about a child's development and activate necessary interventions (Milman et al., 2018).

In South Africa, there is currently no comprehensive management information system with up-to-date information on ECCE service providers. Household survey data to effectively track ECCE access is also limited.[10] In the context of the function shift, however, the DBE undertook a Census of early childhood development programmes in 2021/2022 to track the geographical spread of, and access to ECCE programmes (Department of Basic Education & The Lego Foundation, 2022). The Census also collected basic information relating to registration status, materials, infrastructure, and human resource capacity. This Census in addition to recent efforts to obtain better programme quality measures[11] and measure early learning outcomes (see Giese et al., 2022) are important developments. But moving beyond these 'static' snapshots of the system will require planning for a measurement system that supports continuous quality improvements (i.e., learning about what is working and what is not). An measurement system could course corrections in processes and procedures with the goal of better child development outcomes (Cavallera et al., 2019). Continuous improvement will also require a culture shift from compliance monitoring towards ongoing quality improvement, reflection, and shared learning (Nores & Fernandez, 2018).

While a chasm has existed between the limited availability of any information systems in ECCE in South Africa and what would be required for effective management, the large application system established for the COVID-19-related relief package implied that systems can be implemented. The recent Census of early childhood development programmes also helps in establishing the substance for an early childhood development management information system (ECD-MIS). Recently, tools have been developed to help monitor early learning programme outcomes and guide programme improvement (see Snelling et al. (2019) for the Early Learning Outcomes Measure (ELOM)). Pockets of Information Technology excellence to support early childhood development also exists in the NGO sector. Raikes, Sayre, and Davis (2021) cite a case study from 'Grow ECD' – a franchise of South African ECCE programmes – which has been using a data-driven approach to ensure ECCE facilities meet service delivery standards.

Partnerships to strengthen the delivery of ECCE services

Over the COVID-19 pandemic period, NGO networks working for systemic change in the ECCE system have accomplished remarkable efforts with the support of private philanthropy. Much has been learned about the type of capacity required to implement innovative support projects in the sector. Even before the pandemic, NGOs have had a history of trialling new systems and engaging in capacity-building initiatives to support improved efficiencies in ECCE programming (Ilifa Labantwana, 2014; Impande, 2022).

Building a stronger ECCE system requires strengthening partnerships and dialogue between private players and government. Philanthropic support and NGOs in the sector are a significant resource to tap into in experimenting with new operating models, developing innovative financing models, and unlocking capacity-building opportunities as private sector excellence is imparted to public systems (Nores & Fernandez, 2018). Where ECCE human resource shortages are evident in government, integrated service departmental teams could also be augmented by NGOs working on early childhood development.[12]

There are two key approaches to strengthening partnerships. The first is through longer-term financial commitments and the second is through measurement (and more broadly documentation of experiences). In low-to-middle-income countries, it is evident that where donors and funding agencies commit longer-term resources (at least five years), this tends to result in improved continuity of activities and enables higher impacts (Hartmann & Linn, 2008; Cavallera et al., 2019).[13] Longer-term investment from philanthropy and international donors is also more likely if progress measures can be shown, including programme impacts on child developmental outcomes. 'On the ground' experiences of NGOs and private sector partners also need to be clearly documented and made more widely available to feed into broader debates about ECCE programme development (Cavallera et al., 2019). Fostering collaborations with researchers can help to facilitate improved documentation and enhance the development of a policy-relevant research repository from which policymakers can draw (Raikes, Sayre & Davis, 2021).

Conclusion

As the ECCE sector in South Africa rebuilds and recovers from COVID-19, it is imperative that the focus is not simply on replicating the ECCE system that was already in place prior to the pandemic. We need to build back better to ensure that the system is stronger, more comprehensive, and more sustainable.

The troughs in ECCE attendance observed over the first two years of the COVID-19 pandemic highlight the need to address conditions in this quasi-market that leave it vulnerable to economic and health shocks. The COVID-19 crisis revealed that this requires increased government oversight and more public financing to support a largely private and informal ECCE sector. Addressing financial sustainability will require accelerating the registration of ECCE programmes, increased subsidies and substantially more public spending on ECCE. However, finance alone is a necessary but insufficient condition for sustained access to quality ECCE. Government must build capacity through training ECCE practitioners and expanding the ECCE workforce of government officials. There is also an immediate need to develop information systems to support increased accountability for integrated service delivery in early childhood development and to establish a structure to support continuous improvement cycles.

Finally, the significant efforts of NGOs and philanthropy to counter fragility in ECCE operations and encourage quality improvements over the COVID-19 pandemic period further demonstrates the importance of partnerships to strengthen the delivery of ECCE services. The key to improved partnerships will be the transparent and effective leadership of government in shaping a cohesive vision and path forward. While advocacy and civil society groups demonstrated the capacity to fight for just and fair support for the ECCE system, the legal battles and associated costs that ensued during the pandemic could have been avoided through improved stakeholder consultation and transparent leadership from government. As the oversight function for ECCE shifts to the DBE in 2022, there is an opportunity for new leadership to chart a course of collaboration and trust with private providers and key NGO stakeholders. This will provide the first foundational layer for a more sustainable, capable, and accountable ECCE system.

Notes

1 This chapter was produced with funding from the Early Learning Programme supported by the Allan Gray Orbis Foundation Endowment.
2 The Department of Social Development has been responsible for the overall oversight and coordination of early childhood development until the child enters formal schooling, whereas the Department of Basic Education has been responsible for grades R – 12.
3 If young children were not attending ECCE programmes, respondents were also asked to provide reasons for this. Respondents were also asked to report on their current ability to afford ECCE fee payments and whether an open and affordable ECCE programme existed within 5km of where they live.
4 Own calculations using the General Household Surveys 2017 and 2018.
5 Mass looting and insurrection attempts in mid-July 2021 in two very populous provinces, KwaZulu-Natal and Gauteng, are also likely to have affected access to ECCE as general safety concerns and related economic impacts limit the demand for outsourced childcare.
6 The reason for this approach is largely due to public relief finance for ECCE having been redistributed from a public fund earmarked to support youth employment.
7 After accounting for the ECD conditional grant, it is stated that a subsidy value of R17.50 for 717 767 children is anticipated in 2023/24 (National Treasury, 2021, p. 328). Subsidies are typically provided for 264 days in a year.
8 Across national government and 9 provincial governments, there were just 119 fulltime equivalent DBE staff and 729 Department of Social Development (DSD) staff dedicated to ECCE (Biersteker & Picken, 2016). The ratio is obtained by identifying the number of children enrolled in programmes in the same year from the General Household Survey.

9 See Montecinos, Gonzalez and Ehren (2021) for a discussion on systems established in Chile to establish more horizontal and vertical accountability in schooling and early childhood development.
10 The General Household Survey in South Africa is only useful in tracking patterns in children's access to early childhood development, without any indicators of programme quality.
11 Various stakeholders have worked together in the past two years to undertake an Early Childhood Development audit and index of early learning.
12 For example, Ilifa Labantwana and partners engaged in improving district-based information and workflow management systems as well as developing improved and simplified measures for registration and standard operating procedures (Ilifa Labantwana, 2014).
13 In Bangladesh, Child Development Centres were established as public-private partnerships, focused on the assessment, diagnosis, and management of a range of neurodevelopmental disorders in children (Khan et al., 2018). The Bangladesh Rural Advancement Committee (BRAC) – an NGO, and donors formed a consortium which pooled funds and had common reporting requirements. An important aspect of the consortium has been to improve the predictability of resource flows – securing financing for longer periods (Hartmann & Linn, 2008).

References

Ally, N., Parker, R., & Peacock, T. N. (2022). Litigation and social mobilisation for early childhood development during COVID-19 and beyond. *South African Journal of Childhood Education*, 12(1), s1054, doi.org/10.4102/sajce.v12i1.1054

Bassier, I., Budlender, J., & Zizzamia, R. (2021). *The labour market impact of COVID-19 in South Africa: An update with NIDS-CRAM wave 3* (NIDS-CRAM Wave 3 Policy Paper Series No. 2). Retrieved from https://cramsurvey.org/wp-content/uploads/2021/02/2.-Bassier-I.-Budlender-J.-Zizzamia-R.-2021-The-labour-market-impact-of-COVID-19-.pdf

Biersteker, L., Dawes, A., Hendricks, L., & Tredoux, C. (2016). Center-based early childhood care and education program quality: A South African study. *Early Childhood Research Quarterly*, 36, 334–344, doi.org/10.1016/j.ecresq.2016.01.004

Biersteker, L., & Picken, P. (2016). *National Audit of Government Officials Responsible for the Overseeing, Management and Implementation of Early Childhood Development Programmes from Birth to Four Years*.

BRIDGE, Ilifa Labantwana, National ECD Alliance (NECDA), The Nelson Mandela Foundation, Smartstart, South African Congress for Early Childhood Development. (2020). *The Plight of the ECD Workforce: An urgent call for relief in the wake of covid-19*. Retrieved from https://www.bridge.org.za/wp-content/uploads/2020/04/Final-report-The-plight-of-the-ECD-workforce-1.pdf [Accessed August 2020]

Brooks, L., & Hartnack, A. (2021, 9 July). Covid children's project teaches crucial lessons. *Mail and Guardian*. Retrieved from https://mg.co.za/education/2021-07-09-covid-childrens-project-teaches-crucial-lessons/

Carter, J., & Barberton, C. (2014). *Developing appropriate financing models to enable the scale-up of ECD services. Technical report*. Ilifa Labantwana: Cape Town. Retrieved from https://www.cornerstonesa.net/ri-policy-research-development-

and-advice/19-developing-appropriate-financing-models-to-enable-the-scale-up-of-ecd-services

Casale, D., & Shepherd, D. (2022). The gendered effects of the Covid-19 in South Africa: Evidence from NIDS-CRAM waves 1–5. *Development Southern Africa* (published online 4 February 2022), doi.org/10.1080/0376835X.2022.2036105

Cavallera, V., Tomlinson, M., Radner, J., Coetzee, B., Daelmans, B., Hughes, R., Pérez-Escamilla, R., Silver, K. L., & Dua, T. (2019). Scaling early child development: what are the barriers and enablers? *Archives of Disease in Childhood*, 104(1), S43–S50, doi.org/10.1136/archdischild-2018–315425

Couchenour, D., & Chrisman, K. J. (2016). Accountability in Early Care and Education. In D. Couchenour & K. J. Chrisman (Eds). *The SAGE Encyclopedia of Contemporary Early Childhood Education (Vols. 1–3)*. Thousand Oaks, CA: SAGE Publications, Inc., doi.org/10.4135/9781483340333

Daniels, N. (2021, 13 May). Preschool teachers angry over slow lockdown relief payments. *IOL*. Retrieved from https://www.iol.co.za/capetimes/news/preschool-teachers-angry-over-slow-lockdown-relief-payments-d556df53-2767-4a82-9632-d573e50ab235 [Accessed 15 July 2021]

Dano, Z. (2021, 21 April). *ECD stimulus fund payments are three weeks overdue, says CECD. IOL*. Retrieved from https://www.iol.co.za/education/early-learning/ecd-stimulus-fund-payments-are-three-weeks-overdue-says-cecd-e6895c62-b7da-4d1a-9c28-aa81f12e556c [Accessed 15 July 2021]

Department of Basic Education. (2019). A 25 year review of progress in the basic education sector. Retrieved from https://www.education.gov.za/Portals/0/Documents/Reports/DBE 25 Year Review Report 2019.pdf?ver=2019-12-13–133315-127 [Accessed 12 January 2020]

Department of Basic Education. (2020). *Action Plan to 2024 Towards the realisation of Schooling 2030. Pretoria*: Department of Basic Education.

Department of Basic Education. (2021). *Joint Press Statement: Early Childhood Development (ECD) function shift. South African Government*. Retrieved from https://www.gov.za/speeches/joint-press-statement-early-childhood-development-ecd-function-shift-16-mar-2021-0000 [Accessed 15 July 2021]

Department of Basic Education. (2015). *The South African National Curriculum Framework for children from Birth to Four*. Pretoria: Department of Basic Education. Retrieved from https://www.unicef.org/southafrica/media/911/file/SAF-national-curriculum-framework-0-4-En.pdf

Department of Basic Education, & The Lego Foundation. (2022). *ECD Census 2021. Because Children Count. Summary of Key Results*. May 2022. Pretoria: Department of Basic Education. Retrieved from https://www.education.gov.za/Portals/0/Documents/Reports/ECD%20Census%202021%20-%20Summary%20of%20Key%20Results.pdf?ver=2022-05-24-091002-577 [Accessed 15 July 2022]

Disaster Management Act: Regulations: Alert level 4 during Coronavirus COVID-19 lockdown, Pub. L. No. 44838 11 July 2021 (2021). Retrieved from https://www.gov.za/covid-19/about/coronavirus-covid-19-alert-level-4#schools

Department of Co-operative Governance. (2021). *Disaster Management Act: Regulations: Alert level 4 during Coronavirus COVID-19 lockdown*. Pub. L. No. 44838 11 July 2021. Pretoria: Department of Co-operative Governance. Available: https://www.gov.za/covid-19/about/coronavirus-covid-19-alert-level-4#schools.

Department of Social Development. (2021a). *ECD Employment Stimulus Relief Fund (ECD-ESRF) supported by the Presidential Employment Stimulus.* Retrieved from https://www.dsd.gov.za/index.php/latest-news/21-latest-news/328-presidential-employment-stimulus-for-early-childhood-development-ecd-services [Accessed December 2021]

Department of Social Development. (2021b, April 16). *Update On Ecd Stimulus Employment Relief Fund from The Department of Social Development.* Retrieved from https://www.dsd.gov.za/index.php/latest-news/21-latest-news/345-update-on-ecd-stimulus-employment-relief-fund-from-the-department-of-social-development [Accessed 15 July 2021]

Desmond, C., Viviers, A., Edwards, T., Rich, K., Martin, P., & Richter, L. (2019). Priority-setting in the roll out of South Africa's National Integrated ECD Policy. *Early Years*, 39(3), 276–284, doi.org/10.1080/09575146.2019.1572074

DGMT. (2020). *Digital food vouchers for social relief of distress.* Cape Town: DGMT. Retrieved from https://dgmt.co.za/food-vouchers/ [Accessed December 2020]

Fukkink, R. G., & Lont, A. (2007). Does training matter? A meta-analysis and review of caregiver training studies. *Early Child Research Quarterly*, 22, 294–311.

Ghordan, P. (2016). *Budget Speech (Minister of Finance, South Africa).* Pretoria: National Treasury. Retrieved from http://www.treasury.gov.za/documents/national budget/2016/speech/speech.pdf.

Giese, S, Dawes, A., Tredoux, C., Mattes, F., Bridgman, G., van der Berg, S., Schenk, J., & Kotzé, J. (2022). *The Thrive by Five Index Report.* Cape Town: Innovation Edge. Retrieved from https://www.thrivebyfive.co.za/wp-content/uploads/2022/04/Index-report-50-page.pdf [Accessed 1 August 2022]

Giese, S., & Budlender, D. (2011). *Government funding for early childhood development.* Learning brief No. 1 (November 2011). Cape Town: Ilifa Labantwana. Retrieved from https://ilifalabantwana.co.za/wp-content/uploads/2017/06/Government-funding-for-ECD-in-South-Africa-summary.pdf

Hartmann, A., & Linn, J. F. (2008). *Scaling up. A framework and lessons for development effectiveness from literature and practice* (Working Paper 5). Washington D.C.: Wolfensohn Center for Development at Brookings.

Ilifa Labantwana. (2014). *Key findings from a review of ECD Centre Registration and Funding Systems in KwaZulu-Natal (Lessons from the Field, No. 2).* Retrieved from https://ilifalabantwana.co.za/wp-content/uploads/2014/06/Lessons-from-the-Field-Key-findings-from-a-review-of-ECD-centre-registration-and-funding-systems-in-Kwazulu-Natal.pdf

Impande. (2022). *Impande ECD Action Areas.* Retrieved from https://www.impande.org.za/what-we-do/ [Accessed 15 July 2022]

Kerr, A., Ardington, C., & Burger, R. (2020). *NIDS-CRAM sample design and weighting* (NIDS-CRAM Wave 1 Technical Report B). Retrieved from https://cramsurvey.org/wp-content/uploads/2020/07/REPORT-B-CRAM-Sample-Design-and-Weighting-in-the-NIDS-CRAM-survey_v7.pdf

Khan, N. Z., Sultana, R., Ahmed, F., Shilpi, A. B., Sultana, N., & Darmstadt, G. L. (2018). Scaling up child development centres in Bangladesh. *Child: Care, Health and Development*, 44(1), 19–30, doi.org/10.1111/cch.12530

Kotze, J. (2015). The readiness of the South African education system for pre-grade R year. *South African Journal of Childhood Education,* 5(2), doi.org/10.4102/sajce.v5i2.388

Milman, H. M., Castillo, C. A., Sansotta, A. T., Delpiano, P. V., & Murray, J. (2018). Scaling up an early childhood development programme through a national multisectoral approach to social protection: lessons from Chile Crece Contigo. *British Medical Journal*, 363, k4513, doi.org/10.1136/bmj.k4513

Montecinos, C., González, Á., & Ehren, M. (2021). From hierarchy and market to hierarchy and network governance in Chile: Enhancing accountability, capacity and trust in public education. In M. Ehren & J. Baxter (Eds.), *Trust, Accountability and Capacity in Education System Reform*. Global Perspectives in Comparative Education (pp. 201–221). Oxfordshire, United Kingdom: Routledge. DOI: 10.4324/9780429344855-10

Motshekga, A. (2021, 19 June). *Minister Angie Motshekga: Basic Education sector's response to the impact of Coronavirus COVID-19 on schooling*. Retrieved from https://www.gov.za/speeches/minister-angie-motshekga-basic-education-sector's-response-impact-coronavirus-covid-19 [Accessed December 2021]

National Treasury. (2021). *Vote 19 Social Development*. Retrieved from http://www.treasury.gov.za/documents/national budget/2021/ene/Vote 19 Social Development.pdf

Naudeau, S., Kataoka, N., Valerio, A., Neuman, M. J., & Elder, L. K. (2011). *Investing in Young Children. An Early Childhood Development Guide for Policy Dialogue and Project Preparation*. Washington D.C.: The International Bank for Reconstruction and Development / The World Bank. DOI: 10.1596/978-0-8213–8526-5

Neuman, M. J., & Devercelli, A. (2013). *What Matters Most for Early Childhood Development: A Framework Paper*. Systems Approach for Better Education Results (SABER) Working paper series, no. 5. Washington, DC: World Bank. Retrieved from https://openknowledge.worldbank.org/handle/10986/20174

Neuman, Michelle J., McConnell, C., & Kholowa, F. (2014). From early childhood development policy to sustainability: The fragility of community-based childcare services in Malawi. *International Journal of Early Childhood*, 46(1), 81–99, doi.org/10.1007/s13158-014-0101-1

Nkgweng, T. (2020, August 21). ECD workers slam Social Development's decision to employ 36 000 youth compliance monitors. *SABC News*. Retrieved from https://www.sabcnews.com/sabcnews/ecd-workers-slam-social-developments-decision-to-employ-36-000-youth-compliance-monitors/ [31 August 2021]

Nores, M., & Fernandez, C. (2018). Building capacity in health and education systems to deliver interventions that strengthen early child development. *Annals of the New York Academy of Sciences,* 1419 (1), 57–73, doi.org/10.1111/nyas.13682

Nutbrown, C. (2018). Leadership in Early Childhood Education and Care. In C. Nutbrown. *Early Childhood Educational Research: International Perspectives*. London: SAGE Publications Ltd. DOI: 10.4135/9781526451811

Parliamentary Monitoring Group. (2022, 14 March 2022). *Question NW487 to the Minister of Social Development*. Retrieved from https://pmg.org.za/committee-question/17956/?utm_source=transactional&utm_medium=email&utm_campaign=searchalert

Raikes, A., Sayre, R., & Davis, D. (2021). Mini-review on capacity-building for data-driven early childhood systems: The consortium for pre-primary data and measurement in Sub-Saharan Africa. *Frontiers in Public Health*, 8, 595821, doi.org/10.3389/fpubh.2020.595821

Republic of South Africa. (2015). *National Integrated Early Childhood Development Policy.* Pretoria: Government Printers. Retrieved from https://www.gov.za/sites/default/files/gcis_document/201610/national-integrated-ecd-policy-web-version-final-01-08-2016a.pdf

Richter, L., Biersteker, L., Burns, J., Desmond, C., Feza, N., Harrison, D., Martin, P., Saloojee, H., & Slemming, W. (2012). *Diagnostic Review of Early Childhood Development.* Pretoria: Department of Performance, Monitoring and Evaluation & Inter-Departmental Steering Committee on Early Childhood Development.

Richter, L. M., Behrman, J. R., Britto, P., Cappa, C., Cohrssen, C., Cuartas, J., Daelmans, B., Devercelli, A. E., Fink, G., Fredman, S., Heymann, J., Boo, F. L., Lu, C., Lule, E., McCoy, D. C., Naicker, S. N., Rao, N., Raikes, A., Stein, A., ... Yoshikawa, H. (2021). Measuring and forecasting progress in education: what about early childhood? *Npj Science of Learning,* 6(1), 27, doi.org/10.1038/s41539-021-00106-7

Richter, L. M., Daelmans, B., Lombardi, J., Heymann, J., Boo, F. L., Behrman, J. R., Lu, C., Lucas, J. E., Perez-Escamilla, R., Dua, T., Bhutta, Z. A., Stenberg, K., Gertler, P., & Darmstadt, G. L. (2017). Investing in the foundation of sustainable development: pathways to scale up for early childhood development. *The Lancet,* 389(10064), 103–118, doi.org/10.1016/S0140–6736(16)31698-1

Skole-Ondersteuningsentrum NPC and Others v Minister of Social Development and Others. (2020). (24258/2020) ZAGPPHC 267 (GP) (6 July 2020).

SmartStart. (2021). *Smartstart Annual Report 2019–2020.* Retrieved from https://www.smartstart.org.za/2021/03/15/annual-report/ [Accessed December 2021]

Snelling, M., Dawes, A., Biersteker, L., Girdwood, E., & Tredoux, C. (2019). The development of a South African Early Learning Outcomes Measure: A South African instrument for measuring early learning program outcomes. *Child: Care, Health and Development,* 45(2), 257–270, doi.org/10.1111/cch.12641

South African Government News Agency. (2020, 19 February). *Bill to make early childhood development compulsory.* Retrieved from https://www.sanews.gov.za/south-africa/bill-make-early-childhood-development-compulsory   [Accessed March 2020]

Taylor, N., & Draper, K. (2014). *NEEDU National Report 2013: Teaching and Learning in Rural Primary Schools.* Pretoria: National Education Evaluation and Development Unit.

United Nations Children's Fund. (2019). *A World Ready to Learn: Prioritizing Quality Early Childhood Education.* New York: UNICEF. Retrieved from https://www.unicef.org/media/57926/file/A-world-ready-to-learn-advocacy-brief-2019.pdf

Valerio, A., & Garcia, M. H. (2013). Effective Financing. In P. R. Britto, P. L. Engle, & C. W. Super (Eds.), *Handbook of Early Childhood Development Research and its Impact on Global Policy* (pp. 467–486). Oxford, United Kingdom: Oxford University Press.

Vegas, E., & Santibanez, L. (2010). *The Promise of Early Childhood Development in Latin America and the Caribbean. Latin American Development Forum.* Washington D.C.: The World Bank. Retrieved from https://openknowledge.worldbank.org/handle/10986/9385

Wills, G., & Kika-Mistry, J. (2021a). *Early Childhood Development and Lockdown in South Africa: 2021 Quarter 1 Update on Attendance Trends* (NIDS-CRAM Wave 4 Policy Brief, No. 12). Retrieved from https://cramsurvey.org/wp-content/uploads/2021/05/12.-Wills-G.-_-Kika-Mistry-J.-2021.-Early-childhood-

Development-and-Lockdown-in-South-Africa-2021-quarter-1-update-on-attendance-trends.pdf

Wills, G., & Kika-Mistry, J. (2021b). *Early Childhood Development in South Africa During the COVID-19 pandemic: Evidence from NIDS-CRAM Waves 2–5* (NIDS-CRAM Wave 5 Policy Paper, No. 14). Retrieved from https://cramsurvey.org/wp-content/uploads/2021/07/14.-Wills-G-_-Kika-Mistry-J.-2021-Early-Childhood-Development-in-South-Africa-during-the-n-COVID-19-pandemic-Evidence-from-NIDS-CRAM-Waves-2-5.pdf

Wills, G., & Kika-Mistry, J. (2021c). *Supply-side and Demand-side Approaches to Financing Early Childhood Care and Education in South Africa* (Ilifa Labantwana and ReSEP ECD Working Paper Series, ECD WP 003/2021). Retrieved from https://ilifalabantwana.co.za/wp-content/uploads/2021/11/Supply-side-and-demand-side-approaches-to-financing-early-childhood-care-and-education-in-South-Africa-V08.pdf

Wills, G., & Kika-Mistry, J. (2022). Early childhood care and education access in South Africa during COVID-19: Evidence from NIDS-CRAM. *Development Southern Africa* (published online 15 February 2022), doi.org/10.1080/0376835X.2022.2028607

Wills, G., Kika-Mistry, J., & Kotze, J. (2021). *Early Childhood Development and Lockdown in South Africa: An Update Using NIDS-CRAM Wave 3* (NIDS-CRAM Wave 3 Policy Papers No. 12). Retrieved from https://cramsurvey.org/wp-content/uploads/2021/02/12.-Wills-G.-Kika-Mistry-J.-Kotze-J.-2021-Early-Childhood-Development-and-lockdown-in-South-Africa-An-update-using-NIDS-CRAM-wave-3.pdf

Wills, G., Kotze, J., & Kika-Mistry, J. (2020). *A sector hanging in the balance: Early childhood development and lockdown in South Africa.* (NIDS-CRAM Wave 2 Policy Paper No. 15). Retrieved from https://cramsurvey.org/wp-content/uploads/2021/05/15.-Wills-G.-Kotze-J.-Kika-Mistry-J.-2020-A-Sector-Hanging-in-the-Balance_ECD-and-Lockdown-in-South-Africa-1.pdf

Wotipka, C. M., Rabling, B. J., Sugawara, M., & Tongliemnak, P. (2017). The Worldwide Expansion of Early Childhood Care and Education, 1985–2010. *American Journal of Education*, 123(2), 307–339, doi.org/10.1086/689931

12 Tracking the pulse of the people

Support for democracy and the South African government's response to COVID-19

Cindy Steenekamp

Introduction

Democracy is in recession worldwide (EIU Democracy Index, 2021; Varieties of Democracy, 2022). The decline in levels of democracy and freedom has been coupled with a decline in support for democracy as citizens are becoming increasingly critical of political authority, state institutions, and democratic systems (Lührmann & Rooney, 2021). In many ways, the outbreak of COVID-19 late in 2019 has exacerbated these pre-pandemic trends. Many established democracies in the West adopted technocratic-style approaches to manage the public health crisis, while younger and 'flawed' democracies as well as many 'hybrid' and authoritarian regimes relied on more coercive measures to manage society (EIU Democracy Index, 2021). As a result, the pandemic has

> entrenched divisions between those who favour the precautionary principle and expert-driven decision-making (and have tended to support government lockdowns, green passes and vaccine mandates), and, on the other hand, those who favour a less prescriptive approach and more freedom from state interference (and have been more hostile to what they see as the curtailment of individual freedoms).
>
> (EIU Democracy Index, 2021:3)

The negative impact of the pandemic on the levels and quality of democracy globally has been well-documented through metrics generated by organisations such as Varieties of Democracy (V-Dem), Polity IV, Freedom House and *The Economist* Intelligence Unit (EIU), to name a few. These macro-level data include established measures to assess the status and strength of democracies, however, they are not the only means to study democracy. Democracy entails government by the people and relies on the attitudes and acceptance of its citizenry for survival (Claasen, 2020:118). The strength, stability, and durability of a democratic regime requires sufficient public or popular support, which translates into legitimacy for the political system and its incumbents (Lipset, 1959; Easton, 1965, 1975; Klingemann, 1999;

DOI: 10.4324/9781003294931-12

Bratton & Mattes, 2001; Norris, 2011). When democratic governments are unable to secure or maintain popular support, they are vulnerable to political, economic, or social crises and increased risk of democratic breakdown (Mishler & Rose, 1999). Thus, the analysis of citizens' attitudes – utilising individual or micro-level data – toward the political system and its various parts, their political behaviour, and their endorsement of a democratic political culture, is just as significant in the assessment of democracy as macro-level studies.

The purpose of this chapter is to track popular support for democracy in South Africa during an unprecedented public health crisis. More specifically, this chapter will utilise data from the two most recent rounds of the Afrobarometer to measure citizen support for and evaluations of democracy and prominent political actors since the onset of the global pandemic as well as public opinion relating to the South African government's response to COVID-19 by means of a fivefold analytical framework, namely, political community, regime principles, regime performance, regime institutions, and political actors.

Measuring popular support for democracy

In his seminal contribution to the study of political support for democracy, David Easton (1965, 1975) identified the importance of both attitudes and actions towards political objects. In other words, while some citizen evaluations relate to the performance of political institutions and actors, others appear to be more closely related to 'basic aspects of the system' (Easton, 1975:437). As a result, Easton distinguished between two models (types of support) and three levels (objects of support) of support for democracy. Popular support for democracy is characterised as being either diffuse or specific in nature. Diffuse support is defined as the 'evaluations of what an object is or represents – to the general meaning it has for a person – not for what it does' and is based on the reservoir of attitudes that sustains support for the political regime when demands are not met (Easton, 1975:444). In this way, diffuse support is more stable and durable than specific support. Specific support, on the other hand, relates to the 'satisfactions that members of a system feel they obtain from the perceived outputs and performance of the political authorities' (Easton, 1975:437). Specific support is conditional and based on the capacity and effectiveness of political authorities to deliver outcomes, and thus far more likely to fluctuate than diffuse support. These two models or types of support for democracy represent two different modes of orientation to the three levels or objects of the political system: the political community, the political regime, and political authorities. This distinction (and measurement) of support for democracy is important because it is possible for a political regime to persist without specific support for political authorities; however, it will not survive without diffuse political community and regime support (Easton, 1965, 1975; Dalton, 1999:59).

In a significant advancement of the study of political support, Pippa Norris (1999) retained the two models or types of political support but considered them to be 'a continuum from the most diffuse support for the nation-state down through successive levels to the most concrete support for particular politicians' (Norris, 1999:9–10). Norris (1999:10–13) also expanded upon Easton's three objects or levels of political support to form five distinct objects of support, ranging from most diffuse to most specific support. The first object – political community – was conceptualised much the same as Easton in that it relates to a basic attachment to the nation and refers to sentiments of national pride and identity. The second (regime principles) and third (regime performance) objects relate to what Easton termed 'political regime'. Regime principles represent the core values and basic principles of democratic regimes, such as 'freedom, participation, tolerance and moderation, respect for legal-institutional rights, and the rule of law' (Norris, 1999:11), while regime performance taps into evaluations of the performance of political systems. The fourth (regime institutions) and fifth (political actors) objects relate to what Easton termed 'political authority'. The regime institution object aims to measure generalised support for various political or state institutions, including 'governments, parliaments, the executive, the legal system and police, the state bureaucracy, political parties, and the military' (Norris, 1999:11). The fifth object – political actors – refers to specific support for political authorities, including the performance of individual political leaders and evaluations of the political elite (Norris, 1999:12).

This fivefold framework serves as a useful analytical tool since the support for one object of support is likely to predict changes that may occur in other objects. Similarly, by understanding support for the various objects of democracy, we are able to assess the strength and quality of democracy based on the extent to which support is long lasting and stable (diffuse) or dependent upon and influenced by short-term specific evaluations or pressures, such as the onset of the COVID-19 pandemic.

Support for democracy in South Africa: A macro-level overview

Before an analysis of popular support for democracy, it would be useful to map some of the macro-level trends relating to the overall quality of democracy in South Africa just prior to the outbreak of the pandemic to present. There are three broad schools of macro-level data available: the first focuses on qualities of government and government performance (such as Polity IV),[1] the second includes various political rights and civil liberties indicators (such as Freedom House),[2] while the third utilises a combination of institutional, and rights and freedoms measures. The EIU Democracy Index,[3] for example, utilises a range of indicators measuring electoral process and pluralism; the functioning of government; political participation; political culture; and civil liberties to classify countries as a 'full' or 'flawed' democracy, 'hybrid' regime, or 'authoritarian' regime and generate an index score out of 10, where 10 reflects high levels of democracy. Just prior to the pandemic in 2019, South Africa was classified as a 'flawed' democracy and ranked 40 (out of 167 countries) with an overall score of 7.24 (out of 10). Although South Africa was still classified as a 'flawed democracy' in 2021, it dropped to 44 (out of 167 countries) in the global rankings and the overall index score declined to 7.05 due to the weaker scores on the functioning of government and civil liberties indicators.

Another example is the Liberal Democracy Index by V-Dem.[4] This Index includes the liberal model (see the black line in Figure 12.1), which assesses constitutionally protected civil liberties, strong rule of law, an independent judiciary, and effective checks and balances that, together, limit the exercise of executive power (V-Dem Codebook, 2022:49). The Index also takes the level of electoral democracy into account (see the dark grey line in Figure 12.1), which includes the core value of making rulers responsive to citizens, achieved through electoral competition for the electorate's approval under circumstances when suffrage is extensive; political and civil society organisations being able to operate freely; elections are clean and not marred by fraud or systematic irregularities; and elections affect the composition of the chief executive of the country. In between elections, there is freedom of expression and an independent media capable of presenting alternative views on matters of political relevance (V-Dem Codebook, 2022:43). Since the first democratic elections in South Africa in 1994, the Liberal Democracy Index score (see the light grey line in Figure 12.1), ranging from 0 to 1, increased from 0.29 in 1994 to 0.59 in 2021, despite a gradual decline from 0.67 in 2012.

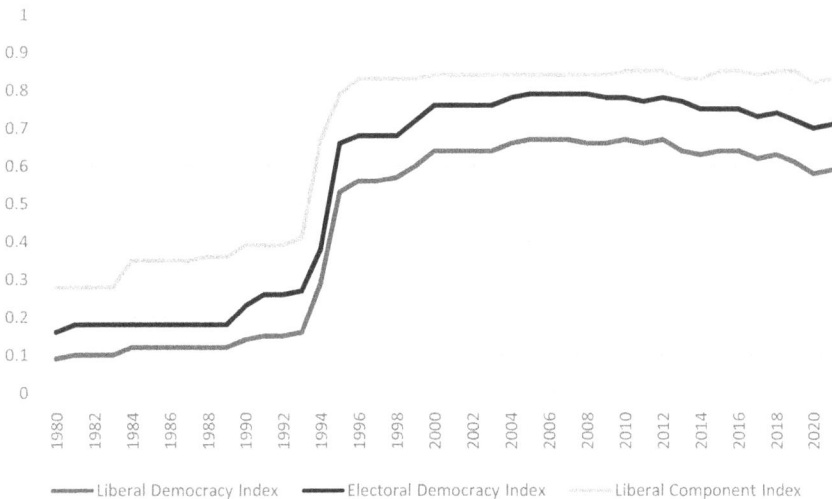

Figure 12.1 Liberal democracy index in South Africa, 1980–2021.

It is interesting to note that the Liberal Democracy Index score declined from 0.61 prior to the pandemic in 2019 to 0.58 in 2020 (the lowest level since 1998) before increasing slightly to 0.59 in 2021.

The macro data illustrates that the democratic political system and its constituent institutions are in place and function formally in South Africa and the ideal of liberal democracy has somewhat been achieved despite a gradual decline since 2012. These findings are not surprising as one would expect that the state machinery and institutional frameworks in a stable democracy would only be minimally affected during times of crisis. Popular support for democracy, however, is equally as important for political systems as it legitimates the regime and those who govern but is far more susceptible to internal and external pressures, such as a global pandemic. The following section tracks citizen support for and evaluations of democracy and prominent political actors since the onset of the global pandemic as well as public opinion relating to the South African government's response to COVID-19.

Tracking public opinion in South Africa since the onset of the pandemic

In an attempt to contain the outbreak and slow the spread of COVID-19 in South Africa, President Cyril Ramaphosa declared a national state of disaster on 15 March 2020 (Ramaphosa, 2020a). The government's initial Coronavirus/COVID-19 Emergency Plan included, amongst others, a travel ban and visa cancellations for visitors from countries considered to be high risk, enhanced testing of and self-isolation or quarantine for South African citizens returning from high-risk countries, the discontinuation of all non-essential travel by government employees across all spheres, the closure of several land and sea ports, the closure of schools, and limiting contact amongst people by discouraging non-essential domestic travel and prohibiting gatherings of more than 100 people. By 23 March 2020, President Ramaphosa announced a national lockdown for 21 days, which was later extended to 30 April 2020 (Ramaphosa, 2020c).

The national lockdown imposed stringent restrictions on travel and freedom of movement by closing all non-essential businesses and requiring South Africans to remain at home, except to buy food, seek medical care, or collect social grants (Ramaphosa, 2020b). In addition, anyone suspected of having COVID-19, or who had been in contact with someone who tested positive for COVID-19, was required to undergo testing, treatment, isolation, and/or quarantine or face potential imprisonment, a fine, or both for non-compliance (Labuschaigne, 2020:23–24). The government also introduced various mandatory public health social measures, such as wearing a suitable face mask or covering and maintaining a distance of at least 1.5 metres from others when leaving home for essential goods. One of the most controversial regulations, however, was the prohibition of the sale and transportation of cigarettes and alcohol (Ramaphosa, 2020c).

Initially, South Africans strongly supported the government's response to contain the spread of COVID-19. Results from the first wave of an online research survey[5] to track and monitor public opinion, perceptions, and behaviours in response to COVID-19 conducted by Ipsos at the end of March 2020 revealed that the majority of citizens (59%) either completely or somewhat agreed that the South African government had been open and honest about the extent of the coronavirus outbreak, while 60% were either very or somewhat confident that the government was prepared to effectively deal with coronavirus. In addition, the vast majority of South Africans supported the government ban on any travel to and from affected countries (92%), precautions being put in place on public transport systems to prevent the spread of coronavirus (94%), and the imposition of mandatory quarantine for those infected with coronavirus (93%). South Africans also placed a high degree of confidence in medical professionals (89%), traditional forms of media, such as radio (85%), television (85%), and newspapers (78%), and government health officials (77%) as accurate sources of information on COVID-19 (IPSOS, 2020a).

In April 2020, findings from a telephonic survey conducted in 20 African countries[6] showed that 83% of South Africans were very (55%) or somewhat (28%) satisfied with the government's response to COVID-19. Of the 20 countries surveyed, the South African government was ranked 6th, and the level of satisfaction amongst South African citizens was notably higher than the other Southern African countries (Mozambique, Zambia, and Zimbabwe) polled. Similarly, 83% of South Africans indicated that they trusted the information from government about the coronavirus completely (52%) or mostly (31%). This level of trust was significantly higher than their Southern African counterparts and ranked the South African government 4th best on the continent (IPSOS, 2020b).

Public opinion surveys conducted in 18 African Union Member States in August 2020[7] revealed that satisfaction with the government response to COVID-19 in South Africa was relatively high but declining. A total of 70% of South Africans indicated that they were very (42%) or somewhat (28%) satisfied with government's response, marking a 13% deficit from four months prior. Satisfaction was slightly lower among women and those living in urban areas. Comparatively, the South African government ranked 11th out of 18 participating African countries and citizen satisfaction levels dropped below those in Mozambique (72%), Zambia (73%), and Zimbabwe (73%). Levels of trust in various individuals and organisations' handling of the pandemic in South Africa were relatively high. South Africans placed the greatest degree of trust in their own family doctor (82%), followed by the Ministry of Health (77%), hospitals, clinics, and medical facilities (72%), and the Presidency (71%). Only 37% of South Africans trusted traditional healers a great deal or a fair amount. By this stage, respondents were also asked about their views on relaxing restrictions. Respondents were provided two statements and asked to indicate which was closer to their view: (1) loosening restrictions now puts too many people at risk of contracting COVID-19 and we need to wait at least two more weeks, or (2) the health risks are minimal if people follow social distancing rules, and we need to get the economy moving again. The majority of respondents (57%) indicated that we need to get the economy moving. This sentiment was strongest amongst men, those aged between 18 and 35, those living in rural areas, and those households in the highest income bracket (PERC, 2020).

By the last quarter of 2020, the economic impact of national lockdowns and restrictions on movement had started to take its toll. According to the Quarterly Labour Force Survey (QLFS), for example, unemployment in South Africa increased from 30.8% to 32.5% between quarters 3 and 4 of 2020 (StatsSA, 2021a). This phenomenon was not unique to South Africa and many public opinion polls began to shift their focus to tracking the socio-economic perceptions of citizens globally, in addition to continued support for and adherence to public health social measures. The results of a Global Predictions (2021)[8] survey conducted in 31 countries worldwide from 23 October to 6 November 2020 showed that 60% of all respondents believed it was unlikely that their economy would fully recover from the effects of the pandemic in 2021. South African respondents were even more sceptical as three-quarters (76%) agreed. Almost all South African respondents (95%) also agreed that 2020 was a bad year for South Africa, an increase of 14% from 2019, while 57% indicated that income inequality was likely to increase. South Africans were, however, more optimistic about the global outlook as 57% agreed that the global economy would be stronger in 2021 than in 2020 (IPSOS, 2021).

Results from the last two rounds of the Afrobarometer survey[9] conducted in South Africa provide good insights into the perceptions and opinions of South Africans prior to the outbreak (August and September 2018) and after the first two waves (May and June 2021) of the pandemic (Afrobarometer 2022). Of particular importance is the measurement of South Africans' popular support for democracy as well as government's handling of the COVID-19 pandemic (in the case of the latter survey) by way of Norris' (1999) fivefold analytical framework.

Political community

The first object of political support – political community – relates to a citizen's basic attachment to the nation and refers to sentiments of national pride and identity. South Africans in both rounds of the survey were asked to express their identity by choosing between being a South African and being a member of their ethnic group (see Table 12.1).

Table 12.1 illustrates how strong sentiments of national pride more than halved between 2018 and 2021 in South Africa. Almost a third of South Africans (31.4%) expressed a strong attachment to their national identity pre-pandemic, while only 15.2% shared the sentiment in 2021. Although the majority of citizens (51.5%) in 2021 are equally attached to their national and ethnic identities, an increase of 9.4% from 2018, the declining levels of national pride do not bode well for the levels of diffuse support for democracy in South Africa.

Regime principles

Another measure of diffuse support for democracy is the core values and basic principles of democratic regimes, i.e., regime principles. South Africans in the latest two rounds of the Afrobarometer survey were presented with three statements about democracy and asked to indicate which came closest to their opinion (see Table 12.2). The majority of South Africans (53.8%) indicated that democracy is preferable to any other kind of government in 2018. By 2021, however, only 38.9% of respondents preferred democratic governance; a decline of 14.9%. The decline in support for democracy was not coupled with an increase in support for non-democratic alternatives, but apathy regarding the system of governance. In 2018, a quarter of South Africans (25.4%) indicated that it did not matter to them what kind of government is in place. This sentiment increased by 15% (to 40.4%) in 2021. Alarmingly, indifference about the system of governance in South Africa surpassed citizens' support for democracy as a preferred regime type in 2021.

With regards to the South African government's response to COVID-19, the majority of citizens found it difficult to comply with government restrictions, yet overwhelmingly supported government's temporary limit on the freedom of movement and the curtailment of individual freedoms when faced with an emergency like the global pandemic. Data from the latest (2021) round of

Table 12.1 Sentiments of ethnic versus national identity[10]

	2018	2021
I feel only (ethnic group)	14.0	14.9
I feel more (ethnic group) than (national identity)	9.5	14.9
I feel equally (national identity) and (ethnic group)	42.1	51.5
I feel more (national identity) than (ethnic group)	8.6	6.0
I feel only (national identity)	22.8	9.2

Source: Author's compilation utilising Afrobarometer data, 2018 and 2021 rounds.

Table 12.2 Support for democracy in South Africa

	2018	2021
Democracy is preferable to any other kind of government	53.8	38.9
In some circumstances, a non-democratic government can be preferable	18.5	19.0
For someone like me, it doesn't matter what government we have	25.4	40.4

Source: Author's compilation utilising Afrobarometer data, 2018 and 2021 rounds.

the Afrobarometer showed that South Africans believed the government was justified in temporarily limiting democracy or democratic freedoms to manage COVID-19. More specifically, the majority of South Africans supported censoring media reporting (51.1%), the use of police and security forces to enforce public health mandates such as lockdown orders, mask requirements, or restrictions on public gatherings (71.5%), and postponing elections or limiting political campaigning (61.5%). In a similar vein, almost three-quarters (73.5%) of South Africans agreed (31.6%) or strongly agreed (41.9%) that even though the lockdown or curfew had negative impacts on the economy and people's livelihoods, they were necessary to limit the spread of COVID-19. Despite the support for these new regime principles, the majority of respondents (59%) found it difficult (28.8%) or very difficult (30.2%) to comply with the lockdown or curfew restrictions imposed by the government.

Regime performance

Citizen evaluations of and their satisfaction with democracy are also important indictors of their diffuse support for the regime and regime performance object of support. The data in Table 12.3 reveals that South Africans believe the country to be a democracy, but with major problems. This sentiment increased from 43.8% in 2018 to 47.0% in 2021. The data also shows that more (by 4.4%) South Africans believe South Africa is not a democracy and fewer (by 5.5%) believe South Africa to be a full democracy in 2021. Similarly, South Africans' satisfaction with democracy has decreased between both rounds under investigation. Levels of satisfaction were low in 2018 where less than half (42.1%) of respondents were 'fairly satisfied' (30.4%) or 'very satisfied' (11.7%) with the way democracy works in South Africa. By 2021, less than a third of respondents (31.4%) were either 'fairly satisfied' (23.5%) or 'very satisfied' (7.9%) with democracy; a decline of 10.7%. The implications of these findings are cause for concern as they are symptomatic of a decline in diffuse support for democracy in South Africa.

In terms of regime performance as it relates to the government's management of the public health crisis, the majority of South Africans (58.5%) indicated that government was managing the response to the pandemic 'fairly well' (35.2%) or 'very well' (23.3%), while an even higher percentage (71.7%) believed that the government was doing 'fairly well' (31.6%) or 'very well'

Table 12.3 Assessment of democracy in South Africa

	2018	2021
Not a democracy	8.9	13.3
A democracy, with major problems	43.8	47.0
A democracy, but with minor problems	30.3	27.7
A full democracy	15.2	9.7

Source: Author's compilation utilising Afrobarometer data, 2018 and 2021 rounds.

(40.1%) at keeping the public informed about COVID-19. In addition, just over a quarter (27.3%) of respondents reported receiving some form of assistance from the government (food, cash payments, relief from bill payments, or other assistance) that they did not normally receive prior to the pandemic. In contrast to citizen evaluations of and their satisfaction with democracy during the pandemic, the South African government fared favourably with regards to the management of the public health crisis.

Regime institutions

In order to gauge generalised support for various political or state institutions – specific support for democracy – respondents in both rounds were asked to indicate the extent to which they trust parliament. The data revealed that confidence in regime institutions is low and declining. Less than a third of South Africans (32.1%) trusted parliament in 2018, which declined to 27.6% in 2021.

Much the same as support for regime institutions, specific support for regime institutions' response to the pandemic was low. Table 12.4 illustrates high levels of distrust in official public health statistics related to COVID-19 and the government's ability to provide a safe vaccination for citizens. The majority of South Africans (57%) did not trust the official statistics provided by government on the number of infections and deaths due to the COVID-19 pandemic at all (34.7%) or even a little bit (22.3%). Even more (63.6%) did not trust the government to ensure that any vaccine for COVID-19 that is developed or offered to South African citizens is safe before it is used in the country, while fewer than 40% indicated that they were likely (16.7% somewhat likely and 23.2% very likely) to get vaccinated if a vaccine for COVID-19 became available and the government said it is safe. Similarly, more than half of South Africans (55.3%) believed that the benefits of government programmes to support people during the pandemic were unfairly distributed (by favouring certain groups or regions). Despite these low levels of trust in regime institutions, there was support for some government decisions relating to the pandemic. For example, 66% of South Africans either somewhat (22.2%) or strongly supported (43.8%) the government's decision

Table 12.4 Support for regime institutions' response to COVID-19

	Trust	Do not trust
Degree of trust in the official statistics provided by government on the number of infections and deaths due to the COVID-19 pandemic	33.2	57.0
Degree of trust in the government to ensure that any vaccine for COVID-19 that is developed or offered to South African citizens is safe before it used in the country	25.9	63.6

Source: Author's compilation utilising Afrobarometer data, 2018 and 2021 rounds.

to close schools in an effort to limit the spread of COVID-19, however, 66.5% believed the period during which schools were closed was either somewhat (14.8%) or much too long (51.7%).

Political actors

The fifth object of political support measures specific support for political authorities, including the performance of individual political leaders. Respondents in both rounds of the Afrobarometer surveys were asked to indicate the extent to which they trust the president (see Table 12.5). Trust in the President was low but consistent in 2018 (38.2%) and 2021 (38.1%). It is, however, interesting to note that when respondents were asked to rate the performance of the President over the previous 12 months, the majority (56.5%) either approved (37.0%) or strongly approved (19.5%) in 2018. Despite a slight decline of 2.4% in 2021, the majority (54.1%) of South Africans either approved (37.9%) or strongly approved (16.2%) of President Cyril Ramaphosa's performance during the outbreak and the first two waves of the pandemic.

While specific support for democracy in relation to political actors yielded mixed results, support for political actors and their response to COVID-19 is less auspicious. For example, 61.7% of South Africans were somewhat (20%) or very worried (41.7%) that politicians were using the pandemic as an opportunity to increase their wealth or power, or to permanently restrict freedoms or political competition, while the vast majority of respondents (78%) indicated that a lot (64.6%) or some (13.4%) of the funds and resources that were available to the government for combatting and responding to the COVID-19 pandemic were lost or stolen due to corruption among government officials.

Overall, a review of the micro-level data provides interesting, and sometimes conflicting, insights into citizen's support for democracy and their views on how government has handled the COVID-19 pandemic, especially in relation to the various objects of political support. The data reveals worrying signs for diffuse support for democracy, which is a prerequisite for the persistence of democracy as the preferred regime type in South Africa, and support for regime principles and regime performance in response to COVID-19 was mostly positive. On the other hand, specific support for democracy and the manner in which regime institutions and political actors responded to the global pandemic were generally low and declining.

Table 12.5 Trust in political actors

	2018	2021
Institutional trust or confidence in the President	38.2	38.1
Approval of the President's performance over the past 12 months	56.5	54.1

Source: Author's compilation utilising Afrobarometer data, 2018 and 2021 rounds.

Explaining popular support for democracy in South Africa since the onset of the pandemic

There are a number of possible explanations emanating from the literature as to why citizens support the models and objects of democracy or not. Apart from cultural approaches that focus on social capital theory (Putnam *et al.*, 1993; Putnam, 2000, 2002) or post-materialist theory (Inglehart, 1977, 1997, 2018) to explain declines in civic engagement or the changing value orientations within society, most scholars cite economic and political performance as the most significant factors in shaping support for democracy. On the one hand, socio-economic changes associated with modernisation have been linked to increased support for democracy (Lipset, 1959), while other studies have stressed economic wellbeing by focusing on macro-economic and social indicators and the evaluations of citizens thereof (Kornberg & Clarke, 1992; Clarke *et al.*, 1993; Weatherford, 1987, 1992). On the other hand, there is evidence that suggests support for democracy is based on political factors, such as institutional arrangements (Anderson & Guillory, 1997; Norris, 1999), presidential and parliamentary approval or political trust (Newton, 1999, Miller & Listhaug, 1999), and the functioning of political institutions in shaping support for democracy by addressing issues relating to corruption, responsiveness, and accountability (Anderson & Tverdova, 2003, Linde & Peters, 2020).

Studies undertaken in Africa suggest evidence of both the institutional and performance explanation. Bratton and Mattes (2001:448) argue that the nature of democratic support in Africa is either intrinsic or instrumental. Intrinsic support is based on support for democratic values, including political freedoms, civil liberties, and equal rights, while instrumental support is considered a means to an end for citizens, resulting in the alleviation of poverty or improved standards of living, for example (Steenekamp & Musuva, 2022). Intrinsic support is unconditional support for democracy and the inculcation of democratic values that can sustain the political regime under any circumstance, while instrumental support is conditional support for democracy that can be withdrawn by citizens depending on the government's capacity to deliver various economic and political goods (Steenekamp & Musuva, 2022). In terms of the implications for democracy, the distinction between the nature of democratic support being intrinsic or instrumental is much the same as the distinction between the two models or types (diffuse and specific) of support for democracy.

An analysis of political governance and policy regulations and enforcement, the socio-economic context, and impact of COVID-19 on the economy, as well as reports of irregular expenditure relating to COVID-19 measures by various government agencies and public officials, would support a combination of the institutional and performance explanations for the levels of democratic support in South Africa prior to the onset of the pandemic until present.

When declaring a National State of Disaster on 15 March 2020, President Cyril Ramaphosa announced the establishment of a National Coronavirus Command Council (NCCC) to lead government's emergency response plan to manage COVID-19 in South Africa (Ramaphosa, 2020a). The South African government, on the recommendation of the NCCC, introduced a five-level COVID-19 alert to manage the gradual easing of the extended national lockdown, which came to an end on 30 April 2020, with level 5 including the most prescriptive restrictions and level 1 including the most relaxed restrictions. The swift and decisive action by the South African government was internationally lauded and initially widely supported by the public, as evident from the results of the Afrobarometer data relating to regime principles. However, the nature, timeframe, legality, and enforcement of the COVID-19 restrictions raised serious questions about the curtailment of civil liberties in the government's response to the COVID-19 pandemic and the implications for diffuse and intrinsic democratic support.

The five-level COVID-19 alert system was in effect for more than two years, from 26 March 2020 to 22 June 2022, which was significantly longer than COVID-19 restrictions in the majority of other countries and subject to a myriad of legal challenges (*BusinessTech*, 2021). Since the downgrade of each alert level was accompanied by an easing of various restrictions, some argued that the numerous iterations of the COVID-19 policy regulations were evidence of the government's responsiveness to the criticism and concerns of its constituents (Singh, 2020:441). However, others, including Dr Glenda Gray, a member of the Ministerial Advisory Committee (MAC) and chairperson of the South African Medical Research Council (SAMRC), described aspects of the phased approach as 'nonsensical and unscientific' because the relaxation of alert levels often introduced conflicting, confusing, and sometimes irrational regulations (Karrim and Evans, 2020). During lockdown level 4, for example, Trade and Industry Minister, Ebrahim Patel, introduced regulations relating to the sale of clothing, footwear, and bedding which effectively excluded the sale of summer goods (South African Government, 2020b). More specifically, the regulations prohibited the sale of open-toe shoes and permitted the sale of short-sleeved shirts only as 'undergarments for warmth' (South African Government, 2020b). Less than a month later, the Gauteng Division of the High Court found some lockdown regulations, such as those relating to funerals, the operation of public transport, limiting exercise, and prohibiting certain sectors (informal) and industries (hairdressers and salons) from resuming business to be irrational (Labuschaigne, 2020:26–27). In the court's view, according to Labuschaigne (2020:27), this 'smacks of a paternalistic approach, rather than a constitutionally justified one'.

Similarly, serious concerns about the legality, governance, and implications for democratic practice were raised about the NCCC and the National Joint Operations and Intelligence Structure (NATJOINTS), the latter described as 'an entity established by a Cabinet memo without basis in legislation' (Merten, 2020a). While the NCCC was responsible for the political governance and management of COVID-19, NATJOINTS, consisting of soldiers, police and intelligence agents, was established to 'operationalise the directive' of the NCCC (Merten, 2020a). The militarised response was evident as the SANDF was bestowed with additional powers and deployed with a mandate to support the South African Police Service (SAPS) in enforcing the national lockdown regulations (Staunton *et al.*, 2020:8). There were subsequently multiple reports of the excessive force utilised by these security agencies, including the death of several citizens, the use of rubber bullets, and allegations of abuse (Haffajee, 2020).

Apart from the political governance and enforcement of COVID-19 regulations, the impact of the pandemic on the economy and the socio-economic context needs to be considered given the instrumental nature of support for democracy in South Africa. Although even the most well-resourced countries experienced stagnation and decline as a result of the global pandemic, emerging economies like South Africa, have borne the brunt and are likely to experience longer-lasting consequences. A review of selected macro-economic indicators shows that the gross domestic product (GDP), GDP per capita, and GDP per capita purchasing power parity (PPP) all declined between 2019 and 2020 (World Bank, 2022). By November 2020, the main budget balance had a deficit of almost R440 billion, which marks a 77% increase from the same time in 2019 (*Business Insider*, 2020) and recorded a shortfall of more than R550 billion or 11.2% of GDP on its main budget for the year at the end of March 2021 (Naidoo, 2021). The gross loan debt as a percentage of GDP stood at 70.7% in the 2020/2021 financial year and is projected to stabilise at 75.1% in 2024/25 before gradually declining, depending on how well and quickly major reforms and fiscal consolidation are implemented to stabilise debt (South African Treasury, 2022:87). To further compound matters, credit rating agencies, Moody's and Fitch dropped South Africa two and three notches, respectively, below investment grade status in November 2020 and maintained negative outlooks, while Standard and Poor's (S&P) held a stable outlook with a 'junk' rating (Stoddard, 2020). From the data above, it is clear that the pandemic had had a considerable impact on an already depressed economy and further calls into question the appropriateness of the extent and length of the five-level COVID-19 alert system adopted by the South African government.

Apart from the severe economic stress, there were a multitude of socio-economic factors at play. South Africa is one of the most unequal societies in the world, despite its status as a higher-middle-income country (World Bank, 2021). In September 2021, StatsSA announced an adjustment of the national poverty lines to include an amount of R624 per person per month on the food poverty line, which is also known as the extreme poverty line, and is defined as 'the amount of money that an individual will need to afford the minimum required daily energy intake' (StatsSA, 2021c:3). Almost half of the adult population in South Africa live below the food poverty line (Toyana, 2021). Similarly, the rate of unemployment continued to increase.

Approximately 15% of the work force, or 2.8 million people, lost their jobs between February and June 2020, while a third of the work force are estimated to have lost their income temporarily due to furloughs during the hard lockdown (Visagie & Turok, 2021:52). By the third quarter of 2021, the official unemployment rate was 34.9% (or 14.3 million adult South Africans) and marked the highest unemployment rate since the start of the QLFS (StatsSA, 2021b). The expanded or unofficial unemployment rate, which includes those who have stopped looking for work, increased by 2.2 percentage points between the second and third quarters of 2021 and stood at 46.6% (StatsSA, 2021b). Despite the dismal unemployment rate, some gains were recorded in the informal sector with the addition of 9,000 jobs (StatsSA, 2021b). The resilience of the informal sector, which accounts for approximately a third of the labour force in South Africa, is all the more admirable given the abundance of social and economic hardships. For example, almost 15% of all households in South Africa are located in informal settlements, which often lack running water, electricity, and proper sanitation, while the vast majority of South Africans rely on various forms of public transport that are often overcrowded (StatsSA, 2021d). While many of the public health social measures such as hand washing and social distancing were both effective and cheap measures at preventing the spread of the virus in other parts of the world, they assume a 'universal capacity to change behaviour and overlook the vast inequalities in infrastructure access' in South Africa (de Groot & Lemanski, 2020:261). Given the socio-economic reality of many South Africans, the political governance of COVID-19 remains questionable and is likely to continue to erode support for democracy. This is because citizens in new or young democracies, such as South Africa, are more likely to evaluate and support democracy based on its performance or what it can deliver rather than rely on their experience of democracy and deeply entrenched democratic values, as is the case for citizens in more established democracies. The government's failure to deliver basic economic goods, coupled with the dire economic outlook, could explain the low and declining levels of support for regime institutions since 2018 and result in South Africans' loss of faith in democracy.

The instrumental nature of support for democracy in South Africa could also, in part, explain the consistent levels of institutional trust in the President and support for his performance since the onset of the pandemic. In an attempt to provide some economic relief and mitigate the impact of COVID-19, President Ramaphosa announced an economic stimulus package to direct resources to the pandemic response and support the functioning of the economy on 21 April 2020 (Ramaphosa, 2020d). The stimulus package amounted to roughly 10% of South Africa's GDP and included an R500 billion social support and economic relief fund, funded in part by loans from the World Bank and International Monetary fund (de Villiers *et al.*, 2020:802). The social relief and economic support package involved: a significant increase in the health budget; relief of hunger and social distress; support for businesses and workers; and a phased reopening of the economy (Ramaphosa, 2020d). More specifically, the government increased existing social grants (child support, old age, disability, foster care, and care dependency) by offering top-ups to the value of between R250 and R300 a month for six months to the total value of R41 billion (de Villiers *et al.*, 2020:802). The government also introduced a Social Relief of Distress grant to the value of R350 per month, which can take the form of cash, food parcels, or vouchers to purchase food (South African Government, 2022).

While the short-term relief for millions of South Africans, especially those most vulnerable in society, was welcomed, several concerns about the relief package were raised. First, the relief package did not include a strong economic stimulus allocation and came at the cost of long-term benefits aimed at improving the standard of living and development needs in the country. In the same vein, the failure by government to deliver on long-term development goals may be blamed on the reallocation of these funds (de Villiers *et al.*, 2020:802–803). Second, if the economy is not significantly stimulated, citizens may become more dependent upon the state, which will inevitably deepen levels of poverty and inequality (de Groot & Lemanski, 2020:261). Third, these short-term relief measures are being funded by medium- to long-term loans, which could result in a debt crisis if public spending is not significantly decreased, national revenue increased, and business confidence and direct foreign investment encouraged (de Villiers *et al.*, 2020:804). And finally, while support for the ruling African National Congress (ANC) declined from 53.91% in the 2016 municipal elections to 45.59% in the 2021 municipal elections (Electoral Commission of South Africa, 2022a), the results could have been far worse in the absence of these short-term relief measures, which may have partly been utilised as a calculated electoral campaign tool.

While it may be cynical to raise the opportunistic merits of the short-term economic relief measures introduced in May 2020, electoral support for the ruling party has steadily declined from 69.69% to 57.50% between the 2004 and 2019 national and provincial elections (Electoral Commission of South Africa, 2022b). At the same time, the results from the Afrobarometer data showed low and declining specific support for political actors since the onset of the pandemic. A possible explanation for these findings is that much of the dissatisfaction amongst voters is based on the perceptions of mismanagement and pervasive corruption that plagues public office. The establishment of a R500 billion social support and economic relief fund was no exception. In a presentation to Parliament on 20 October 2020, a mere six months after the announcement of the COVID-19 relief fund, the Special Investigating Unit (SIU) reported the investigation of R10.5 billion (or 67% of the expenditure to date) in potentially corrupt pandemic scandals (Merten, 2020b). The SIU reported that most of the irregular spending was at the provincial government level, where more than 75% of funds made available for COVID-19 measures amounting to R7.254 billion are thought to have been misappropriated predominantly in Gauteng (R4.339 billion), Eastern Cape (R1.802 billion), and KwaZulu-Natal (R533 million).

At the national level, about a third of COVID-19 funds spent (or R158 million) were under investigation, including R220 million spent on water tanks by the Department of Basic Education (Mertens, 2020b). In addition, the Office of the Auditor-General identified approximately 80,000 COVID-19 transactions during a real-time audit for review. These transactions include, but are not limited to, the overpricing of Personal Protective Equipment (PPE), the procurement of non-essential goods under COVID-19 emergency provisions, and the use of service providers not registered for VAT or who were in the de-registration process but still awarded contracts (*BusinessTech*, 2020). There were also several high-profile corruption scandals relating to senior public officials. In June 2021, the President placed Health Minister, Zweli Mkhize, on leave after he was implicated in a R150 million COVID-19-related communications tender. The minister resigned on 6 August 2021 (Ellis, 2021). In addition, the President's spokesperson, Khusela Diko, took special leave after allegations surfaced relating to the Gauteng COVID-19 tenders of Royal Bhaca Projects headed by her husband, Madzikane II Thandisizwe Diko, to the value of R125 million (*IOL*, 2020). The chronic misappropriation of public resources has devastating effects on the lives of the most vulnerable in society, the economy, as well as the legitimacy of government as citizens continue to lose confidence and faith in political institutions and public officials (i.e., specific support for democracy). This crisis of legitimacy has serious implications for the objects, models, and nature of political support in South Africa.

Conclusion

The outbreak of the COVID-19 pandemic late in 2019 has quickly become the most significant socio-economic and political challenge in contemporary history. The global response included the swift withdrawal of civil liberties as nation after nation closed their borders and restricted the movement of people through lockdowns of an unprecedented nature. While the South African government had a few months head start to learn from other nations and prepare a response to the pandemic, it was evident that the socio-economic reality of overcrowding in informal settlements, lack of access to running water and proper sanitation, and a population plagued by chronic illness, TB and HIV would devastate an already weakened public healthcare system. In many ways, President Ramaphosa was left with the impossible decision to prioritise the public health crisis and buy as much time as possible to slow the spread of COVID-19 at the expense of a flailing economy. The speed and decisiveness with which the national lockdown was implemented and the government's 'following the science' approach received widespread international acclaim as an example of good governance.

Times of crisis, however, can place even the most stable of democracies under stress. A review of macro-level data prior to the outbreak of the pandemic and again in 2021 reveals that the democratic political system and its constituent institutions are in place and function formally in South Africa. However, a review of micro-level data shows a decline in both diffuse and specific types of support for democracy. South Africans have become increasingly critical of the various objects of support, including regime principles, regime performance, regime institutions, and political actors, since the onset of the pandemic. It is encouraging that the public onion data relating specifically to the government's handling of COVID-19 reflects a more positive evaluation on most measures. However, the normalisation of emergency powers, the extension of state authority into the private lives of citizens, the criminalisation of non-compliance with public health social measures, and the militarisation of the state's response to COVID-19 are detrimental to the intrinsic nature of political support. On the other hand, the contraction of the economy, unsustainable government debt, a decline in revenue, high levels of poverty, inequality and unemployment, and widespread corruption, mismanagement, and dysfunctional public administration are all likely further erode the instrumental nature of political support in South Africa.

Notes

1 The Polity IV Project is housed at the Center for Systemic Peace in Virginia, USA. https://www.systemicpeace.org/polityproject.html.
2 Freedom House is a non-profit, majority U.S. government funded organisation in Washington, D.C., that conducts research and advocacy on democracy, political freedom, and human rights. The chapter draws on data from the Freedom in the World Project. https://freedomhouse.org/reports/freedom-world/freedom-world-research-methodology.
3 The Democracy Index is housed at *The Economist* Intelligence Unit (EUI). https://www.eiu.com/n/campaigns/democracy-index-2021/.
4 The Varieties of Democracy (V-Dem) Research Project is based at the V-Dem Institute at the Department of Political Science, University of Gothenburg, Sweden.
5 The Ipsos Coronavirus public perceptions and behavioural responses survey was conducted in 32 countries, each with approximately 1000 respondents aged between 16 and 74. The South African wave included interviews with 1008 participants via the Ipsos online panel. It is important to note that the results were weighted to South Africans who have access to the internet either at home and/or on their mobile phones. The sample is therefore more urban, more educated and/or more affluent than the general population and should be viewed as reflecting the views of the more 'connected' segment of the population. The online survey had a credibility interval of +/−3.5% as there were more than 1000 respondents.
6 The fieldwork in South Africa was conducted by Ipsos, took place from 2 to 6 April 2020, and included interviews with 1099 respondents aged 18 and older in Durban, Johannesburg, and Pretoria. The data is representative of the populations in the urban areas included and unweighted.

7 The fieldwork in South Africa was conducted by Ipsos, took place from 3 to 17 August 2020, and included telephonic interviews with 1395 respondents. Samples were drawn to be nationally representative and weighted by gender and region.

8 The online survey was conducted by Ipsos on its Global Advisor online platform. The total sample included 23 007 respondents from 31 countries, including 500 from South Africa aged between 18 and 74. The sample in South Africa is more urban, more educated, and/or more affluent than the general population and the results reflect the views of the more 'connected' segment of the population.

9 Afrobarometer is a pan-African, nonpartisan survey research network that provides reliable data on Africans' experiences and evaluations on democracy, governance, and quality of life. The fieldwork was conducted by Plus 94 Research, who interviewed a nationally representative, random, stratified probability sample of 1 829 adult South Africans between 30 July and 26 September 2018 (Round 7) and 1 600 adult South Africans between 2 May and 12 June 2021 (Round 8). Both rounds yield results within a margin of error of +/−2.5 percentage points at a 95% confidence level.

10 Percentages do not total 100% as respondents could also 'refuse' to answer or 'not know' (not reported).

References

Afrobarometer. (2022). Survey resources and data. Retrieved from https://www.afrobarometer.org/surveys-and-methods/survey-resources/

Anderson, C.J. & Guillory, C.A. (1997). Political institutions and satisfaction with democracy: A cross-national analysis of consensus and majoritarian systems. *American Political Science Review*, 91(1), 66–81.

Anderson, C.J. & Tverdova, Y.V. (2003). Corruption, political allegiances, and attitudes toward government in contemporary democracies. *American Journal of Political Science*, 47(1), 91–109.

Bratton, M. & Mattes, R. (2001). Support for democracy in Africa: Intrinsic or instrumental? *British Journal of Political Science*, 31(3), 447–474.

Business Insider. (2020). *SA's budget deficit is now 77% bigger than this time last year, new figures show*. Retrieved from https://www.businessinsider.co.za/state-of-the-budget-shows-sas-revenue-shortfall-hurting-as-expenditure-rises-2020-12 [Accessed 18 June 2021].

BusinessTech. (2020). *R10.5 billion under investigation for 'Covidpreneur' looting in South Africa*. Retrieved from https://businesstech.co.za/news/government/442058/r10-5-billion-under-investigation-for-covidpreneur-looting-in-south-africa/ [Accessed 18 June 2021].

BusinessTech. (2021). *Government faces mounting court challenges to South Africa's new lockdown rules*. Retrieved from https://businesstech.co.za/news/business/502287/government-faces-mounting-court-challenges-to-south-africas-new-lockdown-rules/ [Accessed on 28 January 2022].

Claasen, C. (2020). Does public support help democracy survive? *American Journal of Political Science*, 64(1), 118–134.

Clarke, H.D., Dutt, N. & Kornberg, A. (1993). The political economy of attitudes toward polity and society in Western European democracies. *Journal of Politics*, 55(4), 998–1021.

Dalton, R.J. (1999). Political support in advanced industrial democracies. In: P. Norris (Ed.) *Critical Citizens: Global Support for Democratic Government*. Oxford, U.K.: Oxford University Press.

de Groot, J. & Lemanski, C. (2020). COVID-19 responses: Infrastructure inequality and privileged capacity to transform everyday life in South Africa. *Environment and Urbanization*, 33(1), 255–272.

de Villiers, C., Cerbone, D. & van Zijl, W. (2020). The South African government's response to COVID-19. *Journal of Public Budgeting, Accounting and Financial Management*, 32(5), 797–811.

Diamond, L. (2015). Facing up to the democratic recession. *Journal of Democracy*, 26(1), 141–155.

Easton, D. (1965). *A Systems Analysis of Political Life*. New York, U.S.A: Wiley.

Easton, D. (1975). A re-assessment of the concept of political support. *British Journal of Political Science*, 5(4), 435–457.

Electoral Commission of South Africa. (2022a). *Municipal Elections Results Dashboard*. Retrieved from https://results.elections.org.za/dashboards/lge/ [Accessed on 28 January 2022].

Electoral Commission of South Africa. (2022b). *National and Provisional Elections Results Dashboard*. Retrieved from https://results.elections.org.za/dashboards/npe/app/dashboard.html [Accessed on 28 January 2022].

Ellis, E. (2021). *Exposed and tarnished by the Digital Vibes scandal, Zweli Mkhize goes down fighting*. Retrieved from https://www.dailymaverick.co.za/article/2021-08-06-exposed-and-tarnished-by-the-digital-vibes-scandal-zweli-mkhize-goes-down-fighting/ [Accessed on 28 January 2022].

Haffajee, F. (2020). *Ramaphosa calls 11 lockdown deaths and 230,000 arrests an act of 'over-enthusiasm' – really!* Retrieved from https://www.dailymaverick.co.za/article/2020-06-01-ramaphosa-calls-11-lockdown-deaths-and-230000-arrests-an-act-of-over-enthusiasm-really/ [Accessed on 12 May 2021].

Inglehart, R. (1977). *The Silent Revolution: Changing Values and Political Styles among Western Publics*. Princeton, U.S.A: Princeton University Press.

Inglehart, R. (1997). *Modernization and Postmodernization: Cultural, Economic, and Political Change in 43 Societies*. Princeton, U.S.A: Princeton University Press.

Inglehart, R. (2018). *Cultural Evolution: People's Motivations Are Changing, and Reshaping the World*. Cambridge, U.K. & New York, U.S.A: Cambridge University Press.

IOL. (2020). *Khusela Diko takes leave after R125m PPE tender scandal linked to husband*. Retrieved from https://www.iol.co.za/news/politics/khusela-diko-takes-leave-after-r125m-ppe-tender-scandal-linked-to-husband-cfd793c8-99dc-4416-87f0-fd32ef6f18b7 [Accessed on 12 May 2021].

IPSOS. (2020a). Coronavirus: Opinion and Reaction (South Africa Report). Retrieved from https://www.ipsos.com/sites/default/files/ct/news/documents/2020-04/coronavirus_online_polling_south_africa_wave_1.pdf [Accessed on 17 February 2021].

IPSOS. (2020b). Responding to COVID 19 in African Countries: Analysis and Report of Survey Findings. Retrieved from https://www.ipsos.com/sites/default/files/ct/publication/documents/2020-05/responding-to-covid-19-in-african-member-states-may-5-2020.pdf [Accessed on 17 February 2021].

IPSOS. (2021). Global Advisor 2021 Predictions. Retrieved from https://www.ipsos.com/sites/default/files/ct/news/documents/2020-12/global-predictions-2021-ipsos.pdf [Accessed on 17 February 2021].

Karrim, A. & Evans, S. (2020). *Unscientific and nonsensical: Top scientist slams government's lockdown strategy.* Retrieved from https://www.news24.com/news24/SouthAfrica/News/unscientific-and-nonsensical-top-scientific-adviser-slams-governments-lockdown-strategy-20200516 [Accessed on 12 May 2021].

Kornberg, A. & Clarke, H.D. (1992). *Citizens and Community: Political Support in a Representative Democracy.* New York, U.S.A: Cambridge University Press.

Klingemann, H.D. (1999). Mapping political support in the 1990s: A global analysis. In: P. Norris (Ed.) *Critical Citizens: Global Support for Democratic Government.* Oxford, U.K.: Oxford University Press.

Labuschaigne, M. (2020). Ethicolegal issues relating to the South African government's response to COVID-19. *South African Journal of Bioethics and Law,* 13(1), 23–28.

Linde, J. & Peters, Y. (2020). Responsiveness, support, and responsibility: How democratic responsiveness facilitates responsible government. *Party Politics,* 26(3), 291–304.

Lipset, S.M. (1959). Some social requisites of democracy: Economic development and political legitimacy. *American Political Science Review.* 53(1), 69–105.

Lührmann, A. & Rooney, B. (2021). Autocratization by decree: States of Emergency and democratic decline. *Comparative Politics,* 53(4), 617–649.

Mechkova, V., Lührmann, A. & Lindberg, S.I. (2017). How much democratic backsliding? *Journal of Democracy,* 28(4), 162–169.

Merten, M. (2020a). *Lockdown level 4: The curfew – and other crackdowns – raises disturbing questions for South Africa's democracy.* Retrieved from https://www.dailymaverick.co.za/article/2020-04-30-the-curfew-and-other-crackdowns-raises-disturbing-questions-for-south-africas-democracy/ [Accessed 18 June 2021].

Merten, M. (2020b). *Covid-19 corruption: Two-thirds of contracts are under investigation.* Retrieved from https://www.dailymaverick.co.za/article/2020-10-20-covid-19-corruption-two-thirds-of-contracts-are-under-investigation/ [Accessed on 18 June 2021].

Miller, A. & Listhaug, O. (1999). Political performance and institutional trust. In: P. Norris (Ed.) *Critical Citizens: Global Support for Democratic Government.* Oxford, U.K.: Oxford University Press.

Mishler, W. & Rose, R. (1999). Five years after the fall: Trajectories of support or democracy in post-communist Europe. In: P. Norris (Ed.) *Critical Citizens: Global Support for Democratic Government.* Oxford, U.K.: Oxford University Press.

Naidoo, P. (2021). *South Africa's main budget gap at 11.2% of GDP, beating forecast.* Retrieved from https://www.news24.com/fin24/Economy/south-africas-main-budget-gap-at-112-of-gdp-beating-forecast-20210505 [Accessed on 18 June 2021].

Newton, K. (1999). Social and political trust in established democracies. In: P. Norris (Ed.) *Critical Citizens: Global Support for Democratic Government.* Oxford: Oxford University Press, 169–187.

Norris, P. 1999. Institutional explanations for political support. In Norris, P. (ed.) *Critical Citizens: Global Support for Democratic Government.* Oxford, U.K.: Oxford University Press.

Norris, P. (2011). *Democratic Deficit: Critical Citizens Revisited.* Cambridge, U.K.: Cambridge University Press.

Parliamentary Budget Office. (2021). *Social grant performance as at end March 20/21.* Retrieved from https://www.parliament.gov.za/storage/app/media/PBO/National_Development_Plan_Analysis/2021/june/03-06-2021/May_2021_Social_Grant_fact_sheet.pdf [Accessed on 28 January 2022].

PERC. (2020). Responding to COVID-19 in African Countries: Cross National Findings. Retrieved from https://www.ipsos.com/sites/default/files/ct/publication/documents/2020-09/data-cross-national-survey-31-august-2020.pdf [Accessed on 14 August 2021].

Putnam, R.D. (2000). *Bowling Alone: The Collapse and Revival of American Community.* New York, U.S.A: Simon & Schuster.

Putnam, R.D. (2002). *Democracies in Flux: The Evolution of Social Capital in Contemporary Society.* New York, U.S.A: Oxford University Press.

Putnam, R.D., Leonardi, R. & Nanetti, R. (1993). *Making Democracy Work: Civic Traditions in Modern Italy.* Princeton, U.S.A: Princeton University Press.

Ramaphosa, C. (2020a). *Measures to combat Coronavirus COVID-19 epidemic.* Retrieved from https://www.gov.za/speeches/statement-president-cyril-rama-phosa-measures-combat-covid-19-epidemic-15-mar-2020-0000 [Accessed on 12 May 2021].

Ramaphosa, C. (2020b). *Escalation of measures to combat COVID-19 epidemic.* Retrieved from http://www.dirco.gov.za/docs/speeches/2020/cram0323.pdf [Accessed on 12 May 2021].

Ramaphosa, C. (2020c). *Extension of Coronavirus COVID-19 lockdown to the end of April.* Retrieved from https://www.gov.za/speeches/president-cyril-ramaphosa-extension-coronavirus-covid-19-lockdown-end-april-9-apr-2020-0000 [Accessed on 12 May 2021].

Ramaphosa, C. (2020d). Further economic and social measures in response to the COVID-19 epidemic. Retrieved from https://www.thepresidency.gov.za/speeches/statement-president-cyril-ramaphosa-further-economic-and-social-measures-response-covid-19 [Accessed on 18 June 2021].

Singh, J.A. (2020). How South Africa's Ministerial Advisory Committee on COVID-19 can be optimised. *South African Medical Journal*, 110(6), 439–442.

South African Government. (2020a). *About alert system.* Retrieved from https://www.gov.za/covid-19/about/about-alert-system [Accessed on 12 May 2021].

South African Government. (2020b). *Regulations and Guidelines – Coronavirus Covid-19.* Retrieved from https://www.gov.za/covid-19/resources/regulations-and-guidelines-coronavirus-covid-19 [Accessed on 12 May 2021].

South African Government. (2022). *Social relief of distress.* Retrieved from https://www.gov.za/services/social-benefits/social-relief-distress [Accessed 28 January 2022].

South African National Treasury. (2022). *Government debt and contingent liabilities. Budget Review 2022.* Retrieved from http://www.treasury.gov.za/documents/national%20budget/2022/review/FullBR.pdf [Accessed on 15 February 2022].

Statistics South Africa. (2021a). *Quarterly Labour Force Survey (QLFS). Quarter 4: 2000.* Retrieved from http://www.statssa.gov.za/publications/P0211/P02114th Quarter2020.pdf [Accessed on 28 January 2022].

Statistics South Africa. (2021b). *Quarterly Labour Force Survey (QLFS). Quarter 3: 2021.* Retrieved from http://www.statssa.gov.za/?p=14957 [Accessed on 28 January 2022].

Statistics South Africa. (2021c). *National Poverty Lines, 2021.* Retrieved from http://www.statssa.gov.za/publications/P03101/P031012021.pdf [Accessed on 28 January 2022].

Statistics South Africa. (2021d). *General Household Survey (GHS) – 2020.* Retrieved from http://www.statssa.gov.za/publications/P0318/P03182020.pdf [Accessed on 28 January 2022].

Staunton, C., Swanepoel, C. & Labuschaigne, M. (2020). Between a rock and a hard place: COVID-19 and South Africa's response. *Journal of Law and Biosciences*, 7(1), 1–12.

Steenekamp, C. & Musuva, C. (2022). Political culture in Africa: A comparative analysis of democratic values in South Africa and Kenya. In: U. van Beek (Ed.) *Democracy under Pressure Resilience or Retreat?* Palgrave Macmillan (forthcoming).

Stoddard, E. (2020). *Junked: Fitch and Moody's downgrade South Africa's credit ratings further.* Retrieved from https://www.dailymaverick.co.za/article/2020-11-22-junked-and-fitch-and-moodys-downgrade-south-africas-credit-ratings-further/ [Accessed on 12 May 2021].

The Economist Intelligence Unit. (2020). *Democracy Index 2019: A Year of Democratic Setbacks and Popular Protest.* Retrieved from https://www.eiu.com/topic/democracy-index/ [Accessed on 12 May 2021].

The Economist Intelligence Unit. (2020). *Democracy Index 2021: The China Challenge.* Retrieved from https://www.eiu.com/n/campaigns/democracy-index-2021/ [Accessed on 18 June 2021].

Toyana, M. (2021). *South Africa's poverty threshold increases while social grants fail to keep pace.* Retrieved from https://www.dailymaverick.co.za/article/2021-09-09-south-africas-poverty-threshold-increases-while-social-grants-fail-to-keep-pace/ [Accessed on 25 January 2022].

Varieties of Democracy (V-Dem). (2022). *Codebook. Version 12.* Retrieved from http://www.v-dem.net/static/website/img/refs/codebookv12.pdf [Accessed on 25 January 2022].

Varieties of Democracy (V-Dem). (2022). *Graphing Tools.* Retrieved from http://www.v-dem.net/graphingtools.html [Accessed on 25 January 2022].

Weatherford, S.M. (1987). How does government performance influence political support? *Political Behavior*, 9(1), 5–28.

Weatherford, S.M. (1992). Measuring political legitimacy. *American Political Science Review*, 86(1), 149–166.

World Bank. (2021). *The World Bank in South Africa – Overview.* Retrieved from https://www.worldbank.org/en/country/southafrica/overview#1 [Accessed on 18 June 2021].

World Bank. (2022). *World Bank Open Data.* Retrieved from https://data.worldbank.org/ [Accessed on 25 January 2022].

Index

For Product Safety Concerns and Information please contact our EU
representative GPSR@taylorandfrancis.com
Taylor & Francis Verlag GmbH, Kaufingerstraße 24, 80331 München, Germany

www.ingramcontent.com/pod-product-compliance
Lightning Source LLC
Chambersburg PA
CBHW060238220326
41598CB00027B/3978

* 9 7 8 1 0 3 2 2 8 0 0 9 7 *